MW01273172

TWO TRUTHS

DANA C CARVER

Two Truths Copyright © 2020 by Dana C Carver. All Rights Reserved.

All rights reserved. No part of this book may be reproduced in any form or by any electronic or mechanical means including information storage and retrieval systems, without permission in writing from the author. The only exception is by a reviewer, who may quote short excerpts in a review.

Cover designed by Create Space

This book is a work of fiction. Names, characters, places, and incidents either are products of the author's imagination or are used fictitiously. Any resemblance to actual persons, living or dead, events, or locales is entirely coincidental.

Dana C Carver
Visit my website at www.danaccarver.com

Printed in the United States of America

First Printing: Nov 2020
Amazon Publishing

ISBN 978-0-473-44054-1

For my parents
who have always supported my search for Truth

I'm a traveller of both time and space
To be where I have been
To sit with elders of the gentle race
This world has seldom seen
They talk of days for which they sit and wait
All will be revealed

JAMES PATRICK PAGE & ROBERT PLANT 1973

Table of Contents

PROLOGUE

Lake Tahoe, California

The first thing Renee noticed was the birds. They rose in a flutter, a sea of black in the sky. Next came the rumble, and the empty chair ahead swung on its cable. Then came a deafening wall of whiteness, rushing like frothy water beneath her dangling legs, engulfing the skiers below.

Renee had known something was going to happen. She'd felt it coming for weeks, like a flu hovering at the back of her throat.

She looked up the mountain.

The ridge was a snowless, dark line. Bare now, except for the silhouette of a black figure framed by the empty blue sky.

It was him. He was waiting.

Her heart pounded as the lift came to a stop. She slid off the chair, the slope looming long and steep ahead.

She started with an awkward pace, each step lighter as she drew nearer, her loneliness evaporating.

Bearded, he stood in a large rawhide coat, a gun held firmly against his side, three dead rabbits draped over his thick arm.

Scraping her hair from her eyes, she faced him, a strange lightness creeping up her spine and settling in her shoulders.

"Never sneak up on a hunter," he said, his lips moving without disturbing his mustache.

"I didn't. You were watching me."

His teeth chattered. *Surely he was too strong to be cold?*

"I've been cold since I turned sixty," he said, reading her mind. "But better to be in the mountains cold than at home by the fire."

A tear fell then. It was what she would remember most, the way it ran, slow and heavy, down the white stubble of his cheek, leaving a silver trail. She clasped his steel-cold fingers and brought his hand to her flushed cheek. It smelled of gunpowder and the moist earth and feces of the rabbits.

"You are warm," he sighed. "One of the wonders of youth."

There was comfort in the thickness of his voice, and she could feel his pulse, fast and strong.

"Are you God?" she asked.

Tilting his head back, he chuckled. "No, I am not God. My name is Ernest. I'm a hunter, a writer, and once a soldier. And I'm dying from this cold."

"I'm Renee," she said. "And I'm no one."

He smiled. "You are more important than you know."

She moved closer to him, compelled to keep him warm. He spread his arms so she could nestle her head in his armpit, and intertwined, they walked over the ridge to a cabin on the far slope.

Inside, a rough wooden table was pushed against the far wall. Beside it was a fireplace. Three black pots hung from its mantel and antlers were mounted above. Beyond was a bed with a red woolen blanket at its foot.

"I've dreamed about this place," she said. "About you."

"Yes," he said, shivering. "I know."

"Come," she said. "I'll make a fire."

There was kindling neatly splintered in an iron bowl beside the hearth. She stacked the sticks and held a match to them until they began to crackle and smoke, then laid a log across their flames.

He lay down with the coat beneath his head and one arm splayed out beside him. His face flickered yellow and black with the flames. She sat next to him and he took her hand in his, filling her instantly with light.

"Why am I here?" she asked.

"In time it will make sense."

"Shouldn't I be afraid?"

"You know when to be afraid and when not to," he said. "Don't your parents speak to you about your gifts?"

What gifts?

But she didn't ask, afraid to break the moment.

"Never mind," he said. "Whatever they tell you is useless. They only know half the Truth. And there's nothing more dangerous."

"Will *you* tell me?"

"You can't go on the journey if you already know the Truth. And the Truth will mean nothing to you if you don't go on the journey. So, you see, I can't tell you."

"Will I see you again, after this?"

"Maybe. There is so little time."

"Then tell me something," she said. "So that one day I'll know this happened, that you were real."

He moved closer. She could see the embers of the fire in his eyes.

"You will have three daughters," he said.

Daughters? Her father wouldn't be pleased.

"The first will be dangerous and bright with fire, burning anything feebler than she. The second will be unpredictable, weak in integrity and dramatic like water out of a floodgate. And the third will be as soft and light as the wind, so buoyant you'll struggle to touch her, so wise you won't understand her." He paused. "And you, you will be the earth that grounds them, the fertile foundation from which they will thrive."

Renee took his hands and placed them over her heart, yearning again for the lightness to fill her.

His fingers were huge and rough. They stretched across her collarbone, curling over her shoulders. When she closed her eyes, light wrapped around her back, up her neck, and down her spine.

"Beauty is where the Truth lies," he said softly. "Find it. Embrace it."

PART I

Death

1

Sara
Cincinnati Ohio

There had been rumors they planned to bury Mr. Weishaup's body in the backyard.

"Like a dog," Sara had whispered to her sister that morning as they brushed their teeth. "I hope we get to watch."

She hadn't thought they'd really be lucky enough to watch a backyard burial, but standing with her sister in the foyer of the Weishaups' huge Victorian home beneath eerie modern paintings of the Grim Reaper and various superheroes rolling in the hay, she thought it might be possible.

She took in the high, ornate ceilings, the thickly carved mahogany doors, and the smooth marble statues. There was an abundance of plants, the room alive with green. Ferns sat on end tables, succulents grew in pots behind doors, potted ivy dangled from bookcases. In the corners of the room, stone golems followed her with their eyes. She fished her phone out of her pocket and took a photo of one of the golems.

"Sara," her mother said, snapping her fingers. "Put your phone away. We talked about this."

A giant mirror hung high on the far wall, tilted so Sara could see herself from above, her short, thick hair sprouting in black clusters, her dark blue eyes set in pale skin. Next to her, tiny and olive skinned, Hadley stared up beneath blond waves, her hazel eyes so close to the color of her skin, she appeared like an unfinished painting, light and washed out.

Sara shared the photo quickly, listened for it to send, and slipped her phone back in her pocket.

Mrs. Weishaup approached them, speaking to Sara's mother. "I don't think I've met your daughters, Renee, have I?"

"No, sorry. This is Hadley and Sara, our two youngest."

"And how old are you girls?"

"Seventeen," Sara said, her phone buzzing in her pocket with incoming likes.

"Thirteen," Hadley whispered.

"She's very small for her age," her mother said when Mrs. Weishaup's face reflected doubt.

"Yes, I'd say! I would have guessed *ten*. It'll catch up with you sooner or later though. Everything always does. After all, look at George!" Mrs. Weishaup let out a high-pitched cackle. "Caught up with him, all right, all that snooping around! Now he's dead! Hah! Now come, let's go see the fool while we still can."

The lounge was heavy with the smell of ham and brewing coffee. A few people were milling around a claw-footed table with a white lace cloth, picking fruit off a platter with toothpicks. On the far side of the room, the casket loomed, Mr. Weishaup's white profile visible through the ferns and flowers.

Sara approached the casket and peered in. His cheeks were pink, his hair silvery white. He smelled like baby powder and dill pickles.

She considered the strangeness of dressing a dead man. Was it a job she could do one day? She liked the idea immediately. Would it require much schooling? Surely only a little.

She fished out her phone again, staring at the stillness of his chest, willing it to rise, just once, and startle her. Imagine capturing that on Instagram!

"Ever seen a dead man before?"

She looked up into a pair of brown eyes beneath a pile of curly orange hair.

"No," Sara said, clicking the photo so it captured the girl hovering above the dead body. "It's *lit* though."

"I hadn't either before today. How do you know my dad?" Her upper lip was larger than the lower one, casting a shadow over her mouth.

"This is your dad?" Sara asked, lowering her phone.

"Was my dad, yeah. You don't have to post everything you see, you know."

"Sorry," Sara said, studying the girl. Had she met her before? Sara guessed they were probably the same age.

The girl shrugged and wrinkled her freckled nose.

"I'm Penny." She stuck her hand across her father's body. "You're one of Scott Morgan's daughters, aren't you?"

"Yeah," she said, shaking her hand. "I'm Sara."

Penny's grip was strong. Sara could feel the hold around her fingers after she pulled her hand away. It left a warm, tingly sensation.

"I know your dad. He was around a lot."

"Yeah?" Sara didn't pay much attention to what her dad did.

"Would you like a drink?" Penny asked, moving around the casket accompanied by a wonderful smell of apples and roses.

"Not really."

"I don't mean some lame punch. I mean a drink."

Sara couldn't believe her luck. "Fuck, yeah. If there's one going."

The girl frowned. "You should lose the foul language. It's terribly ordinary."

Sara tried to think of a smart response but couldn't.

"I like your hair though. It's cool." The girl leaned into Sara, her curls brushing Sara's neck, the smell of fruit and flowers engulfing her. "If anyone asks, I'm giving you a tour of the house, okay?"

Sara glanced behind her, looking for her mother or Hadley. When she couldn't find either, she nodded and followed Penny toward the stairs.

Sara stood on the balcony of Mr. and Mrs. Weishaup's bedroom, swiping through the likes and hearts from her golem post. She could hear the fumbling of Penny's fingers and the rustling of her skirt as she picked the lock on the liquor cabinet. Sara couldn't imagine why she would find the soft sounds arousing. She kept her eyes on her phone, trying to look preoccupied.

Finally, Penny appeared with a rocks glass in each hand and handed Sara one, the smell of Band-Aids filling her nostrils.

"Whiskey?"

"Scotch. Some single barrel stuff my dad always raves about. Figured today's as good a day as any. Don't post it, okay?"

Sara put her phone back in her pocket.

"You go to Indian Hills?"

Sara nodded, taking a sip. "Not you though. I'd have noticed you."

"Home schooled. My mother's paranoid, completely wacko."

Sara noticed a painting over the bed of Batman and the Grim Reaper wrestling in a field. "You do those paintings?"

"How'd you know?"

Sara shrugged. "You look like the arty type."

"What do you think of them?"

"I think you might be as wacko as your mom."

Penny laughed, her large upper lip curling back to reveal straight white teeth and a dark pink tongue.

"See that door?" Penny pointed to a door half hidden by ferns on the other side of the room. "It's the library. There's a pool table in there. Wanna game?"

The library was grand, with dark walnut bookshelves, ornate mahogany furniture and a marble hearth, but it was in complete disarray. The pool table was indiscernible beneath piles of books and folders. Papers were crumpled and gathered in heaps on the floor, and the air was stagnant and sour.

Penny hesitated in the doorway, her knuckles white around the Scotch bottle. Sara noticed her shirt had slipped from her shoulder, the purple satin of her bra bold against her freckled skin.

"This isn't right," Penny said. "My father is meticulous. He lectures my mother when she puts a fork in the spoon tray."

Penny moved further into the room, setting the Scotch bottle on an empty bookshelf. "Should we clear this table?" She kicked some wads of paper to the floor and lifted her dress, using it to wipe a layer of dust. Sara looked for a glimpse of purple satin to match the bra.

"I'm not wearing any," Penny said.

"What?"

"Underwear."

Sara's face grew hot. She tipped her glass back and finished the Scotch in a large gulp.

"Well, you were looking."

"I wasn't looking."

"Yes, you were." She came to Sara and put her finger under her chin and brought their lips together, her mouth soft and fuzzy, the apple-rose shampoo tingling Sara's nose. Then she pulled away quickly, leaving Sara standing with her lips still pursed.

Sara fought the instinct to pull her phone out like she usually did in awkward moments. Instead, she lifted the bottle of Scotch off the shelf and refilled her glass.

"There's something you should know," Penny said.

"That you're into girls?"

"No, this is serious," Penny said, moving toward the leather chairs by the window and sitting down. "My dad didn't die of cancer. He was murdered."

"Murdered?"

"He told me a few weeks ago that he was afraid something might happen to him. He said he'd discovered something important and was on a mission to expose it. He said if he was killed everything I needed to know would be in the library." She paused for a second. "But he was always so paranoid and nervous that I didn't take him seriously, you know? I didn't believe him and now he's dead."

Sara held up the bottle. "You should have another drink."

"You have to listen to me. Our fathers worked together, and whatever's going on, your dad's part of it."

Penny was gravely serious, and despite the images downstairs of Spiderman humping the Grim Reaper, Sara was inclined to believe her. But she was feeling awkward about the kiss, and the room was starting to spin so she laughed. "You think my dad killed your dad?"

"No. I think your dad's next."

"Oh," Sara said, finally sitting down, her legs like noodles. "Have you checked here like he said?" She looked about the disheveled room.

Penny nodded. "I couldn't find anything. But the thing is, it was in perfect order when I looked the other day. Nothing out of place."

"So, you think someone ransacked it? Like in the movies?"

"It could have been my mother. I don't know."

"What do you want me to do?" Sara asked, hoping it didn't involve too much thinking. Or walking. She wasn't feeling very steady.

"Has your dad said anything to you?"

Sara shook her head.

"Are you sure?"

"Hundo P."

"I don't understand text talk. I was home schooled."

"It's not text talk, it's slang."

"Whatever. Think. Is there anything he's said?"

"If something was up, he wouldn't tell me. He'd tell Brett."

"Is that your brother?"

"No, my older sister. His favorite."

"Well you have to talk to her."

"Brett's a bitch. She hates me."

"You have to try!"

"We might be going to New Zealand."

"What? When?"

"Don't know. Dad mentioned it last week. We're having some dinner discussion about it on Sunday. I don't even know where it is."

"It's down by Australia," Penny said. "When was this decided?"

"He mentioned it a few days ago. We're supposed to have some stupid family meeting about it. Do they speak English there?"

"Of course they speak English there. It's part of the Commonwealth."

Sara didn't know what the Commonwealth was. "What else do you know about it?"

"It's a long way away. I'm surprised you haven't googled it. You could use your phone for something useful, you know."

Sara shrugged. "How far away?"

"You couldn't get any further away without going to the South Pole. It would be a good place to hide."

"Hide from what?"

"That's what you have to find out. You've got to talk to your sister."

The door flew open and Mrs. Weishaup came in.

"There you are!"

She glanced at the bottle of Scotch and moved across the room to Penny, pulling her out of the chair. "Come along! Back to the party. Lord! You girls reek of booze. Come to think of it, I'll have some myself." She hurried them out of the library, picking up the Scotch bottle on the way, and pushed them through the bedroom and into the hallway. "You girls go on. I'll close up the cabinet."

A group of women in flowered dresses stood at the bottom of the stairs. "Penny, darling! There you are!" They waved her down.

"My father's sisters," Penny explained, rolling her eyes.

Sara followed her down the stairs. The house was swarming with black suits and dresses. Empty lipstick-stained glasses cluttered the hutch and the side table. Through the archway, she could see food steaming in large warmers on the dining room table. She noticed the casket had been closed.

"How are you holding up, dear?" an aunt asked, wrapping her arms around Penny.

"Come, have some punch," another one said.

Penny leaned into Sara, apple and rose enveloping her. "Please talk to Brett?"

Sara nodded, "Heard."

"And don't talk to anyone else," she whispered.

And she was gone, orange hair into the crowd.

2

Hadley
Cincinnati, Ohio

It was all wrong. Everyone was lying.

Hadley didn't care about the lying. It was the darkness in her father's eyes, the fear behind his words that worried her.

They weren't going to New Zealand for his work. He was afraid of something, running from something. And her mother's sabbatical was just a way of finding opportunity in an unfortunate situation. That was what her mother always did, tried to make the mess of her father into an opportunity.

"It's just for six months," her father said. "An adventure."

Behold, he travaileth with iniquity, and hath conceived mischief, and brought forth falsehood.

They were having dinner. Her father had skyped Brett in and placed the tablet on the table in front of her empty chair.

"But *why?*" Brett's image screeched from the laptop, her mouth forming the words slightly after they were spoken. "Why *New Zealand?*"

"Work calls!" He forced a smile that didn't raise his eyebrows. "It's a temporary placement. It'll be fun. We can be a family again."

"But I'm about to get tapped, Dad. Then initiation. I would miss everything. Have you forgotten?"

Sara dropped her fork loudly on the table. "I'm not going. *No* way."

"Well, we're going, girls. We leave next Thursday."

"Next *Thursday*?" Sara pushed against the table and scooted her chair back. "You can't be serious."

"As for your initiation." He looked toward the tablet. "You can't go ahead with it. You need to leave before they tap you."

"Dad, you're making no sense," Brett said, leaning into the screen so her face filled the square.

"You can still get out of it. You haven't tossed any bones yet," her father said.

"Tossed any bones?" Sara got out of her chair. "Dad, you're being so extra tonight."

"Get *out* of it?" Brett wailed. "But this is what you wanted for me! This is why I came to Yale. Dad, what's going *on*?"

"I can give you more Truth than you'll find in the Order. Walk away, come to New Zealand and I'll explain everything."

"Why do I have to go to New Zealand for you to tell me?"

"Because it'll be safer there."

Hadley noticed he said safer. Not safe.

"I thought we were going for your work," Sara said. "What's safe got to do with it?"

"*You* stay out of it," he snapped.

"So, I don't have any say in this?"

"None of you have any say in this."

The room was growing small. Hadley could feel a vision coming on. They happened at times like this, when people around her were fearful. Or they happened in times of joy, when people were hopeful and happy.

She was running, dark sand hard against the bare soles of her feet. She was cold, wet strands of her hair clinging to her cheeks and neck. She was breathless, her lungs tight, her legs burning. But she couldn't stop, *wouldn't* stop.

She looked behind her into the thick fog. What was she running from?

She turned back around, realizing the fear she felt was the fear of loss, the fear of something getting away. There was a figure in the fog ahead of her, a blur of height wrapped in whiteness. She saw the flash of a bare foot, a glimpse of an ankle. She reached toward the fog.

"Hadley?"

She blinked and saw her father standing over her.

If there be a prophet among you, I the Lord will make myself known unto him in a vision and will speak unto him in a dream.

"Hadley, I asked you what you thought? About us going to New Zealand."

"I don't want to go," she said, blinking again as the vision faded.

Her father's face drooped, his frown lines setting in. He shook his head. "Where's the get up and go in this family? Renee, tell them. Tell them how lucky they are to have this chance."

Hadley's mother smiled at her, then looked into the screen across the table. "It's a fabulous opportunity, girls. We'll be back before you know it."

She was lying, about the fabulousness of it. And she was wrong about them all returning. Hadley knew they wouldn't all come home, and that those of them that did would return changed. But there was no way of explaining this to her parents. There was never any explaining anything to anyone.

I myself alone bear your cumbrance, and your burden, and your strife.

3

Brett
New Haven, Connecticut

Brett's conversation with her father was playing through her mind. His frantic breathing, the way his words toppled over each other, the way he'd begged her to leave school. It was the begging that had made her hang up. Was it part of his plan for her, some kind of test?

"What's wrong?" Noel asked, clicking the end of his pen.

"You're doing it again." She glared at him.

He put the pen down and closed his textbook. "What were you just thinking about?"

"Nothing," she said. "It's late. I'm too tired to study."

"You want a cup of coffee?"

He asked the question with a raise of his thick eyebrows, trying, as he often did, to tempt her with his charm.

She glanced at her watch. It was two in the morning.

"Maybe we should get some sleep," he said. "We can take turns; one of us keep watch."

"I don't plan on being asleep when they come."

He lowered his voice. "Maybe they aren't going to come. Maybe we should consider that?"

"My father taught me a person creates her own destiny, and I've done what's necessary. They'll come."

"It seems to me *he* created your destiny."

She glared at him again.

"I'm not afraid of you, you know."

She could see the nerve it took him to say this. It was as subtle as the narrowing and fluttering of one eyelid, but as obvious as if he'd quivered.

Why would her father have created her destiny just to try and destroy it now?

"What if only one of us gets tapped?" he asked. "Have you thought about that?"

What he was really asking was whether they'd still be friends when she got in and he didn't. Everyone knew she was first on the list. Or had been. The list had been created at the beginning of the semester, and her father's call had only come last week. She was nervous. A feeling she wasn't accustomed to.

"You've got more of a chance," she lied. "You're a man."

"But your mother's a Morgan."

"My mother's a dissenter Morgan. They say that's worse than being a gentile."

"They say you look like her."

Brett didn't like her mother. She was like a layer of skin that Brett couldn't quite shed, half attached, dry and scaly. Still, Brett appreciated the beauty her mother had bestowed upon her. Beauty was power. And their beauty, with its chiseled cheekbones and stoic jaw, was classic. The thin dark eyebrows, yellow hair streaked with gold and skin that was brown all year long made them both look younger than they were. But youth did not demand respect, and so it was their eyes that saved them. Their narrow, blue-black eyes.

"And anyway," Brett said. "The Morgan's were never Bonesmen, only their partners."

"But your father's a patriarch."

What would he think if he knew her father had called her last week and begged her to drop out of school and move to New

Zealand, giving up everything she'd worked for? She guessed Noel would probably start asking the same questions she'd been asking herself. Mainly, who had her father betrayed?

"Don't overestimate my chances at getting tapped," she said.

"You have nothing to worry about. I'm the one that should be worried."

"You speak five languages. You're top of our class. You'll get in somewhere. Scroll and Key, they'll definitely want you."

"Well, second best isn't good enough. It's Claw and Bones or nothing."

Should she comfort him? No, she wasn't good at consoling, and besides, she had doubts he'd get in as well. After all, nepotism ran deep in the Order. They rarely tapped a student without at least a distant tie to a major family. Noel was a nobody, a nobody with a lot of talent and intelligence, but still a nobody.

"I'm going to ask you something personal," he said, his eyelid twitching.

"Don't bother."

"No. I want to ask."

Not the least bit curious, she reopened her textbook.

"As long as I've known you, I've never heard of you going out on a date."

She knew where he was headed and was disinterested. She turned a page.

"So," he said, "does that mean you've never had a boyfriend? Never had sex?"

She appreciated the fact he hadn't used the word *virgin*. She despised the word.

"No," she said without looking up. "No to both."

"Is it by choice?" he asked. "I mean, you know, so you won't have to reveal anything on initiation night?"

Brett shut the book and looked at him. "How typically male of you," she said, her voice sharp and cold. "To think I consider sex something sacred, something to *wait* for. Should I even bother to explain to you that for a woman sex opens the door to a number of political disasters, pregnancy not being the least of them, and in which case she's ruined no matter what choice she makes?"

Both of his eyelids were twitching now.

"Top of the class, Noel, and you're still an idiot."

He shrugged and looked down at the cover of *Law & Ethics*.

"Besides, I haven't met a man even minutely worth the risk; certainly not you."

But there had been a boy, once. An engineering student who had shared her love for logic and problem solving. She'd often caught him looking at her and, unlike with others, had liked it, had *wanted* him to look.

But her father had warned her about falling in love, about how disruptive it could be, so she'd kept her feelings to herself, convinced she could enjoy his company without it upsetting her study. Except she'd become preoccupied with the wanting of him and found herself checking her phone too frequently, over-analyzing texts and breaking into cold sweats when she ran into him outside class. So, she stopped seeing him, stood him up for dinner at their favorite Mongolian restaurant and changed her phone number.

She wondered where he was now. What had become of him? Did he ever think of her?

Noel was fiddling with the frayed spine of the book. He didn't need to know about Eli. No one did.

"And you're wrong," she said. "About your assumption of initiation night. What they refer to as sexual sharing isn't what you think."

He looked up. "No?"

"It's an orgy."

"Really?"

Brett nodded.

"Did your father tell you that?"

"And the sacrifice isn't made at initiation night like everyone thinks. It's made after."

He was spared more of her enlightenment by a knock on the door. They both jumped, Brett's empty coffee mug crashing to the floor. Their eyes met, and regardless of the fact Noel was only a vehicle to propel her through her academic goals, Brett felt a twinge of intimacy. Everything was about to change, and he was there to share the moment.

She took a deep breath and went to the door, opening it slowly. Two young men dressed in gray suits stood in front of her. She recognized one from her International Trade class, but she didn't know his name. The air was cool and brisk in the hallway, and it wafted in with the smell of burned toast. There was always someone burning toast in the dormitory.

She smiled and stepped aside to let them in.

Simultaneously the young men lifted their right hands and Brett braced herself for what she'd been told was a "thunderous" tapping.

"Noel Soteriades?" asked the man on the left, looking over her shoulder.

Noel rose quickly, shoving his chair back with his knees and stepped forward. The young men came around Brett and into the room. Then, standing erect in front of Noel, they raised their right arms and rigidly slapped Noel on his shoulders with three large whacks.

"Noel Soteriades! Claw and Bones! Do you accept the tap?"

"With respect, sir!" Noel shouted back.

The men nodded in unison and proceeded to hand Noel a small, cream-colored envelope wrapped in a black satin ribbon. "We give you this in utmost confidence. You will honor the seal with privacy."

Cadet-like, they turned quickly on their heels and left the room. As they were closing the door behind them, one of them winked at Brett and flashed her a wry smile.

When she turned back around, Noel was slumped against the desk, staring at the envelope, the fringes of his thick black hair damp with perspiration. Brett was dumbfounded. All her concerns considered, she hadn't expected *this*. She cleared her throat and spread out a wrinkle in her skirt. "Well, open it. What does it say?"

He thumbed the black wax seal, an emblem stamped into it. "I should probably open it alone. It's secret."

So it happened this quickly, the separation from the rest of the world.

"Of course," she said. "I'll go. I'll go get some sleep." She started gathering her books.

"Brett, this is your room." He touched her gently on the shoulder. "*I'll* go."

He slipped the envelope in his pocket and gathered his books into his backpack. She didn't want him to leave. She was seized by a desperate urge to grab him by the shoulders and throw him on her bed. The desire, so unfamiliar, scared her.

"I'll call you tomorrow?"

"Don't bother," she said.

"Brett."

"Go." She pushed him out the door and closed it behind him, listening to his steps in the stairwell fade as he descended. They were ecstatic steps, joyous.

"Shit," she said loudly to the empty room. She rarely used foul language and found the vulgarity soothing. "Shit. Shit. *Shit!*" she said louder.

How could the Bonesmen walk right past her?

Whatever her father had done, it was much worse than she thought.

She went to her desk and sifted through the top drawer until she found a small piece of paper. She fingered it. She'd never planned on calling. But things had changed. She had to know what her father had done. Maybe Hadley would answer. She missed Hadley's voice.

She went to the phone and remembered her father had made her promise to use a payphone. She hesitated before grabbing her jacket and purse and locking the door behind her.

"Hello?"

"Sara. It's Brett."

"Fucking hell. What time is it there?"

"Three in the morning. Watch your language."

"What's wrong? Why are you calling?"

"Is Dad there?"

"You better not be calling from your dorm room. He'll freak."

"I'm on a payphone. Just get him, Sara. Now."

Brett listened as Sara yelled for him. There was music in the background, something Spanish, Flamenco dance music maybe. It was weird not being able to imagine the house they were in.

She pictured Hadley sitting curled on their old pink lounge chair, legs tucked under her, reading their grandmother's Bible. But they wouldn't have taken their furniture with them. It was unlikely they'd even found a house yet. They were probably in a hotel.

"Brett? Is that you?" her father's voice sounded surprisingly close.

"Yes," she said.

"Where are you calling from?"

"A payphone."

"Good girl. Have you thought about what I said? Are you coming out?"

"No, I'm not coming to New Zealand. I'm calling because it's the last Tuesday of April and I haven't been tapped. The Bonesmen came in my room and tapped Noel Soteriades, a *minion* for Christ's sake, right in front of me and barely glanced in my direction. What have you done?"

He exhaled into the receiver, grunted half a word and stopped.

"Dad? You there?"

"They wouldn't shut you out because of me, honey. Just the opposite."

"There's no reason for them to change their minds, Dad. This *has* to be because of you. I can't comprehend what you're doing. You've worked your whole life for this. You've worked *my* whole life for this. You don't really expect me to believe you're accompanying Mom on sabbatical in New Zealand, do you?"

"I love you," he said. "You know that. But unless you skip your graduation and come here, I can't talk to you."

"Why? What's going on?"

"I know your loyalties will always lie with them. I raised you to think that way, so I can't blame you, but I have your mother and sisters to think about now."

"My loyalties? Since when do I have to choose between the societies and you?"

"I'm sorry, Brett, but things have changed."

Something banged on the booth, shaking the phone box. Brett jumped and spun around.

Two figures stood in the darkness.

A flashlight clicked on. She blinked and shaded her eyes. One of the figures thumped on the door.

"Brett? You there?" Her dad's voice sounded far away now.

"Someone's knocking on the phone booth. There's a light shining in my eyes."

"Don't open the door," he said.

"Who is it?" she asked. "What's happening?"

"They always tap the first on the list last. It's them. They've come to tap you."

The door creaked open.

"Listen, Brett. If you do this, if you become one of them, don't tell them where I am. You hear me? When it comes to your sacrifice, please think long and hard about it."

She made out two fingers slipping through the crack.

"Brett Morgan?" a voice asked, the door opening all the way as two hands reached in and slapped her firmly on the shoulders. "Claw and Bones! Do you accept?"

"Yes," she said, startled.

They shoved an envelope in her hand. "We give you this in the utmost secrecy. We ask you to honor it in privacy."

The flashlight clicked off and they were gone.

The phone, still cradled in the crook of her neck, was silent.

"Hello?" Brett said.

"Brett?" It was Hadley's soft voice.

"Hadley, get Dad please."

"He's gone."

"What do you mean he's gone?"

"He dropped the phone and ran out of the house. Are you coming here? I miss you."

"I miss you too, kiddo."

Someone yelling in the background; it sounded like her mother.

"I have to go," Hadley said.

"Wait, Hadley ..."

"Sorry, Mom says I have to hang up. Bye."

Hadley's voice was replaced with the dull hum of the dial tone.

Brett hung up and studied the envelope in the fluorescent light of the booth. The ribbon was sealed with the infamous emblem of the Illuminati. She fingered the smooth wax, savoring its thickness, before she carefully opened the letter.

PLEASE MEET AT THE CITADEL OF THE ORDER

322 PROSPECT WAY

SATURDAY, MAY 8TH

*BE ADVISED THE REQUESTED INITIATE SHOULD NOT WEAR ANY METAL

4

Renee
Cincinnati, Ohio

Renee was supposed to be in Tahoe. It would be the first time in forty years she wouldn't visit the cabin. And for what? Another ridiculous mission of her husband's.

But she'd decided long ago she didn't want to know about his work. And he'd respected this throughout the years, giving her as little detail about his work as possible, keeping phone calls to the office, being vague about his trips overseas. But this latest move, to take the family out of the country, was different. It was desperate and rash.

"You won't be able to go to Tahoe this year," Hadley said from the window seat. She was propped in the sun reading the Bible.

"It's a nice day. Why don't you go outside and play?"

Hadley ignored her suggestion. "You don't want to go to New Zealand either, do you?"

"Of course I want to go. It'll be an amazing experience."

"But you'd rather go to Tahoe."

Renee's life had revolved around her trips to the cabin for so long she couldn't imagine not going. It was her time for reflection, her annual refuel. "Yes," she said, knowing it was useless lying to Hadley. "I'd rather be going to Tahoe."

She went and sat next to Hadley, placing her hand on her knee. "And why don't you want to go?"

Hadley tucked a red ribbon in the inside spine of the Bible and closed it. "Something bad is going to happen there, Mom."

"What do you mean something bad?"

Hadley shrugged. "I don't know."

"You're just reacting to all that crazy talk between Dad and Brett. It's just grownups playing games, nothing more."

"What do you mean, games?"

"They join groups and have secrets. It's like the club you used to run in your tree house with your friends when you were little. Remember that? You used to make up stories and create little mysteries and solve them. It's just like that, only for adults."

"Why would Brett and Dad want to do that?"

Renee thought about this for a moment and then said, "It makes them feel important."

"But they're already important."

Renee smiled. "I know. It's just not the kind of important they want."

"So, we're going then? For sure?"

"Yes," Renee said, kissing her forehead. "All of this packing hasn't been for nothing, kiddo."

"On Thursday?"

"Yep, in three days."

Hadley's face dimmed and she turned and looked out the window.

Renee moved to comfort her and stopped. She had no honest comfort to give her. Instead she stood, pushing aside her brewing panic, and went to finish packing.

5

Hadley
Matangi, New Zealand

A cold southerly whipped against Hadley's face. She zipped her jacket to her chin, surprised at its fierceness. She'd expected New Zealand to be a tropical island, but instead she'd found it was often cold and wet. But it was a fresh cold and a lush wet. And always green.

She'd never seen such green. Whether it was thick with fog or lying beneath the sharp, hot rays of the ozoneless sky, the country was always a plethora of greens; rolling hills covered in blankets of lime green; forest pines planted in perfect rows beside grassy olive-colored paddocks; tall jade poplars skirted with green privet bushes and the emerald leaves of hydrangea bushes.

And when it rained, the dampness released the fertile smells, cracked open the blades and needles and flowers, permeated the air so Hadley could feel the undergrowth, the shrubbery, the soil in the tiny hairs of her nostrils. She'd never been so aware of the earth and the things that grew from it, and she felt overwhelmingly lucky to be exposed to such rawness, for however short of a time it might be.

For Hadley was sure they would not be in New Zealand much longer. A disaster was pending, something that would send them back to the white concrete and swirling rubbish of Cincinnati sooner than they'd planned. But she didn't want to think about that.

She was helping her father rake leaves in the back garden, enjoying the pungent smell of silage and cow dung wafting from the neighboring paddocks. She was happy working alongside her father, his fear absent for the first time since they had arrived.

She knelt to scoop a pile of leaves and a vision came to her. But not the typical one-dimensional flashback where she saw herself from above. This one came from her own vantage point. She could see her hands, withered with dry white creases across the knuckles and adorned in silver rings. The rings were familiar. She knew she'd grown old with them. One wrinkled hand was patting fresh soil and the other was spreading brittle, fallen leaves. Hadley could see wisps of gray hair falling in front of her eyes. She could feel the wheeze of emphysema.

And with thee will I break in pieces old and young.

She blinked and looked up at her father, the vision fading. She was youthful again, her chest clear and hands plump and pink.

"Something is buried here," she said.

Her father looked at her over his rake, raising his eyebrows.

"I buried something here a very long time ago."

He nodded as he raked, pretending to listen.

"I was an old woman and I buried it by a tree," she said, looking around.

On the other side of the yard, behind the hedge, a tree caught her eye. She dropped her rake and went to it. Her father stopped and leaned against the rake, his beanie low across his forehead, wisps of dark blonde hair poking into his eyes as he watched her. He wasn't a tall man, but from her view he seemed large.

"It was here. I buried it here. We must get a shovel," she said, kneeling and scraping at the dirt with her hands.

Her father didn't move.

41

And thou shalt dig therewith, and shalt turn back and cover that which cometh from thee.

"A shovel!" she shouted.

He looked at her as if to say, *Well, okay then, if it's that important to you,* and leaned the rake against a bush, and went to the garden shed.

She continued to claw at the dirt, the earth working its way into her fingernails. Her father reappeared with a shovel, and she pointed to where she'd scratched the soil. "Dig here!"

He cocked his head, gave a perplexed laugh and began to dig. Hadley watched with anticipation. "It's in a steel box and inside the box is a leather bag," she said. "Keep digging."

His shovel hit something and he pulled back. Hadley clapped her hands in excitement.

"It's probably just a rock, Hads."

"It's not. It's the box. Inside is a leather bag with a book."

Her father put the shovel down and lowered his arms in the hole, grimacing as he fished with his hands. Then he looked at her sideways and pulled out a small gray box.

"See! I knew it was there." Hadley took the box and brushed off the dirt. Its rusted latch snapped off in her fingers. She opened the lid and pulled out a leather pouch.

"What is it?" her father asked.

"A book," she said, untying the pouch and pulling out a small red-bound book with gold writing across the front.

And the Lord said unto Moses, write this for a memorial in a book, and rehearse it in the ears of Joshua.

"Let me see that," he said, taking it from her.

He held it close to his eyes, then began running toward the back door.

"Dad! What're you doing?"

She ran after him into the house and followed him to his study.

He flung open the filing cabinet and took out some papers. He laid them across the desk and set the book next to them, moving his finger back and forth from the papers to the book. "It's the same. This is the same writing. My God, Hadley, how did you know it was there?"

"I just remembered."

"You saw it before?"

"I told you, I buried it there a long time ago."

"We've only been in New Zealand for a week."

"A long time ago, Dad. I lived here a really long time ago."

"What do you mean? How do you know?"

Hadley shrugged.

He set the book down and came to her. "Try to explain."

"I remember things all the time, things from the past."

He took her face in his hands. "And to think, all along it was you. Always so old for your age, so wise. I should have known!"

"Me what?" Hadley asked.

He kissed her forehead. "I must get a hold of Brett. We should have made her come with us. I should have been firmer."

His hands fell from Hadley's face and she saw the fear clouding his eyes. She didn't understand why he would be afraid. The book was good. She knew it was good.

"Can I have the book, Dad?"

"What?" He turned back to his desk and looked for something in the drawers.

"The book, can I have it?"

"No." His voice was strained.

"Why has the book scared you?" she asked.

He ignored her and turned back to the filing cabinet, his fingers fluttering through papers.

While he was distracted, Hadley slipped the book into her pocket.

Men do not despise a thief, if he steal to satisfy his soul when he is hungry.

She backed out of the room and walked down the hall to the bathroom. She sat on the toilet lid and opened the book. God had led her to the book. And if she studied it, she would remember how to read it. She was sure she was able to read it once, a long time ago.

Thou wilt receive my words and hide my commandments with thee.

6

Brett
New Haven, Connecticut

Sleep-deprived, Brett stood in front of the windowless sarcophagus, fourteen classmates lined up single file behind her. The building was huge and grim under the streetlights. Had it always been windowless and enshrined in ivy or had it once been a normal house? Either way, it had been the meeting house for Claw and Bones for decades and was generally regarded with awe.

Although the sun had gone down, there was no breeze, and it was warm for a spring night in New Haven. She'd no doubt they would have had to stand there in the snow if the weather chose, and she was thankful for the still air. Her feet were numb from standing erect, but she wouldn't shift her weight. She was the first woman in the history of Claw and Bones to lead the initiates and she wouldn't have anyone regretting the decision.

A bolt moved on the huge triple-padlocked door. She blinked, her eyes stinging from fatigue. She'd imagined this twice before. She willed it to open.

Someone coughed behind her. Was it Noel? It sounded like him. She hadn't been able to get a good look at the others yet. Was there anyone she knew?

Someone hollered out the window of a car as they drove by. "Fucking Fascists!"

A soda can flew out the window and clinked against the curb. Brett questioned the logic of lining them up on the street. Was it advertising? Did the seniors want everyone to know who this year's initiates were?

Someone nudged her from behind. "Brett, the door's opening."

Slowly and steadily, the gap widened until the door was two-thirds open. There was no one on the other side, only darkness.

She could feel the shuffling anticipation of her fellow initiates behind her.

"What're we supposed to do?" someone asked.

"Wait," someone else said. "They'll let us know what they want us to do."

"They won't leave the door open for long." It was Noel. "It's never supposed to open in the presence of a vandal."

"A vandal?" Someone laughed.

"A *non*-member. A gentile." She thought she recognized something in the voice. There was something familiar in the soft articulation.

A dim light was coming from inside, and Brett could vaguely make out a picture frame on the wall. She glanced at the stone masts on either side of her.

"Wait by the pylons," a young man had told them after he lined them up. She'd thought she recognized him from the student paper but wasn't sure. "Stay single file and wait," he'd said. That had been almost two hours ago.

She'd waited long enough.

She stepped forward, past the masts and up the stone path toward the door. When she reached the steps, she turned and looked over her shoulder.

They were all watching, wide eyed.

"Is someone there?" Noel asked. Although he was in the back, his height made him easily heard.

"Not that I can see," she said.

"How do you know we're supposed to go in?" someone asked.

"I don't."

"Then we should wait," someone else said.

She ascended the thick granite steps and walked through the doorway and onto a Persian rug. The entryway was lit by a single flickering candle mounted to the wall. What she'd thought was a picture frame was the face of a grandfather clock, its pendulum still. The time read four o'clock. Identical clocks lined the walls, leading to a closed door at the end of the hall.

"Hello?" she said, her voice bouncing off the clocks.

Only the soft dancing of the candle answered her.

She turned and walked back out into the dusk light.

"Come on," she said to the line of upturned faces. "Let's move in."

"Are they in there?"

"Somewhere."

"But you didn't see them?"

"No."

"What did you see?"

"A hallway of clocks."

"What the hell," Noel said. "Let's go."

"I'm going to wait until I'm invited." It was the boy standing in front.

"You've been invited," the girl behind him said. "What do you call the letter you got?"

"I'm going to wait until someone instructs me," he said.

"*I'm* instructing you," Brett said loudly.

"Who are you? You're not a Bonesman."

"Until you move, no one else can."

"Go," someone said. "You can trust her." That voice again, so familiar.

47

"Yeah, go. They wouldn't open the door unless they wanted us to go in."

Reluctantly the boy in front moved forward, stopping at the bottom of the steps. "Are you *sure*?"

"No, I'm not sure," she said, turning around and reentering. "But when a door opens, you enter."

As the last of them stepped inside, the door closed behind them and the one at the end of the hall opened simultaneously. Brett could see tall shadows crowded behind the door, candles flickering behind them. She approached the door, her eyes adjusting to the new light. She saw the shadows wore hooded cloaks and on the floor was a glossy coffin. The lid was propped open with a stick. It was empty and lined in red velvet.

"Remove your shoes and get in," a voice said from beneath a hood.

She slipped out of her heels and set them neatly against the wall. She stepped into the coffin, the velvet soft beneath her stocking feet, and lay back against the pillow. The fabric smelled like lavender and nutmeg. They closed the lid and she was swallowed by darkness.

She wasn't afraid. She'd heard about this ritual. She knew by being there she was being accepted.

She felt the pressure of her body pressing into the velvet as the casket was lifted. It rocked rhythmically as they carried her. She was lifted higher and the casket tipped at an angle, so her feet slipped toward the front. Then three rocks and a jolt, three rocks and a jolt, until the casket came to a halt.

She could hear a soft hum, like a generator or a badly wired fluorescent bulb. As it grew louder, she realized it was chanting. It was too muffled for her to understand but she could tell it was

German. The lid opened, and she could see the shadows of candles flickering against the wall.

"Brett Morgan," said a cloak looming above her. "Today you are being reborn into society. From here forward, as a sister of the Order of Claw and Bones you will strive for excellence and nothing less. You will do as the Order deems necessary in all political matters. You will rise from the death of your life among the Masses and enter the world of Truth. You will no longer be a victim."

She thought of her father. He'd lain in this coffin, heard these words spoken to him. But as far as she knew, he'd never learned the Truth. She wanted to sit up and tell them not to make false promises. But this was the only way she knew to the Truth. Silly game or not, she had no other option but to play it.

"Come," the cloak said. "Enter your new life, Knight Brett."

She climbed out and stood in front of the group. Someone held out a cloak to her and she slipped it on. Then she was handed a polished, white femur. She held the bone by the ball and examined it. She saw her name etched along its length.

"You shall throw this into the pile," the cloak said. He pointed to a red blanket lying in the middle of the room. It was heaped with bones, all femurs. "And in so doing become a Bonesman."

She gave it a toss and it landed with a clunk on top of the others. Immediately, six hooded members closed the lid on the coffin and hoisted it on their shoulders, off to collect the next greenhorn.

Once the other initiates had been transported downstairs in the coffin, been cloaked and hooded, and tossed their bones in the pile, they followed the seniors and the patriarchs into an adjoining room. It had been hard to see the others in the dim light beneath her hood.

The room was dark, but not in the warm, simmering way the other room had been. The room was dark because the floor, the walls, and the ceiling were covered in black velvet. Fluorescent lights hummed in the ceiling and filtered an eerie green glow across the velvet. In the middle of the room was a large pit sunk a foot into the ground and filled with smooth mud spread neatly to each corner, like a giant unbaked cake.

Brett had heard rumors of the mud pit and had come prepared.

"Hang your robes on the hooks," a patriarch said, nodding his hood toward a row of wooden stakes sticking out of the wall, "and take your clothes off." It was a severe voice, deep and refined.

Brett took off her cloak and hung it on a hook, careful not to turn her back on him as she did. She stepped to the edge of the pit, looking directly into the shadows beneath his hood, careful not to show defiance but strategic in showing her deliberation. She unzipped her dress and let it fall to the floor.

She'd worn nothing underneath.

"Good," the man said, with one swift rise of a cloaked arm. "The rest of you, out of your clothes and into the mud. Become the animals you are. Be not ashamed. For it is those who suppress their savage nature that are ruled by it. In the Order, barbarism should be acted out, released, examined in the controlled midst of your brothers and sisters."

Brett stepped in, the mud softer than she'd expected and much colder, icy goo seeping between her toes. She knelt and scooped mud in her hands, squeezing it so it oozed and splattered. The others were climbing in now, one girl rapidly smearing mud over her breasts and legs. Most of the boys had erections, a few embarrassed, others clearly not.

"What do they want us to do?" one of the girls asked her.

"Whatever you feel like."

"I *feel* like putting my clothes back on and going home."

"Then do that," Brett said.

Brett could feel someone looking at her and turned. Because of the nudity, the mud, the entire strangeness of the scene, it took her a moment to realize who the boy was.

"Eli," she said, a flush coming over her, the mystery of the familiar voice unveiling itself.

"Hello, Brett," he said.

He'd changed since she'd seen him, but she wasn't conscious of his thinned hair and his broadened shoulders. She was distracted by his nudity, her eyes lowering to the trail of fuzz beneath his navel. She looked away.

"You. I ..." she stammered. "I didn't know you aspired for the Order."

"We never had a chance to discuss it."

How long had he waited beneath the red lights of the restaurant that night? How many times had he tried her number before he'd given up?

She crossed her arms over her breasts, "I'm ... It's just ..."

"It's okay," he said. "I know why you did it."

Someone came flying into her then, placing a hand firmly between her legs, and she fell face forward in the mud. She pushed herself up out of the cold goo, momentarily blinded, arms flailing. She could hear Noel laughing, someone else shrieking. She wiped the mud from her eyes and looked for Eli. She wanted to tell him she was sorry, that she'd never stopped thinking of him. She wanted to explain to him why. But she caught a bony elbow with the back of her hand and there were fingers on her breasts, and cocks, two of them, pressed against her leg. She wiped the mud from her eyes. A hoard of arms and legs and chins surrounded her. And everywhere there was hair, mud-caked hair.

She forced herself to smile and slide against the slippery skin and limbs around her. Someone began to howl, a deep hollow

51

moan filling the room. It came from outside the pit. Someone else joined in. Another joined and another, until Brett, too, threw her head back and let out a wail. Each cry joined the others, some angry, some melancholy, a few full of anguish, others ecstatic. Soon the noise became one warped echo of emotion, resonating within the black velvet, out the cracks of the fused windows.

So this is what they heard every spring from the top of Weir Hall, the infamous Yale howling. This is what it was.

After they emerged from the mud, they were hosed down with cold water, followed by ten minutes in a warm shower. She was aware of Eli but avoided eye contact, her mind full of questions she was afraid he might read on her face. How had she missed his political interests? Was he a nobody, driven by his own will, or had he been cultivated like her? If only she'd known! If only she hadn't ended things before they discovered this commonality! What could it have been? This made her angry at her father, sent her teeth grinding at what she'd given up.

At midnight they were marched upstairs to room 333, the sanctum of the Claw and Bones hall. On the west wall hung, among other pictures, an old engraving representing an open burial vault, in which, on a stone slab, rested four human skulls grouped about a crown and bells, an open book, several mathematical instruments, and a handful of withered claws. On the arched wall above the vault were large words in a language she didn't recognize.

Encompassing a wooden podium, two circles of chairs were set up, one within the other. The new knights were told to take their seats in the innermost circle. They waited as the seniors came in, dressed in expensive, plain clothes, and seated themselves in the outer row of chairs. Next came the patriarchs and matriarchs. Shameless and proud, they marched before her: CIA and FBI officials, members of the Senate and the Supreme Court as well as the presidential cabinet, ambassadors, directors of the Federal Reserve Bank, they were all there. As they grouped around the circled chairs, firm and proper, Brett found herself smiling. They'd all watched her strip and slither in the mud, and they'd once done the same. How superbly ridiculous and extraordinary.

A hooded figure carried a briefcase into the center of the circle and placed it firmly on the podium, snapping open the gold latches with his thumbs.

"Tonight, we welcome the country's best and brightest youth to the rest of their lives." The voice was light and feminine. "Lives which, with the help of the brotherhood of Claw and Bones, will be full of power and affluence." He lifted his hand as if to toast, but there was no glass.

"Every society has the haves and the have-nots," he continued. "But there are also the have-mores. And on behalf of my fellow patriarchs," he nodded to the back row, "and our seniors, soon to graduate and begin making decisions that will change this country, this world, and the entire future of mankind," he gestured with both hands to the chairs, "we welcome you juniors to the have-mores."

He called Brett forward and she stood and faced him.

He held out his hand and she took it. "Knight Brett, we welcome you to Claw and Bones," he whispered, his breath smelling of red wine. He pressed two fingers into her palm and then circled her ring finger with his own, following it with two strong shakes. "This is the secret handshake of our brotherhood." He repeated it and then nodded for her to reciprocate the gesture, which she did swiftly and nodded back. Then, stepping back and reaching into his briefcase, he withdrew five thick stacks of cash. He held it in front of her, cleared his throat and said in a full voice, "In the foyer you will find a German-made, Kattenvenne grandfather clock engraved with your name. By accepting this gift," he gave the cash a quick wave, "along with the clock, you will swear not to discuss the Order with gentiles; and you will agree to leave the room if ever the Order is brought up in the company of vandals. Do you swear?"

"I swear," she said.

And with that he handed her fifteen thousand dollars.

7

Renee
Matangi, New Zealand

Scott was having another nightmare, his head thrashing against the pillow. They'd begun a few months ago and had become more frequent since they'd arrived in New Zealand.

Renee moved to wake him and stopped.

What was he saying? Something about Brett?

"Don't do it," he mumbled, his lips half buried in the pillow, his neck twisted so his Adam's apple caught the melon-colored glow from the nightlight.

She leaned in close. "Don't do what?"

"Tell them," he said. "Don't tell them." He flipped his chin to the other side of the pillow, his mouth distorted.

"Don't tell them what?"

"Where I am, who you are."

"Who is?"

"All of us. Who we all are. Who *they* are."

"Brett," she said. "What about Brett?"

"Save her," he said. "From the lies."

Save Brett? As if I could have any influence!

Renee hadn't had a real conversation with her daughter in years.

As a toddler, Brett had been affectionate. Renee could remember how she would crawl onto Renee's lap and bury her head in her chest, looking up at her with soft appreciation. And she'd been observant, interested in the world around her. Not the mobile tinkling above, or the rattle from her grandmother, but the rays of light coming in through the curtains and the crinkles in her hands and the sounds from the neighbors' backyard.

But then Scott had begun to cultivate her, the moments of affection and observation dropping away as she became buried in books and lessons and goals. By the time Brett started school, she'd lost interest in the beauty of the world and, with that, her mother. Renee resented Scott for this change, for his devotion to something all-consuming and pointless.

He sat up, his forehead hitting Renee in the shoulder. "She's wrong. Brett is wrong. I was wrong."

"About what?"

He blinked, his eyes focusing. "I was dreaming?"

She nodded. "About Brett."

He dropped his head into his hands, sweat glistening on his brow.

"What's wrong with Brett?" She asked, placing her hand gently on his damp back.

He shook his head together with his hands. "You never wanted to know."

"Not when it was about you," she said, colder than she meant to. "But if it's about Brett, I want to know."

He lifted his head and looked at her. She couldn't remember the last time they'd looked each other in the eye.

"What is it?"

"There's nothing you can do," he said, falling back onto the pillow. "And I wouldn't know where to start."

"Can you make it right?"

"I'm trying," he said, rolling toward the wall. "That's why we're here."

8

Sara

Matangi, New Zealand

Sara hated New Zealand. The dampness, the thick cow-shit air, the low gray cloud that hovered over their street, the racks of drying underwear set up in people's houses like staple furniture, the sticky pungent smell of roasting lamb, the airy-sweet ice cream, the white cheese, the insects that buzzed about her head at night and stuck to the ceilings during the day. Hadn't they heard of screens?

And the kids at school asked her the stupidest questions. Had she met Post Malone? Did she know Katy Perry? And the uniforms. Whoever heard of uniforms for a public school? And public schools with no boys. Ridiculous.

Sara blamed the fact there were no boys at her school on her obsession with Penny. If there had been boys to flirt with, she wouldn't be thinking of the girl with red hair. It had taken her by surprise, the obsession. What was it with the strange longing? Why couldn't she shake it? Every minute of every day she thought of her, dreamed of their next encounter, schemed excuses to text her. If only she had her number.

She played the day of their meeting over and over in her head. Had she drunk too much and looked stupider than normal? Was stupider even a word? And if it wasn't, had she used it? She replayed every glance, every smile. The way Penny had come around her Dad's casket and stood so close Sara could smell her.

She could still remember the apple rose of her hair. She'd sniffed all the shampoos at the Four Square (what kind of name was that for a grocery store?) trying to find it. But it wasn't how Penny smelled or the kiss that had moved Sara, it was the way she'd looked at Sara like a confidant. The way she'd looked at her at the bottom of the stairs before she disappeared into the crowd. Had these been signs Penny felt real affection for her? She must have felt something, she'd kissed her! But Sara was unconvinced. Penny had said, after all, that she was just playing. Or had she?

If only Sara hadn't drunk so much and could remember it all clearly. She should have tried to get in touch with Penny before she left, said goodbye. But they'd packed up so quickly. Sara hadn't appreciated what was happening until they were on the plane and the flight attendant was welcoming her onto the "seeven-seeven-seeven" and offering her a cup of tea with milk. What kind of people put milk in hot tea?

"A lot of people," her father had said. "This will be good for you, seeing a bit of the world."

She hadn't responded.

In fact, she hadn't spoken to her father since they'd left.

"You're being unreasonable," her mother said from across the living room (the girls at school called it a lounge). Her face was half hidden by a damp pink sleeve of Hadley's sweatshirt (known as a *jersey*) hanging off the clothes rack (clothes *horse*). "It's not fair, you being angry at him. It's his job. It's what pays for your phone and those horrible black nails."

"*I* pay for my black nails," Sara said, un-liking a post she'd changed her mind about.

"With money we give you for doing the dishes, something kids didn't get paid for in my day."

"*Still* not talking to him." She added an emoji.

"You hated Indian Hills. I thought you'd love an excuse to take a year off, have an adventure."

"*Not* loving it."

She was angry about Penny, of course, because *he* had moved her away from the most exciting person she'd met, well, *ever*. They'd apparently moved to New Zealand for his work. But he wasn't working. He was in his office all the time, staring out the window, and didn't go anywhere.

"Have you met any new friends?" Her mother asked.

"What do *you* think?"

"I don't know. That's why I'm asking."

"Maybe I would if there were some boys at school." When her mother didn't comment, she looked up from her phone and said, "Brett would like it here."

"Oh?" Her mother raised her eyebrows. "Why's that?"

"They're all boujee."

"Boujee?"

"Snobs."

"Did you say Brett?" Her father came gliding into the room in his office chair, the wheels babumping across the seams in the hardwood floor. "Have you talked to her?"

"Why would I talk to her? She hates me."

"Brett doesn't hate you, honey," her mother said.

"Oh, I wouldn't be so sure about that," her father said, scratching his head and studying his fingernails.

"Scott!" Her mother exclaimed, standing.

"It's nothing Sara should take offense to," he said, flicking whatever he'd found beneath his nails across the room. "Brett was bred to hate. I'm afraid it's who she is now."

Her mother widened her eyes with that you-need-to-stop-talking-about-this-in-front-of-the-children look.

"No, keep going, Dad. This is the first interesting thing you've said in weeks." Realizing she was speaking to her father, she placed her hand over her mouth and sunk into the pillows of the couch, fumbling with her phone.

Her father pushed against the wall and sent his chair spinning toward her. "Ha! Lovely to have you back." He came to a stop at the couch and reached into the depths of the pillows, took her face in his hands, and kissed her forehead.

She wiped away the moisture from his lips, surprised. He usually only showed that kind of affection to Brett. "What's gotten into you?" She asked, sinking further into the couch. "You're so *extra* lately."

"Extra what?" Her mother asked.

Sara rolled her eyes. "Just *extra*. You know, dramatic and weird."

"Yes, I know," her father said, placing his fingers beneath his chin in thought. "I *am* weird at the moment. I'm dismantling."

"What does that even mean?" Sara asked.

"See, even us oldies have special words," he smirked.

"So, what does it mean then?"

Her mother gave her father another warning look, which he dismissed with a shake of his head. "My purpose has been stripped from me, broken into pieces, so that I must rebuild. I'm preparing for the rebuild."

Sara pictured her father in bits on the floor of the garage, his shadow sifting through them, trying to reassemble himself.

"Everything I was taught was wrong," he continued, pushing off the couch and rolling, babump-babump, to the window.

A small gray bird landed on a branch on the other side of the glass. It cocked its head and looked at him. "How do you find new beliefs to reconstruct yourself?" He tilted his head to mirror the bird. "What do you replace fifty years' worth of indoctrination with?"

"Scott, come away from the window," her mother said. "Don't you have work to do?"

But her father just continued to stare at the little gray bird, scratching his head.

Hadley appeared at his side wearing a pair of red sunglasses and lay her hand on his knee. "It's okay, Dad. It's not your fault." Sara hadn't known she was in the room.

"Should we have a treat?" Her mother clapped her hands, the bird flying away in a startle. "I made some Anzac biscuits."

"What are *they*?" Hadley asked.

"Tooth breaking tasteless cookies the girls at school rave about," Sara said, grimacing.

"It's probably too late," her father said, spinning his chair around.

"Too late for cookies?" her mother asked.

"Too late for everything."

9

Brett
New Haven, Connecticut

Brett was summoned back to Weir Hall the day after their initiation.

The building was different during the day, the stone steps white in the sunlight and the ivy lush and inviting. She entered through the same door she had the night before, the grandfather clocks no longer lining the entryway, and made her way to the door at the end of the hall.

There was a couch and a potted plant where the coffin had been, and beside it a door with frosted glass. A shadow moved behind the glass and the door opened, a woman in a suit and red glasses appearing.

"Brett," she said, putting her hand out. "Margaret De Payen. Please come in."

They exchanged the secret handshake and Brett followed her in.

She motioned for Brett to sit in a seat across from a large desk.

"I trust you found the initiation enlightening?"

"Entertaining, at least," Brett said, sitting down.

The woman frowned.

"I'm sorry." Brett said, finding herself. "It's just I didn't work the last ten years for rituals and dances. I did it to learn the Truth, and I didn't learn anything at initiation."

"Interesting," De Payen said. "That you thought we'd reveal the Truth at initiation."

"I didn't expect that," Brett said. "It's just you asked if I found initiation *enlightening*. And I didn't."

"Do you know why we've summoned you today?"

"To discuss my sacrifice."

"Yes," De Payen said. "More specifically, to *request* your sacrifice."

"You want me to give up my father."

The woman's eyebrows rose above the red frames of her glasses. "Yes, that's right. Your father has become a threat."

"What's he done?"

"It's not what he's done, it's what he's *planning* to do."

"Which is?"

"I can't tell you the details. All I can say is that he's scheming against us."

"And what do you want from me?"

"We want you to tell us where he is."

"I would think an organization linked to the Order wouldn't need me to find out where my father is."

"We don't. It's your loyalty and dedication we're after."

"So, you're asking me to choose between the societies and my father?"

The woman nodded.

"But Claw and Bones and my father are one and the same. He's the reason I'm here at Yale. He's been preparing me for the Order, molding me for this day since I was five years old. How can I possibly turn against him?"

"Sometimes that's just how it works."

The memory of her father's franticness came to her again. *"If you do this, if you become one of them, don't tell them where I am."*

"Can I talk to him first?" Brett asked.

"No. If you want to continue on your journey, become part of the Order, you must have *no* contact with him."

"Isn't that sacrifice enough?"

"Yes. But your progression will be much slower."

Her father had told her there were many steps and that each involved a test. She'd never dreamed one day the test would involve turning on him. Had he known it was a possibility?

"If you ask us to let him live, we will," De Payen said. "It's your choice."

"Let him *live*?"

"We've already tried reasoning."

"You're going to *kill* him?"

"It's the best option," she said. "The cleanest way to protect the Order."

Brett sat back in her chair, gripping the arms.

"It's not our preferred option, but it's necessary for the greater good."

Her father had referred to the greater good frequently. *"I know you're tired, just keep going. It's for the greater good." "I know I'm away a lot, but it's for the greater good." "We aren't just doing this for you, or for me, but for the greater good."*

"And if I don't agree?"

"There will be no consequences if you ask us to keep him alive."

Brett came forward in her chair. "Then why in the world would I agree?"

"Because there will be great rewards if you allow us to kill him."

Brett fell back into the chair again. "I can't make that decision without knowing what he's done."

"He's a nuisance. It will be much better if he's exterminated."

As if her father were a cockroach! Surely the woman was bluffing.

"Brett?"

"You're asking me to order my father's death."

"We'll manage him alive if that's what you choose."

"How kind of you."

"This isn't a joke, Brett."

"So, I just give you a nod of my head and away you go?"

"Basically."

"With a fancy handshake and a candle thrown in?"

The woman nearly smiled, humor lighting her eyes momentarily. "I'll take your sarcasm as a no then," she said. "That's fine. You can go."

"I'm not saying no," Brett said. "I'm saying I need time to think about it."

"Unfortunately, we must be quick, before the damage is done."

A memory came to Brett, of her father instructing her to turn down an invitation to the Senior Prom. *"There will be many tests as you make your way toward the goal of Truth,"* he'd said, pulling her toward him and hugging her. *"Many sacrifices."* She could remember fighting tears of disappointment as he held her against his chest. *"Some will be obvious, others only clear after you've passed them."*

"These rewards you mentioned," Brett said. "What are they?"

"Those details aren't up to me alone. They'll be decided by the board of patriarchs."

"So, I just have to trust you that this is the right move?"

"I assure you it is."

Brett tried to picture her father but could only summon a prototype of his image, the details of his face obscure. What color were his eyes? Blue-green or blue-gray? She'd seen him on Skype the week before, why couldn't she remember?

"I understand your hesitation. It's okay if you're not ready."

"You infer one day I'll find it easy to support murder," Brett said.

"Making difficult decisions quickly is a skill you'll learn."

"I'd think part of that skill would involve having decent information to base a decision on, not just blind loyalty."

"Blind loyalty is the first step toward that information."

"And the Truth that I'll learn," Brett said. "It'll be worth it?"

"Your father thinks so. He's willing to risk his life for it."

Brett put her head in her hands. "So, what is he up to then? Can you please just tell me one thing that makes sense?"

De Payen sat back in her chair and looked out the window, the sunlight revealing the tiny gray roots of her hair. "We never shared the Truth with your father," she said. "He didn't pass the final test."

"So how is he risking his life for it then?"

"He's gone and found it out on his own," De Payen said, still looking out the window.

"And?"

"And now he wants to use it against us out of spite. He's personalized the situation and lost perspective. His anger has made him unstable."

He'd seemed unstable the last few times Brett had spoken to him, an irrational, altered version of himself.

"Go to him if you want," De Payen said, turning back to Brett. "He will tell you the Truth. But the Truth will offer you nothing outside the system it belongs in." She placed her elbows on the desk and leaned toward Brett. "Stay with us and you'll reach places your father never did. Show us your loyalty and you'll become what he wanted for you both."

10

Hadley
Matangi, New Zealand

Someone banged on the door.

"Hadley, come on, we have to go." It was her father. "I'll start the car."

"Where are we going?"

"Just get your coat."

"I've already got my coat on."

"Well, get your sister and make sure she wears her coat."

Hadley opened the door and saw him heading down the hallway toward the garage. She ran her finger along the rough leather of the book in her pocket.

"Where are we going?" Hadley hollered after him.

"Auckland."

"Auckland?" Sara asked from the back seat a few minutes later. "Where's Mom?"

"I don't know. She can meet us there."

"Why don't we call her?"

"She didn't take her phone. You know how she is with her phone."

"But why are we going to Auckland?"

"I have a friend at the embassy. I need to show him something."

"Why do *we* have to go?"

Her father didn't answer. He scrolled through his phone, steering the car with his elbow. It was strange seeing him drive sitting on the right side of the car. He lifted his phone to his ear and began to talk. Hadley would wish later she'd paid attention to his words. It was the last time she would hear him speak without the distractions of the ghosts and angels.

That's when Hadley saw the man. They were driving past a dairy farm and he was standing under a drooping willow tree where the road began to dip. He looked out of place, smooth and pale instead of freckled and weathered. He stood very still, only his hands moving, his white fingers kneading the air, his eyebrows drawn together in concentration.

As they drove past, the man looked up and winked at Hadley, his hands catching some kind of light and reflecting it toward her. She blinked at the brightness and looked away. When she glanced back, he was looking at her, his hands a strange, glaring white.

And the Gentiles shall come to thy light, and kings to the brightness of thy rising.

The car sank as it descended into the dip and her father gasped. She turned to see the huge grill of a cattle truck filling up the windshield. Her father pressed hard on the brakes, his body lurching forward against his seat belt. Tires squealed and Sara shrieked behind her. There was a deafening crash of glass and metal and Hadley was thrown forward, her seatbelt sharp against her neck. Smoke clouded her vision. Her chest was heavy, and her eyes stung. A cow bellowed and Sara screamed again. Then hands, cold hands, gripped Hadley and pulled under her arms. She tried to cough but the hands were tight around her chest. She was unlatched from her seatbelt and tugged from her seat. She could see nothing but dark gray smoke. The cow bellowed louder and Sara's screaming grew closer. Hadley thumped onto the rough, hard asphalt and caught her breath, coughing in relief. She could taste blood like foil in her mouth.

The Lord hath returned upon thee all the blood of the house of Saul.

Hadley spat, the smoke clearing so she could see the car half-crumpled beside her, smoke pouring out of the mangled engine and blowing away from her in the wind. Sara was sitting upright in the back seat, her head hanging forward and a low moan escaping her lips. The right side of the car had been replaced with the twisted white metal of the cattle truck.

A figure was running away in the distance.

Hadley looked down through the smoky haze. Glass was embedded in her hair. She picked a few pieces out and flicked them away from her, then stood slowly and went to the car. She opened the back door, surprised it was still intact, and put her arms around her sister, heaving and pulling until Sara fell out of the door and onto the ground. Then she dragged her, staggering, across the road to the grass. The wind had died, and the air was still. No birds were chirping, and the cows had settled. The only sound was a sizzle coming from the smashed radiator.

Sara grunted, forcing a smile, and spat a wad of blood on the ground. "Fuck," she said as she ran her fingers across her lips and examined the blood. "You okay kid?"

Hadley nodded and went back to the car. She walked robotically, as if someone else was moving her legs. It was like her visions; except she knew it was the present because she could smell the burned rubber and cow dung. She could never smell in her visions; they were always odorless.

She circled the cattle truck until she caught a glimpse of her father's red shirt. It was blurry. She rubbed her eyes and leaned over the crumpled door. Her father's head was gone, the rest of his body upright and buried beneath bull bars. White bits of his spine were poking through his neck, his collar folded and unstained against his shoulder. She could remember him putting it on that morning.

The fathers shall not be put to death for the children, nor the children be put to death for the fathers: but every man shall be put to death for his own sin.

She pitched forward and vomited on the road. She stared at her lunch mixed with the bits of glass and metal strewn about her feet and noticed raisins from the broccoli salad she'd eaten that afternoon. She watched the way the larger pieces of glass reflected the sunshine onto her shins. She slumped against the car, her body limp and heavy, the acceptance of what she'd seen coming slow and thick. She fell to the ground and lay staring dumbly at the bright bits of glass and metal.

He that loveth his life shall lose it; and he that hateth his life in this world shall keep it unto life eternal.

Eventually she wiped her mouth with her sleeve and sat up. She remembered the man with the pale, glowing hands and thought about the cold hands pulling her from the car and the figure she'd seen retreating. She looked up the slope toward the tree.

The man stood beside it.

She pushed her long, wet hair out of her face and turned back to the wreckage. Smoke was rising from the truck and Sara stood behind it, holding her head. A car was coming from the other direction. Sara began waving her hands.

"You go find a phone," Sara yelled. "See if that man up there can help. I'll talk to the driver. Where's Dad?"

Hadley just looked at her.

"Well?" Sara said, moving toward the car. "Where's Dad?"

Hadley looked at the ground.

Sara went around the car, and Hadley watched her climb over the mangled grill and onto the side of the truck and begin prying at the metal. Then she let out a scream.

Fathers, provoke not your children to anger, lest they be discouraged.

Hadley was cold. She thought again of the cold hands that had pulled her out of the car. She stood, leaving Sara and walked up the slope toward the tree where she'd seen the man. Everything moved in slow motion. She saw the man in a driveway, moving toward two ladies who were walking down the driveway toward her. One lady carried a phone. The other was barefoot, an apron tied loosely around her waist. She spoke to the man.

"Are you all right, anyone hurt?"

He pointed at Hadley, tapped his watch and walked past them.

The women saw Hadley and made their way toward her.

"Are you all right, love? Are you hurt?"

She shook her head. "My dad is dead."

"I've called an ambulance." The woman held up her phone. "They'll be here soon. I'm sure he'll be okay."

"He's dead," Hadley said again. "The ambulance won't help. No one got out of the truck. I didn't look in the truck. I should have looked in the truck. That man. Who is that man?"

The lady with the apron went running toward the wreck, the other took Hadley's hand. "What man, dear? Come, sit down. You're bleeding."

"I need to know who that man is. He pulled me from the car."

She could still see him in the driveway, walking away stiffly, no sway to his arms, no hip-swing. "Do you know him?" she asked the lady.

"I thought he was with you, dear."

Hadley shook her head and began to run, stumbling, toward the man. Sirens whined in the distance.

And ye shall chase your enemies, and they shall fall before you by the sword.

It was a long driveway. The woman hollered behind her, telling her to come back. The man had stopped near the house, where the gravel met smooth pavement. He clutched a briefcase to his chest, his arms crossed.

"What do you want?" he asked.

But now that she'd caught up to him, she didn't know what to say. She was faint and short of breath. She stopped and held her head.

"You should lie down. You're hurt."

"Who are you?"

He smiled but his eyes were cold. "I'm a servant of God."

"What were you doing with your hands?"

"God's ways are mysterious."

"Did you pull me out of the car?"

He didn't answer, his smile fading.

"My father's dead, isn't he?"

"Yes. But you, you are alive and might not be for long if you don't have that looked at." He pointed to her head, and she reached up and touched her wet hair. She brought her hand down and saw the thick, dark blood. Her legs collapsed beneath her and she fell to the ground. She could hear the sirens growing closer. The man was leaving her. She could feel him walking into the distance, slipping away.

The woman in the apron was there now, helping her straighten out her legs and roll onto her side. Her voice was quiet and kind.

Brightness enclosed Hadley, swathing her in softness, her body becoming buoyant and light. There was singing too, an old forgotten chime of voice, bell and vibrating string. Surrounding her were fields she'd lived in long ago, fields she'd forgotten about, and an ocean, too, before the fields. The spongy coral was familiar to her, the flowering of the sea anemone. Seaweed brushed against her leg. Except there was no more leg, and then no more body either. Only the memory of her body remained and even that was fading, the lightness seeping into the crevices of her memory. Or was it her memory soaking into the light?

She relaxed into the void, enjoying the gentleness. There was no pressure. The lack of force was blissful, everything light and still. She would stay like this forever. This was where she belonged.

But, like an anvil on her chest, something pushed hard into her, then released. Before she could return to the stillness it pushed on her again, almost through her. Again and again, it pushed and released. Pushed and released. Until the tiring pull of gravity returned with the weight of life. The chimes, the ocean, the fields, the brightness; one by one they disappeared. She reached out to gather them to her and saw she had a hand and there were voices. Heavy voices. Living voices.

"No," she said. But no sound reverberated.

She tried again, the mass of her body severe, her chest heaving as it searched for air. "No!"

But there was no resonance in her throat; no sound at all save the buzz of life around her.

And in those days shall men seek death and shall not find it; and shall desire to die, and death shall flee from them.

11

Renee
Matangi, New Zealand

The sky opened above Renee with a loud crack of thunder and within seconds her hair was matted to her forehead, rain dripping along her cheek bones and collecting in the corners of her mouth. It tasted different than rain in Cincinnati; it was sweet and clean. But with it came a sense of dread, for today was not any day, today was a day of death.

She patted the pocket of her coat, realizing she'd forgotten to bring her phone. She hadn't brought an umbrella either. She'd left the house to be alone, to wander and mourn as she did every year on this day, the anniversary of Ernest's death.

Another crack of thunder shook the sky.

"Death is calling me," he'd said, standing in the cabin in front of the unlit fire. *"And I will go to her this time."*

She hadn't argued with him. Later, she wondered if she should have. It was a day of somber discussions, all of which happened in silence. At the time it had seemed normal.

The rain was getting heavier. She saw a bus shelter across the road and made her way toward it.

What were we doing that day? Was it telepathy? How were we doing it? Am I remembering it right? Did it happen at all?

She ducked into the shelter, the downpour deafening against the tin roof.

She could feel death like she had on this day forty years ago. The rain had come hard and unexpected then too. It had pelted the windows of her father's car as Ernest's death was announced on the radio. She'd cried silently, her father unaware that she'd known the man, the legend.

She stared at the cracked asphalt road from behind the thick gray lines of rain.

Oh God, who is it? Not my girls, not one of my girls, please.

She thought of Hadley, of her tiny hands and small curved nails that never seemed to grow. She pictured her the day before, working in the yard with Scott, her hair untamed in the wind, her mouth serious with concentration. The memory felt warm.

It's not Hadley. The girls are safe. I can feel it.

Every year after Ernest's death, she had visited the cabin in Tahoe, its roof not much different than the shelter she sat under now. On years when she could afford it, she would stay longer and do what she could to maintain the cabin, tightening boards and placing traps to kill the vermin that tried to burrow in the rotten spots of wood.

Rain pelted against the road, the blur of a thousand gray lines. The sense of dread and death was strong.

Who is it? Who has died?

Besides her daughters, there was no one else that mattered to her except her husband, and he mattered less than he should. Their relationship contained only a dim love that hummed like a low wave frequency she couldn't tune into.

Lightening cracked above, splitting the high branches of a tree and sending them crashing onto the road in front of her.

Scott. It's Scott that's died.

The knowing settled into her chest, burrowing itself there. But it did not bring despair, not as Ernest's death had on the same day many years ago.

The rain eased and the sun pushed a ray through the clouds. She closed her eyes against the brightness. Her husband's death would cause her daughters great pain. The political ramifications, the media, the reporters, the lies. Her life, their lives, would soon be thrown to the wolves.

12

Brett
New Haven, Connecticut

"Our mission is accomplished," De Payen said, folding her hands over her knee.

A heaviness came over Brett, like a thick, damp towel. She paused, staring at the woman before asking, "My father is dead?"

"Remember, it's for the greater good."

Brett stared at her lap, the heaviness intensifying. She wanted to lie down.

"You must understand the benefit this mission has created."

"I *don't* understand," Brett said, looking up.

"You'll be rewarded for your loyalty."

"I would hope the least of my reward would be you explaining the *greater* good."

De Payen uncrossed her legs and ironed her skirt with the palms of her hands. "The benefit is twofold," she said. "We have eliminated a threat, and we have gained a loyal member—one we believe will do important things for us."

"Why so vague? I need to know *why* my father was a threat. I did what you wanted." Her words sounded warped inside her head, like someone else was speaking them.

"Allowing him to live, *managing* him, would have required resource better used elsewhere."

"But what was he *doing*?"

"As you move through your indoctrination, you'll come to understand."

"No," Brett said, shaking her head. "No, that isn't good enough. I need to know now."

De Payen stopped smoothing her skirt and clasped her hands together. "He was planning to disclose knowledge that could destroy us."

"Destroy us how?"

"The details will be revealed." She recrossed her legs. "In an accelerated fashion, of course. To honor your sacrifice."

"I want to know *now*."

"Your loyalty will be rewarded, I promise."

Brett opened her mouth to ask how but her lips and tongue were thick and wouldn't form the words.

"You'll learn to live with it," the woman said. "That's your real test."

"What is?"

"Learning to overcome guilt. Our conscience is our greatest barrier to Truth."

Brett dropped her head into her hands.

"Our conscience is merely a desire to avoid guilt, an obsolete emotion. You must see it only for what it is, a neurochemical reaction detrimentally attaching itself to a necessary and rational action."

"But I don't know that it was necessary! I can't *see* the rationale."

"The rationale, is that it's for the greater good."

How had he died? But Brett couldn't bring herself to ask.

"Go now," De Payen said. "And remember what I told you, about the guilt."

Brett got up and stumbled to the door.

"Don't let it win."

Brett stepped from the walls of Weir Hall into bright sunlight and blue sky.

Sun and sky her father would never see again.

She moved quickly down the street and around the corner and fell into the shadow of a building, her legs buckling beneath her. She slid to a crouch, avoiding the eyes of two students walking by. She felt a strange urge to go to them, to ask them to help her. But help her with what? She wanted someone to tell her everything would be okay. But the one person who had always done that for her was dead, at her command.

She thought of Eli, of how they used to sit that first year of college, huddled across the table in the dim restaurant discussing Truth. She wanted to see him, *needed* to see him.

What had he sacrificed? What would he think of hers?

She remembered how they used to talk until the restaurant closed around them, how she would always make the first move to go, reach for the bill, decide who paid, afraid if she didn't that something would happen, something she wouldn't know what to do with. She'd always felt foolish afterward. Why'd she have to control everything? Why couldn't she have just left it and seen what happened? And finally she'd convince herself she was over-analyzing nothing. Who was she to think he felt anything for her?

She needed to know, before they met again within the society. She needed to talk to him as a friend, one last time.

She knew where he lived. He was still in the same apartment. She scrambled to her feet and began to walk.

The door was open. A two-seater couch had been dragged onto the grass in the sun. She could see the drag marks from the legs drawn on the concrete behind it. Eli was propped on the couch, his legs spread the length of it, reading. She noticed he'd put on weight, his book propped on a soft belly, and saw the thin hair she'd overlooked in the mud pit. He'd aged, yet his face was still round and flushed, youthful.

He hadn't seen her. She could walk by, change her mind. But where would she go? She didn't want to be alone. And what if he saw her walking away? How would she explain later if he asked?

"Hello," she said, squinting against the sun.

He looked up and she watched his eyes flicker from surprise to delight to curiosity. "Hi," he said, pulling his shirt from his belly, and shifting himself on the couch, bringing his feet to the ground.

She stood shielding her eyes and looking at him, and he sat with a triangle of shadow across his face, looking at her. She remembered how comfortable they'd been together, how quickly they'd become friends.

She walked across the grass and sat down next to him on the couch. He reached over the arm of the chair and turned back with a beer.

She didn't drink beer, but she took it anyway.

He pulled out another and leaned back into the couch.

It had always been like this with them, a silent kind of understanding, an acceptance of each other's presence.

"You used to drive by here after you stood me up." His voice was confident. She'd always loved his voice, the verbal expression of his intelligence. "Do you remember that? How you used to drive by?"

Had she? She remembered wanting to, but she didn't think she had.

"Twice," he said. "The weeks right after."

"It was immature of me," she said.

He sipped his beer, staring ahead. "To stop talking to me or driving by?"

Both, she thought, but said, "Driving by."

They sat in silence, the sun dropping behind the house and a chill setting in. It was comforting to be with him. Thoughts of her father dropped to a light knowing, her stomach settling.

"I don't know when it happened," she said finally. "But at some point, I fell for you and it became inconvenient. *Quite* inconvenient. You understand, having the same political ambitions?"

Her phone vibrated in her pocket. She fished it out, saw it was her mother and declined the call.

"Is that an apology?" He asked.

"Yes," she said.

"We could have talked about it," he said. "We could have decided *together*."

She looked at him. "I didn't know how to do that."

"Me neither," he said, still not looking at her. "But I wish we had."

She took another sip of beer. "It would have made things worse. Harder."

Her phone vibrated again, lighting up through the thin fabric of her pants. She silenced it.

"We might have discovered we were on similar paths."

"Maybe," she agreed. "But if I had confronted my feelings and found out you felt the same, I would have lost myself in the mutuality of it. It would have weakened me."

He shifted forward on the couch, finally looking at her. "Or it may have *fueled* you. It could have made us both stronger."

It was familiar, looking in his eyes, the gray discs outlined in yellow, the splatter of freckles on the bridge of his nose.

"Maybe we could have found a way to make it work, to make it something different, something extraordinary," he said. "We could have found a way to avoid it ruining things. We're not average people, you know."

Could they still? But she didn't ask, the old fear sending her to her feet. "I should go."

He looked up at her. "Why'd you come then?"

"I was wondering how you went with the sacrifice."

"And yet you're going before you've even asked."

She leaned against the arm of the couch. "So, how'd you find it? The process I mean."

"I refused," he said.

"You *what*?"

"It's an antiquated custom, so I challenged it."

"You did?"

"I've proven myself with my grades, with my choices in life, with my ability to deliver. I shouldn't need to prove anything through some outdated symbolic sacrifice."

Brett tottered on the cushioned arm. "What ... what did they say?"

"They said they'd consider my opinion."

"But how did they react?"

"With no expression, like they always do."

"What do you think will happen?"

"Who knows," he said with a shrug.

"But what if they *cut* you?"

"They won't. My mother's a descendant of the Rothschilds."

So, he was cultivated like her. Of course he was.

But not like her. If he was willing to challenge a custom, he was better than her, stronger.

Her phone vibrated in her pocket again. She fished it out.

CALL ME IMMEDIATELY. IT'S ABOUT YOUR FATHER. THERE'S BEEN AN ACCIDENT.

She put the phone back in her pocket, the beer in her stomach working its way back up and burning her throat. She swallowed and leaned into the couch, sweat dripping from beneath one of her breasts and rolling under the droop of her shirt.

"And you?" Eli asked. "I take it you sacrificed something?"

She nodded.

"Do you want to talk about it?" he asked.

She wiped the back of her hand across her forehead and stood again. "I have to go."

"But you said you came to talk about the sacrifice."

"I just wanted to see you," she said, moving across the grass away from him, her legs in slow motion, detached from her body. "The sacrifice was an excuse."

"I kept the same apartment these past three years," he said. "In case you changed your mind and wanted to find me."

She turned and looked at him, forcing a smile.

He raised his beer in a salute.

If she had known it was the last time she would see him, she would have saluted back.

13

Sara
Cincinnati, Ohio

The church was large and bright with white marble. Sara leaned her head back and looked up at the arched ceiling, a single strand of cobweb hanging in the pink light of a stained-glass window. She thought about posting it, but her mother had made her leave her phone at home. She watched it sway lightly, trying not to think of her father in the casket in front of her.

She'd wished her father dead many times in the past few weeks and now he was.

Dead, like Penny had warned her.

She pulled her eyes from the cobweb and looked around the church, wondering if Penny was there.

"Sara," her mother said, touching her on the shoulder. "Have you decided whether you're going to say anything?"

Sara looked down at her rough, chewed nails beneath black polish. She was weary and disorientated from the flight to Los Angeles, where she'd been keenly aware of her father's body stored below with the luggage.

"It's okay if you don't want to say anything. It's up to you, but I do need to know, honey."

Sara thought of the last time she'd seen Penny. She wished she could remember what Penny had said to her as they parted.

"Sara?"

Sara looked up at her mother, the latest victim of her anger (although she dared not wish her dead). Sara was consumed with the thought that her mother *must* have known about her father's impending death. And that she'd not only failed to protect him but had been absent on the day of his death because she was mourning her long-lost love from the last century whom no one was allowed to talk about but whom everyone was well aware of.

"Okay, honey. How about you give me a thumbs up if you want to speak, otherwise we'll just open the floor to others. Okay?"

Sara nodded and her mother approached the podium. Behind it was a screen with a photo of her father. He was smiling, his bushy blond eyebrows sprouting above his blue eyes, his face larger than the altar, making him seem like God himself.

In front of the podium was the closed casket. The undertakers had not managed to reconstruct him well enough for an open casket. Sara tried not to imagine what he looked like beneath the lid.

Hadley sat next to her, swinging her legs beneath the pew. She'd only been released from the hospital two days before they flew home and had yet to speak a word.

As their mother began addressing the congregation, Sara tried to remember Penny's parting comment on the day they'd met. There had been a request, a plea for her to do something. Had she asked her to talk to her father? Was that it?

Her mother finished talking and the photo of her father was replaced with a recent family photo. It had been taken the summer before, the last time all five of them had been together. Her mother was on the left, with Sara and Hadley in the crook of each arm. Her father stood slightly apart, with Brett close at his side.

Brett!

Sara sat up straight in the pew, her elbow accidently jabbing Hadley's arm.

Where the hell was Brett?

She'd been so obsessed with the thought of seeing Penny she hadn't noticed Brett was missing. Sara looked at the empty seat on the other side of Hadley.

How was it possible Brett had not shown?

Sara remembered the last time she'd heard Brett's voice on the phone. It had been a few days before the accident. She'd sounded scared and angry.

That was what Penny had asked her! She'd asked her to talk to Brett. Penny had thought Brett knew something.

Now Brett hadn't turned up to the funeral.

Sara's mother was looking at her. Sara sat frozen in her seat.

Brett hadn't shown, Hadley hadn't spoken a word since the crash. Would none of her father's daughters speak? The question seemed louder than the organ.

She slumped into the pew, afraid if she spoke to the congregation, they would see in her eyes that she'd known her father was in danger and done nothing.

Dear God, if you please make this moment pass without me having to speak, I promise I will find out what happened to my father and avenge his death.

She wasn't exactly sure what it meant to avenge someone's death, but she was sure it was a worthy offering.

To Sara's surprise, Hadley let go of her hand, stood and approached the casket, placing both hands on the lid and lowering her forehead to the surface. She remained there for a few minutes before kissing the casket and lifting a hand toward Sara.

Sara saw her chance and rose from the pew and went to her. She took Hadley's hand and lowered her lips to the casket lid. The surface was cool and slick. She closed her eyes and placed her forehead on it, mimicking Hadley, and remained there until Hadley squeezed her hand.

Together they returned to the pew.

"Thank you, girls," her mother said, turning her palms upward toward the crowd. "If anyone else would like to offer a tribute to Scott, please come forward."

Sara laid her head back and fixed her eyes on the squares of light checkered across the arched beams of the vaulted ceiling and breathed deeply, whispering to a God she didn't believe in.

Okay then, I'll avenge my father's death.

14

Brett
Cincinnati, Ohio

Brett stood half hidden behind a giant hydrangea bush, a magenta flower tickling her neck as she watched the closed wooden doors of the church.

She'd meant to enter, hadn't considered the possibility she wouldn't. She'd accepted what she'd done, examined her guilt and grief as the matriarch had told her. But here she stood, cowering across the street.

Was it her sisters' grief she was avoiding? Her mother's drilling eyes? Or was it her father's body, presenting the reality of what she'd done in the simplest form?

"You'll learn to live with it," De Payen had said.

The organ chimed loudly, the birds in the surrounding trees fluttering in alarm, petals and leaves dispersing in the sunlight.

"Our conscience is merely a desire to avoid guilt, an obsolete emotion. You must see it only for what it is, a neurochemical reaction ..."

Those words had been playing in her mind. They'd been the clincher for Brett, the deciding factor in her sacrifice. After all, they'd been spoken in her father's own logic. Just as he'd taught her that romantic love was a chemical reaction to force her to find a partner and procreate, something that would distract her from the ultimate prize of power and Truth, so guilt was a barrier. She had to shed it to move forward. Her father would have agreed with her sacrifice.

The doors opened and black-clothed people streamed out of the church. Her mother came out first, stone-faced, followed by Sara, staring at the sky as she walked. Hadley, her tiny blond head hung low and cheeks glistening wet in the sunshine, seemed a crumpled version of herself.

Despair pierced Brett's throat, cut into her ears.

She may have managed to avoid the claws of romantic love, but she'd walked directly into the talons of guilt. In the end, being aware of neurochemicals didn't stop them transmitting.

"Let's go," she said to herself. "You've seen enough."

15

Hadley
Cincinnati, Ohio

The cool, crisp light of mortality was still strong and vivid. So much so, Hadley couldn't bring herself to speak.

She'd been admitted to the hospital for tests and lay in the steel-framed bed, reveling at the weight of life and willing herself to die as the doctors came and went with their pushing and prodding. She wanted to explain to them there was nothing wrong with her brain, it was her soul that was refusing to speak. She was contemplating writing this down for them on the little whiteboard they'd given her, when she heard the misty voice.

Stop.

It was Mr. Ernest, standing behind her mother at the end of the bed. Hadley knew who he was immediately by his gray beard and dark eyes. She'd seen him in photos. His body was large and rotund, and completely transparent.

You must stop wishing for death, he said sternly to her. *The bull will not fight if he knows you want to lose. He is cunning and clever and wants the challenge.*

Hadley was so surprised to hear the spirit speak that she forgave him for speaking of bulls when she was trying to die.

I can hear you, she said without using her voice.

And I can hear you.

Can you help me die? She sat up, suddenly frantic he might disappear and be unable to help.

Her mother came to her side.

"What is it, darling?"

Realizing her mother couldn't hear or see Mr. Ernest, Hadley lay back down and asked the spirit again, *Can you help me die?*

Oh no, death should take you when she's ready and only then.

Death is a girl?

Only something so beautiful could be a woman.

Despite not wanting to worry her mother, Hadley began to cry. Death *was* beautiful and fuzzy, like nothing she'd experienced in life. *Oh I wish I could be an angel too*, she said.

You have been before. And someday you will be again, he said. *Then, while you will marvel at the joy of death, you will wallow in your desire to touch and kiss and love like you did when you were alive. And for the record, I'm not an angel. I'm a ghost.*

Then he began to cry too, his weightless body shaking her small bed as he sobbed. Her mother called the nurses, and they came running and began fussing over the cords and buttons.

Hadley ignored them, fascinated and frightened by the ghost's crying. Surely misery wasn't possible somewhere so beautiful? Surely the soft light that so briefly held her after the accident was too perfect for crying.

Please stop, she said.

Then another voice spoke, a wisp in her right ear, a cool wind tickling her hair. *When you choose death instead of letting death choose you, misery and crying are part of the afterworld, Hadley. The light is not so bright when the longing for life is strong.*

Hadley saw her father perched on the rail of her bed, nearly the same as he'd been in life, except he was transparent like Mr. Ernest, and unlike the ghost, he had wings sprouting from his shoulders.

Ernest ended his own life, her father continued. *That is why he is a ghost and not an angel. That is why you must not do the same, why you must live until your time.*

The nurses left, having found nothing wrong with the equipment or Hadley's vitals.

Her mother sat on the side of her bed and wiped Hadley's bangs from her brow. "Oh, Hadley, why don't you speak?"

Hadley, who had been clutching the whiteboard marker in her hand, carefully began to print in capital letters on the board.

IT'S OKAY MOM I'M FINE. DON'T WORRY.

She set the whiteboard down, reached for her mother's hand and smiled warmly at her.

She couldn't explain the yearnings of her soul to the doctors or to her mother. They wouldn't understand. But she could try to stop wishing for death as the spirits had both suggested. This gave her something to focus on.

A time to be born, and a time to die; a time to plant, and a time to pluck up that which is planted.

PART II

Discovery

16

Renee
Cincinnati, Ohio

Renee opened the door and walked into the classroom, her heels clicking on the wooden floor. She didn't make eye contact with her students. She didn't notice most were young and a few were old or that some hovered over their desks, anxious to learn, and others slouched with boredom. She didn't care one way or the other. She was supposed to be in Tahoe.

She flicked back a strand of silver-blonde hair that had worked itself from her braid and adjusted her glasses on her nose.

"In the back of this syllabus, you'll find a note card," she said, handing a stack of stapled papers to a student in the front row. "Before I begin class, I want you to write down why you've chosen to take this course. I expect sincerity. If you've chosen this class because you thought it would be an easy grade, fine. You aren't required to put your name on it."

She propped herself on the front of her desk and crossed her arms. "And please take special note of the absence policy. I won't be flexible. If you miss more than three classes, you'll fail."

A maple leaf fluttering in the crease of a window caught her eye. She watched it flap in the wind. Ernest had left letters in the window creases of the cottage her parents rented in Tahoe City. Renee would find them in the morning, flapping and wrinkled and scratched with prose. She read these letters each fall when she returned to Tahoe. This year they would go untouched.

A hand rose in the back row. Renee turned from the window and nodded toward it. It was a large hand, dark brown with a pale-pink palm.

"With my game schedule, I'll miss more than three classes."

She followed the long, lean arm toward the voice.

His face was dark and smooth, his skin so flawless his eyebrows looked like mistakes. He was Jonas Powell, the Bearcat's basketball legend. The exception, she was told by the administration, to her absence rule.

Renee didn't agree with the leniency given to athletes. "And why does your schedule demand immunity?" she asked.

"I play for the basketball team," he said, light-green eyes shining back at her.

"All talent should be nurtured. However, my class is about literary theory and you'll put equal time into this class as everyone else does. For every hour of class you miss, you'll show up on Wednesday afternoons or Saturday mornings to make them up."

"I'll look forward to it," he said with a slow, deliberate wink.

His response startled her. It wasn't what he said but the perfectly solid way he'd said it and the smile that followed, telling her not to judge him. She turned away.

"Anyone else with a valid excuse, and by valid I'm referring to a letter from a doctor or a dean, can also make up their hours on these days. But, if you don't have an excuse, you must come to class. A hangover isn't an excuse. And now, starting with you," she said, pointing to a random student. "Tell me who your favorite authors are and why."

The students' voices were a distant murmur as they stood and spoke. Stephen King, John Grisham, Janet Evanovich, Elmore Leonard, Danielle Steele. She nodded at intervals, rose her eyebrows here and there, but she wasn't listening. She'd accepted the mediocrity that came with teaching at a state university long ago.

Why did I agree to fill in for the quarter? I could be reading faded letters by the firelight in Tahoe, sleeping amid the tawny smells of the cabin.

"D.H. Lawrence, Nabokov, Hunter S. Thompson, and always and especially, Ernest."

Renee turned her head slowly toward the voice. Jonas stopped talking and ran a hand over his smooth, brown scalp.

"So, you liked *Hell's Angels*, did you?" she asked him.

"Haven't read that one. I've only read *The Proud Highway*, but I find Thompson's style addictive."

"Arrogant would be a better description. And Ernest, what do you like about him?"

"He was intimate with death. No one writes about death like he does."

"An example?"

"He used life to explain the despair of death."

Without invitation, Jonas stood, taller than the tops of the windows, his shoulders broad, his arms lean and faintly lined with veins.

" 'Dying was not what he feared. But living was the rustle of wild game in the bush and the hot wind of the Sahara on his skin. Living was a warm fire and whiskey welcoming him home from the rain. Living was a boat beneath his feet and sea spray in his eyes and a fish hard against the line. Living was a woman's resistance and her laughter as she surrendered.' "

He nodded to show he was finished and sat down.

He'd quoted the phrase perfectly, so cautious and dry and real that the room and the other students had become a dull white fog, and Renee could only see Jonas, tall and green-eyed in front of her, his tongue licking the corner of his lips, still fresh with Ernest's words.

He began gathering his books. "You'll have to excuse me, I have practice."

He headed for the door, stopping in front of Renee and dropping his note card on her desk. "It's a beautiful verse," he said, leaning into her. "I know I didn't do it justice. But we must pay tribute to beauty as best we can, mustn't we?"

And he left.

After the bell rang and the room emptied, Renee collapsed into her chair and tossed the note cards across the desk so they fanned out in front of her. She sifted through them hastily until she found Jonas's card.

There was only one sentence, written in large, red letters.

I'M TAKING THIS CLASS BECAUSE I WANT TO BE YOUR LOVER

In the corner, in smaller print, was his name.

It wasn't creative or clever. It had been done in a John Irving book. But something in his handwriting told her he expected her to know this. It was the precision, the careful slant of his letters written against the guide of a ruler.

His voice still rang in her ears. *We must pay tribute to beauty as best we can.*

She'd heard something similar before, a long time ago. She stood quickly, gathered the note cards into her briefcase and left the room.

17

Sara
Columbus, Ohio

"Who?" the man behind the desk asked, his face a maze of wrinkles.

"Mrs. Weishaup," Sara repeated.

"Oh, Mrs. Wei*shaup.*" He pronounced it wise-how instead of wise-hop. "You mean Clara."

"Yes, that's it. Clara Weishaup."

"And you are?"

"Sara Morgan."

"Are you family?"

"I'm a friend of her daughter's."

"Right, I see. And the purpose of your visit?"

"To talk with her ... to *visit.*"

"Will there be anything else?"

"Well, I was going to put a show on for her, you know a little circus act or something. You want me to show you?" Sara put her bag down and did a handstand against the wall, her phone falling out of her pocket. She jumped back to her feet and grinned at him, dizzy.

He smiled, his wrinkles pushing aside as he leaned toward her and whispered, "Be careful. Too much sarcasm and they'll keep you here." He winked. "Should I go get Mrs. Weishaup then?"

"Please," Sara said, picking up her phone. "I've come a long way to see her."

"The visiting room is through that door." He pointed. "You can wait for her there."

Sara was surprised to find the room so comfortable, the couches plush and pink in the sunlight, the windows thrown open so she could hear the birds in the tall trees. What would happen if Mrs. Weishaup jumped out of the window and went running into traffic? Maybe she would be in a straitjacket, her ankles chained together and locked.

But Clara entered in a silk blouse, a cashmere sweater draped across her shoulders, the sleeves tied loosely around her neck. A short, wide man followed her into the room and Clara paused as he closed the door, waiting for him to lead the way. He swept his arm toward Sara and nodded. "Have a seat, Clara."

She looked at Sara, then the chair opposite her and then back at the man. He pretended not to notice. She tapped him on the shoulder and gestured toward the chair. He sighed and made his way to it, pulling it out and offering it to her with a tired smile. She nodded at him, smoothed her skirt, and sat.

"I'll be over here if you need anything," he said to Sara.

Sara cleared her throat and smiled at Mrs. Weishaup. "I'm Sara Morgan. We met earlier this year, at your husband's funeral."

Mrs. Weishaup looked over Sara's shoulder and out the window, her hands neatly folded in her lap.

"Scott and Renee's daughter," Sara added.

Clara's eyes were bright and clear but showed no interest.

"Your husband, George, and my father were friends."

Sara saw a flicker of recognition.

"I was the one who drank all the Scotch in your liquor cabinet. You remember, with Penny?"

"I know who you are," she said. "I'm crazy. Not stupid."

"Glad we got that out of the way, then." Sara said. "So, how's Penny? What's she up to these days?"

"I don't know."

"Doesn't she come to visit?"

"Whatever you want to know, I'm not going to tell you."

"I'm just looking for Penny, that's all. Can you tell me how I can get in touch with her?"

Clara stood. "Karl, I'd like to leave now."

"Wait. I'm her friend. I just want to get in touch with her, that's all. I've skipped school to come here, been on a bus for two hours."

"If you can't find Penny, it's because she doesn't want you to."

"She doesn't know I'm looking for her. I've been out of the country and I've just moved back."

"I have nothing to tell you. You'll have to find her on your own."

"I went by your house and it's empty. I looked through the white pages. I searched the internet. I can't find her, Mrs. Weishaup, and I need to see her. It's important."

"Who sent you? The Trilateral Commission? The Calderbergers? I already told you, I'm not stupid."

"No one sent me."

"You met my daughter *once*. Do you even know who you're working for? I bet you don't. Most people don't."

"I'm not working for anyone. Penny would *want* to see me. I know she would."

"Really?" Mrs. Weishaup stared at Sara, her eyes tracing the length of her body. "And why's that?"

"Because she asked me to help her on the day I met her, and I wasn't ready. And, well, now I am."

Mrs. Weishaup threw back her head and laughed. It was more like a cackle than a laugh, and it slowly turned into a strange, guttural howl, her lips forming an oval, her throat stretched and open so the air made a long, hollow echo.

"Oh, now none of that, Clara," the guard said, coming toward her, holding his hands over his ears. "Haven't we talked about this?"

Sara put her hands over her ears too. It was a shattering howl, high pitched, oddly controlled and precise.

"I'll have to take her back to her room, Miss. Sometimes she does this for hours."

"Wait," Sara pleaded. "Please, Clara. Tell me where she is. I swear to you I'm her friend. I can help her."

She stopped howling. "You can't help her, dear."

"Why?"

"Well, because she's dead, of course. She's been dead for months."

Mrs. Weishaup shrugged, as if there were worse matters and tilted her head back and positioned her throat for another howl. The man led her quickly through the door and pulled it closed behind them. Sara could hear the chilling howl weaken in the distance. It seemed to mock her, laughing and singing the words just spoken. *Dead for months. Of course, she's been dead. She's dead, of course. Well, because she's dead. She's dead because for months you were gone, of course.*

Sara didn't know how long she'd been sitting on the couch, listening to these words in her head, before the wrinkled man from the reception desk came and tapped her on the shoulder.

"I brought you a coffee," he said, handing her a warm cardboard cup.

"Thanks. Is she still screaming?"

"Oh, that's not screaming, that's howling. Her screaming is much louder and doesn't last as long. She does both often."

"So, I didn't cause that?"

"It's just what she does. Most people who come to see Clara, they know this."

"I don't really know her. I knew her daughter."

"Lovely girl, her daughter."

"You've met Penny?"

"Only in passing. Hard not to notice all that red hair."

"How often did she come?"

"Oh, she's been here a few times, maybe three? She was here the other day, actually. Brought some flowers."

"What do you mean *the other day*?"

"Well, last week, I guess it was. I had a terrible cold and she offered me a tissue. Nice girl."

"Are you sure it was her daughter? What did she look like?"

"Tall, red hair, big smile, freckles."

Sara put her coffee down and scooted to the edge of the sofa. "And you say this was last week?"

"It was, yes."

"That book I signed when I came in, can I have a look at it?"

"I'm sorry, but the visitors book is confidential."

Sara stood. "Listen, you don't have to give me her address, I just need to know if she's alive."

"Alive?"

"Clara told me Penny's been dead for months."

The man waved a wrinkled hand in dismissal and shook his head. "This is an institution for the mentally ill, dear. They all say things like that. When Clara's in one of her moods, she could say anything."

"Please, will you look?" She walked toward the reception room. "Just tell me what day she signed in? I need to be sure."

He stood and collected her empty coffee cup. "I don't know."

"I'll stand on my hands again," Sara grinned. "Oh, and I can juggle too. Do you have any fruit?

"Come on. I'll see what I can do."

Back at the reception desk, he flipped through the yellowed pages of the register as Sara watched the second hand on the clock tick-ticking, tick-ticking, tick-ticking.

"Last Saturday," the man said, his finger keeping his place in the book, his glasses propped on the end of his nose. "Penny Weishaup. It says right here."

"Can I borrow a piece of paper?"

The man pushed a small pad toward her. She scribbled her name and phone number on it and pushed it back to him. "If she comes back, will you give her this?"

"Certainly."

She stood there with the pen in her hand. "You're not going to tell me anything else, are you?"

"At least you know she's alive."

Sara flashed him her best pout.

"Maybe you should try looking at the university." He was scrutinizing the book again, his finger running along writing she couldn't see. "Yes," he said. "I think you should look at the university."

"Ohio State?"

"Cincinnati. Have a look at the University of Cincinnati."

"Where, at a dormitory? An apartment?"

He closed the book and removed his glasses. "That, I can't tell you."

"It's a big university."

"Ten minutes ago, she was one in seven billion. I've narrowed your search for you by about a hundred and fifty thousand percent," he said. "And I didn't even make you juggle."

Sara opened the door and stepped into the sunlight. "You'll give her the message if you see her?"

"If I see her, I will."

Sara started down the path, catching the faint sound of a high-pitched howl, carried to her by the wind.

18

Hadley
Cincinnati, Ohio

Hadley was on the third floor, crouching at the windows of her mother's office. She was happy to be home and surprised how the house had retained its energy during the months they'd been abroad. The earthen walls were warm against her skin in the afternoon sun, the balconies and verandas teemed with lush green vines, and the tiled floors were slick and cool in the shade of the olive trees. Regardless of Hadley's new obsession with death, life persisted.

Her mother's office was the only room on the third floor. It had a round windowed turret where her mother could work as she looked out over the rooftops. But her mother hadn't worked since her father's death and the room had remained locked and untouched since their return.

Forbidden from its circular views, Hadley sat in the room, hovering in her betrayal. It was here she came to read the Bible for it was the only room with a ceiling of orange and yellow glass, which colored the thin pages when she read in the sunlight. It was here, too, she smiled because something in her heart tugged at the skin around her mouth and not because others expected her to. It was here she felt closest to death.

Her father had let her into the room, opening the door without a key. He stood behind her now. She could feel the faint, misty-moist touch of his hand at her neck. She appreciated the comfort he offered; knew she wouldn't have made it through the last month without him. Still, she wished he would push the door to the room open and leave her alone in the soft, warm tangerine light. But his presence was an appendage, a wing stretching from her back, and she'd no choice in the matter.

There is no wisdom nor understanding nor counsel against the Lord.

Her mother would be home soon, and Hadley waited for the car to pull in the drive. The aerial view would allow a glimpse of how her mother was feeling.

Her mother had been unhappy lately. She'd postponed her annual trip to Tahoe to go to New Zealand and then had to cancel it altogether because of the accident, mostly because Hadley was still not talking. Hadley didn't mean to scare her mother by not talking. She just couldn't bring herself to do it. Everyone thought it was because of the accident, and it was. Except the accident had not made her mute in the way everyone thought. It was her new hollow, breathless need to die that made her speechless. And even if Hadley could speak, she couldn't explain her need for death to anyone. The ghost and angel were her only comfort.

For this cause ought the woman to have power on her head, because of the angels.

Her mother's silver sedan turned the corner onto Rosalind Drive, the windshield grabbing the sun and flashing it into Hadley's eyes. Hadley could see her mother behind the wheel, one hand tapping a finger to music, the other reaching for the garage door opener hanging from the visor. The car disappeared into the stucco garage and the door lowered itself.

The side door of the garage opened, and her mother came out smiling, no sloped shoulders, no wrinkles above her nose, not even a tired frown. Hadley thought this was strange, but she didn't have time to think about it. She had to get out of the room and downstairs before her mother suspected where she was. She hurried out the door, her father shutting it behind her with a click.

The carpet was soft and warm against her bare feet and she took each step deliberately so she could enjoy the fuzzy-furry feeling. Sara came out of the bathroom on the second floor, a towel like a turban on her head, beads of water on her arms.

"Been upstairs again?" She winked at Hadley.

Hadley put her index finger to her lips.

"Don't worry, I won't tell," Sara said.

Since the accident, Sara was kinder to Hadley. Would Brett be the same? She would be home in a few weeks. Hadley wasn't excited about seeing her, not like she used to be. Brett had become aloof since being at university. Her father thought it was his fault. He told Hadley he had, with his living breath, taught Brett many falsehoods.

A false witness shall perish, but the man that heareth, speaketh constantly.

Hadley hurried down the hallway to the stairs leading to the first floor. The stairs were made of wide, slate tiles. They were slick against her feet. Was this the same feeling Jesus felt when he walked across water? She often wondered about Jesus.

With each step she slowly placed her foot heel-to-toe so she could feel the cold work its way across her foot until she landed on the hardwood floor of the foyer.

Her mother came through the door and immediately Mr. Ernest went to her. Usually he held up her mother's shoulders, offering them support and power. But today her mother held them up on her own. Did her mother know the difference between her own strength and Mr. Ernest's? Hadley didn't think so because if her mother knew Mr. Ernest was there, she wouldn't miss him so much.

Her mother came to Hadley and placed both hands on Hadley's face, kissing her on the top of her head.

Hadley smiled at her. Who or what had put such a shine on her face?

The answering machine beeped on the kitchen counter and her mother moved toward it. Hadley listened to the sound of her fancy shoes clicking against the wood floor. It was a happy sound, a home-for-the-day sound, a crisp, clean assurance her mother wasn't an apparition.

Steam was rising from a large pot on the stove. Her mother lifted the lid and sniffed, pressing the button on the answering machine as she did.

The machine clicked on. "This is Mr. Stephenson from Indian Hills. My condolences for the recent loss of your husband. I know these are difficult times for your family, but Sara has not arrived at school today, and I would appreciate it if you would contact us at your earliest convenience."

Her mother's shoulders began to droop, and Mr. Ernest reached and supported them with two transparent white hands. He pushed her to the sunroom and lowered her into the swinging couch. The sun was not yet behind the garage and it shone in her mother's eyes, highlighting the wrinkles around her eyes. Mr. Ernest pointed at the refrigerator, and Hadley opened it and pulled out a bottle of wine.

Hadley liked the way the silver screw disappeared into the bottle and the hollow pop that sounded when she pulled the cork out. She poured a glass and took it to her mother.

"Thank you, darling," she said, taking a sip.

There was a dribble of wine on her bottom lip and Mr. Ernest leaned down and tried to lick it off, but he couldn't. Hadley pulled the sleeve of her shirt over her hand and wiped the wine from her mother's face.

"Your sister," her mother said. "Your unfathomable sister. What're we going to do with her?"

Hadley wasn't sure which sister her mother was referring to. She guessed, because of the answering machine message, it was Sara. Hadley wished she could explain to her mother that Sara was a doer and not a learner and school didn't suit her. She wanted to tell her mother it would be wiser for her to worry about Brett.

On them that know not God, and that obey not the gospel of our Lord ... shall be punished with everlasting destruction ... and from the glory of his power.

But she didn't say this. Instead she sat down next to her mother and rested her head softly on her shoulder.

"Do you know where Sara is?" her mother asked.

Hadley nodded against her shoulder and pointed upstairs.

"She's home?"

Hadley nodded again.

"Oh, thank God. Do you know where she was today?"

Hadley shook her head.

They sat together in silence, Hadley rocked gently by her mother's breaths and the occasional lift of her wine glass. Hadley knew something had happened during the day that made her mother happy but made Mr. Ernest sad. The ghost would talk to her about it later, when her mother was sleeping. He often came to Hadley's room at night and talked to her. And sometimes, when he was sad like tonight, he would cry.

19

Renee
Cincinnati, Ohio

Renee was on the third floor, a collection of short stories spread before her on the desk. She was contemplating doing her first critique in months when Sara shouted up the stairs. "Mom! Some dude in a suit's at the door!"

Several times, Renee had asked Sara not to yell up the stairs. It was a terrible American habit that Renee became conscious of when they lived in New Zealand. She'd always hoped for refinement for her daughters. But for now, Renee was quite happy knowing Sara had gone to school all week.

Renee removed her glasses and looked out over the rooftops of the neighborhood. She wondered, as she often did, what people did with their lives beneath the ceramic, tin and slate of their homes.

Do any of them aspire to greatness? How many of them have known love?

She laughed at the irony of how she respected greatness and love and yet had given up on both.

"Mom!" Sara's voice was closer now. "Are you there? Some dude's at the door."

Renee picked up her empty mug and opened the door. Sara stood disheveled on the stairs, her T-shirt ripped and sagging across her collarbone, her hair matted to one side of her head, her socks mismatched.

Renee touched her warmly on the shoulder. "Next time, can you please come to the room and knock instead of yelling up the stairs?"

Sara rolled her eyes, turned, and started back down the stairs.

Renee watched her lunge down them, skipping every other step in a hurry to get nowhere. She had only compassion for Sara's crudeness. She guessed Sara was mourning Scott's death more than any of them. She'd worshiped her father. And there would be guilt, too, for being angry at him before he died.

Slowly, Renee descended the steps.

As she entered the living room, she saw the front door was open. She approached it expecting a Jehovah's Witness but found a reporter slouched against her trellis. He wore no identification; the greed and curiosity in his eyes gave him away.

"Hi. My name is Jason Storn and I'm a reporter for the *Washington Post.* Could I have a moment of your time, Mrs. Morgan?" He glanced at Sara peering over Renee's shoulder and frowned. "In private."

Renee stepped onto the front porch, closing the door behind her.

"I'm curious about your husband's death, Mrs. Morgan."

"Oh?"

"I've been looking into loose ends in the New Zealand coalition case and it seems some of those loose ends died with your husband. Can you tell me anything useful?"

"I'm not familiar with the New Zealand coalition case."

He looked surprised. "I'm referring to your husband's mission in New Zealand."

"We moved to New Zealand for the family, for a break. I took sabbatical and Scott did menial work for the embassy."

"Working as assistant to the US ambassador is hardly menial, nor is trailing missing fugitives."

114

"Missing fugitives?" Renee laughed.

"That's what his file says."

"What file?"

"His government file."

"Files lodged with the CIA," Renee said. "How would you have seen that?"

"Through a contact."

"And what makes you confident of its validity?"

"The contact is dependable."

Renee shrugged. "I'll have to trust you on that. Either way, I wasn't aware of any mission of Scott's. As far as I know, he was offered a fixed term job at the embassy and thought it would be a good opportunity for the family. It's no more complicated than that."

"So, you knew nothing about his mission?"

"I'm sure you have good intentions, but you're wasting your time talking to me. I'm not interested in any scheme of the government's, even if it was a mission of my husband's."

"Not interested?" he asked. "Or don't know about it?"

"One is a product of the other," Renee said. "Now tell me, who is behind this article?"

"I'm freelancing. I've been following the secret society of Claw and Bones, of which your husband was a member."

"So, you're a young conspiracy theorist." She smiled.

"I'm interested in secret societies."

"If I told you what you wanted to hear, that my husband's death wasn't a car accident but a meticulously planned extermination, it wouldn't matter because you wouldn't find anyone reputable to print it."

"So, he *was* murdered."

"I didn't say that."

"Off the record?"

"I told you I don't know."

"Why wouldn't anyone print it?"

"If it was murder, the people that engineered it are probably the same people that own the press."

"Engineered your husband's death?"

Renee smiled at him warmly. She was trying to be nice, but she could see she was only encouraging him.

"Is this the truth, Mrs. Morgan?"

"Excuse me, I have pressing work."

"But Mrs. Morgan, if what you're saying is true, the public has a right to know about it."

"I don't know if it's true or not. I think it's possible Scott's job overseas involved a mission that I didn't know about. I think it's possible it involved fugitives. I think it's possible, although unlikely, he was murdered. But even if it was true, the public wouldn't do anything about it. It would just be another drama that, at its best, might spawn another terrible action movie and change nothing. I suggest you don't waste any more of your time on this. I don't plan to."

"Shouldn't we let the public decide whether they want to know or not?"

"They don't want to know. They aren't designed to."

"And who is it that designs the public?"

"The same people who own the press and strategically murder politicians."

"Are you mocking me, Mrs. Morgan?"

"I'm mocking the system."

"How about names then? Surely there's someone you know who would talk to me?"

"Have a nice day, Mr. Storn," she said, opening the door.

She paused before stepping inside, curious about what he'd seen in Scott's file, and considered prying. But she changed her mind and closed the door, leaving him on the porch.

Inside, Sara sat on the couch.

"Was that about Dad?" she asked, her mouth full of cookies.

"Yes. Please take your feet off the coffee table."

"How come you talked to him? You never talk to them."

Renee shrugged. "I don't know. I suppose I was sorry for him. Feet please."

Sara rolled her eyes and pulled her feet down.

Would Scott have wanted her to tell the reporter what little she knew? She had no sense of whether he would or not. She'd rarely talked to him about his work.

"Mom?"

"Yes?"

"Why are all these reporters interested in Dad's death? I mean it was a car accident in New Zealand. What do they care about it here?"

"All these reporters?" Renee asked.

Sara waved her hand in the air. "There have been others while you were at work."

"Why didn't you tell me?"

Sara shrugged.

Renee looked at her daughter, slumped on the couch. She'd groomed herself while Renee was talking to the reporter. Her hair now spiked in a hundred different directions, black and thick and glossy; her pale lashes coated in mascara and a dark line drawn beneath them. Renee could still see the baby she'd been. Her pale skin, flushed pink at the cheekbones was still the same, and her eyes full of humor and rebellion. She'd been a defiant baby and slower to develop than her sisters. Renee had always worried about her.

She walked to the couch and kissed Sara on the forehead. She smelled strongly of patchouli. To Renee it smelled of cat urine and brandy. She wrinkled her nose and gently placed her hands on Sara's shoulders. "People love drama, honey. They're just reporters doing their job."

Sara pushed her hands away. "It's *not* just reporters doing their job. I might not be as smart as Brett, but I'm not an idiot. Dad's death was weird. And I was *there*. Where were you?"

"I'm sorry I wasn't there, Sara."

"Just tell me the truth. Who killed Dad?"

"Brett's not smarter than you. There are many types of intelligence."

"Whatever. She's smarter than me all round. Tell me who killed Dad."

"Sara, I've told you before, no one killed your father. They found the cattle truck driver and he was a local farmer. He'd been living in Matangi his whole life. What would that man want with killing your father?"

"I don't know. You tell me. Why were we even in New Zealand in the first place?"

"It was an opportunity for us, a break for your dad, an opportunity for me. You know that."

"You don't care about Dad, that's the problem! You never cared about him."

"I cared about your father."

Sara stood. "You're a fucking liar."

"Don't use that language, Sara."

"When's Brett getting here?"

"Tonight."

"Good."

"It's unusual for you to be pleased to see Brett," Renee said, curious.

"Well maybe she'll tell me what's going on. She was the one Dad told everything after all."

Renee laughed, despite herself. "Do you think Brett is going to confide in *you*?"

Immediately she regretted her choice of words.

"See," Sara said. "So there *is* something I don't know!"

"No, that's not what I meant. I just can't bear to see you set any of your hopes on Brett."

"Whatever. I know you're lying. And I'm not going to school tomorrow, just so you know." She glared at Renee and stomped out of the living room.

Renee let her go. Sara was right, after all. They had gone to New Zealand because Scott had been in trouble. And his strange behavior would not have gone unnoticed. It would be cruel to make her daughter doubt the obvious.

20

Sara
Cincinnati, Ohio

Sara found the Kappa Delta house at the end of Clifton Avenue. It was a low brick dormitory with pink flowers and large green KΔ letters hanging above the door. These same letters had been under Penny's photo in the freshman yearbook she'd found online. Only the name under the photo had said Penny Wilson, not Penny Weishaup, but Sara was certain it was Penny.

She approached the door, her hands shaking at the thought Penny might open the door, might be in front of her, in the flesh. Before she had a chance to knock, the door opened and two girls stepped out, backpacks slung over their shoulders, each preoccupied with her phone.

"Hi," one girl said, looking up. "What's up?"

"Just looking for a friend. Penny, Penny Wilson. She around?"

"She's got an early class on Mondays, I think."

"She skipped this morning," the other girl said. "She's still in bed. You might want to come back later."

"I'm from out of town, don't have much time. Any chance you could see if she's awake?"

"We're late for class but check yourself if you want. Second floor, room eight."

They opened the door wider so Sara could enter. "You have to wear a visitors' pass. Just write your name on a card and pin it to your shirt. We'd do it for you but we're late."

They closed the door behind them, and Sara found herself in a white-tiled foyer next to a green clothed table with blank visitors' passes fanned out next to a pen. The house smelled of fake vanilla, cheap perfume and cooking grease. Other than faint talking coming from the other room, the hall was quiet. There were stairs to her right. She bypassed the table and started up them, her armpits dampening, her heart thumping in her ears.

On the second floor the walls were decorated with composite photos of the sisters. The rooms were neatly numbered, the doors covered in magazine cutouts of celebrities in glittery dresses and young men in their underwear. She found number eight and knocked.

There was a rustle behind the door and the sound of something hitting the wall. Then it was quiet. Sara knocked again.

"Come in." The voice was low and muffled.

Sara opened the door slowly.

It was dark in the room, the only light coming from a small, bubbling fish tank on the far wall, glowing green with algae.

"Who is it?" the voice said from the dark.

Sara wasn't sure which was going to prove worse, that this *was* Penny or that this was a stranger waking up from a hangover.

There was only one way to find out. Sara flipped on the light.

"Ah, Jesus. Turn it off, will you? There's a little light over by the desk."

But Sara was too busy staring at the painting over the bed.

"Did you hear me? Turn it off."

"I liked the one with Spiderman better," Sara said, smiling. "You should have kept that one."

Penny dropped her hands from her eyes and squinted up at Sara. Her hair was short and flattened to her head from sleeping, but it was as red as Sara remembered it.

"Holy shit," Penny said.

"Man, you're a hard person to find."

"Holy shit," Penny said again. "I thought you were in New Zealand."

"I was."

"What're you doing here?"

"I need your help."

"Does your father know you're here?"

Sara moved herself to the end of Penny's bed and sat down. So close, after so many weeks!

"Well, does he know?"

"He's dead," Sara said. "They killed him just like you said they would."

Penny came up out of the sheets, throwing her bare legs over the end of the bed. "Did I tell you or what?"

Sara stared at her legs, pale and freckled, only inches from her own.

"It was awful how it happened," Sara said finally. "There was this dip in the road and the truck, it was like it was waiting for us because suddenly it was there and then Hadley was dragging me out of the car and then the ambulance came, and oh God, they pulled my dad from the car and Jesus his head was gone, completely gone!"

Sara hadn't expected to spill her story but now she had, she wondered if Penny might reach out and comfort her.

Instead Penny jumped out of bed and began pacing the room with her hand on her forehead and her elbow in the air. "I knew it. I told you, didn't I? And you didn't believe me!"

"I didn't have time to believe you!"

"You could have come to me after the funeral. You could have come!" Penny stopped pacing and pointed accusingly at Sara.

"Don't be *salty*. My dad was freaking. He moved us off to New Zealand within weeks after the funeral."

"Never mind," Penny said, pacing again. "Never mind. You believe me now." She stopped pacing. "What do you know? Tell me what you know."

I'm in love with you, and it's killing me. That's what I know.

"I don't know anything," Sara said. "I tried to talk to my dad about it one night, asked him about your father and what they did together. He said it didn't matter, it was all over, that everything was destroyed. Then he started talking about something in Iraq. It didn't make any sense."

"They went to the Middle East together. Did you know that?"

Sara shook her head.

"A week before my father died, they purchased a flight to Baghdad. Something happened there. Tell me what you know."

"I don't know anything. That's why I'm coming to you. He didn't make any sense. My dad said they tried, they were so close, but everything was ruined. He kept saying that. Over and over, he kept saying everything was ruined, shaking his head."

"Okay, who knows you're here?"

"No one. I went to see your mother and she told me you were dead."

Penny waved away the comment. "Lunatic, complete wacko."

"And I found your picture in the freshman yearbook and here I am."

"Okay, listen, Sara." Penny came and knelt on the floor in front of her and took her hands. "There's a lot you need to know and then there's even more we must do. Can I trust you?"

"Hundo P."

"And that means?"

"Yes, totally. Hundred percent."

"Good. You like research?"

"Research?"

"Yes. It's too much for me, all the history and books and names. You're going to have to help me get through it all. We're going to figure it out together, okay?"

"Sure, okay."

"For now, you need to get out of here. I don't want anyone to know we're hanging out together."

Sara pulled her phone out of her pocket. "Give me your number."

"Are you crazy? We can't text. That would be a death sentence."

"Well, how do I get hold of you then?"

"Meet at the Warehouse on Vine Street. Saturday night, ten o'clock."

"What warehouse?"

"It's a dance club in the industrial district," she said, yanking Sara off the bed and pushing her toward the door.

"*Savage.*"

"And don't talk about any of this with your sister."

"Who, Brett?"

"Yes, Brett. You know she's in the same secret society our dads were in?"

"What that stupid Claw and Bones thing?"

"Yeah. It's mentioned a lot in our dads' stuff and the next step for her will be getting into the Order. Don't trust her."

"What's the Order?"

"I don't completely understand. But I know there's a hierarchy of societies and they're powerful and if your sister has been inducted into Claw and Bones then she's moving up the ranks."

"And what do you mean our dads' stuff? Did you find something in the library?"

"Did I ever."

"What? What did you find?"

124

"Folders taped under the pool table. They obviously put them there quickly because there was no order to the papers inside, just random articles and pages ripped from books and written notes. Now go," Penny said, pointing to the door. "And don't trust Brett."

"I've never trusted her."

"Well, make sure you don't mention me to her for any reason and stay off the internet about all this."

Sara opened the door. "See you Saturday?"

"Go," Penny said and pushed her out.

21

Brett
Cincinnati, Ohio

Brett was walking in the crisp morning air listening to *La Princesse Maleine*, her favorite opera. The opera had been written nearly a hundred years before Brett was born, by a woman named Lili Boulanger who had died at 24, leaving the piece unfinished. Brett was nearly that old. It was this fact that made the opera meaningful. It reminded Brett that talent, no matter how remarkable, couldn't escape death. Every note was a message telling her she must approach life with urgency.

She hadn't slept the night before, and the mezzo soprano of the opera soothed her. Being home was unsettling. The simple, incessant chatter of her family left her restless. How could they be so content with their mediocre lives? It astounded her none of them were interested in the Truth. They'd never asked anything about her school or her induction into Claw and Bones. She missed her father's ambition. Yet even he had failed her. Or was it she that had failed him?

She pushed the thought from her mind as she rounded the corner of Rosalind Drive to the sound of the rising soprano. She saw Sara on the far side of the street, her backpack slung over a shoulder, a doughnut in one hand. Noticing Brett, Sara held up her thumb and two fingers in a rude greeting and smiled, a piece of chewed doughnut falling from her chin.

Brett paused the opera and crossed the street. "Since when do you get out of bed before noon?"

"Since when are you interested in what I do?" Sara asked, dropping her napkin on the ground and starting toward the house.

Brett let her go, stooping to pick up the napkin. She didn't really want to know what Sara was up to. It would, no doubt, be something idle.

She'd hoped at least one of her sisters would be interested in the family legacy, but they both seemed indifferent. She didn't understand why her father hadn't tried harder to cultivate them. How long would she have to stay here and witness their purposeless lives?

After a disappointingly average coffee at the local café, Brett returned to Rosalind Drive. Inside the house, the refrigerator hummed, two steel jars on top rattling as they vibrated against each other. A toilet flushed upstairs, and water rushed between the walls. A green triangle was blinking on the stereo. Someone had pushed pause and gone to bed. Idiots.

Brett used the remote to stop the stereo and walked up the stairs. She stopped outside Sara's room and looked at the open drawers and clothes piled on the floor. Cigarette butts cluttered the windowsill, and three old glasses of orange juice, the pulp dry and stuck to the rims, sat on the desk. Headphones, books, pens, and an old box of chocolates littered the floor.

She wandered down the hall to her own room and stood in front of her bookshelf.

"Brett?"

She turned to see her mother standing in the doorway wearing a black silk robe, her hair tied loosely in a ponytail. She'd aged since Brett had been away; lines had appeared around her mouth and eyes.

"How are you?" her mother asked. "We've barely talked since you've been home."

"There's nothing to talk about," Brett said.

"We could talk about your father's death. You know it's ..."

"Don't bore me with emotional discourse. You never loved Dad when he was around. Let's not pretend now."

"Brett!" her mother said moving to sit on the bed.

"It's fine if you didn't love him. I know why you were together."

"I wasn't going to talk to you about your father and me. It's your grief I want to talk about. And why you weren't at the funeral."

"What I don't understand," Brett said. "Is if you married him to carry on the family tradition, then why'd you dissent?"

"I don't want to talk politics with you, Brett."

"Well, there's nothing else I want to talk about."

"I did what I could to get you into Yale. I've supported you, but don't push it on me."

"Do you even know what you're giving up?"

"Is that why you've come home this summer? To finally convert me?"

"You're strong and smart. Glory could be yours."

"*Glory?* What Glory? Glory wouldn't keep a daughter from her father's funeral, only hatred would do that."

"I don't hate my father."

"Then why weren't you there? Where were you?"

An image of De Payen in her red glasses came to Brett. "*Our conscience is our greatest barrier to Truth.*" "*Don't let guilt win.*"

"You're waiting for the letter aren't you, dear?" Her mother asked, her face softening.

Brett raised her eyebrows.

"You think I know nothing, but I haven't escaped it all. I've seen more than I wanted through your father. And now, I suppose, I'll live it through you."

"I won't share it with you, don't worry."

"I'm your *mother*, Brett."

"A painful fact I'm reminded of every time I look at you."

Her mother raised her arms in exasperation and stood. "Okay, you win. I'll go. Just know I love you."

When her mother was gone, Brett pulled the curtains and rested her head on her desk.

How long would she have to stay here? Was there anywhere else she could go while she waited? She couldn't go back to Yale. Yale was done, all tasks for that chapter accomplished. All she could do was wait for the letter.

And why was a letter necessary once one had been initiated and made a sacrifice, especially a sacrifice like hers? But she knew the tradition was that if they wanted her in the Order, she would receive a letter.

Tradition or antiquated custom?

Eli's words rang in her ears. Where was he? What was he doing? Would he get a letter after refusing the sacrifice? The thought was constantly on her mind. If he did, then her father's death was in vain. If he didn't, she may never see him again. She wanted to text him, but she didn't, for fear he was marked now like her father. She wanted to spare him herself, spare him what she was capable of doing for the Truth.

And what if the reward for her sacrifice was something other than becoming part of the Order? What if they had something else in mind for her? She was destined for more than partnership in a law firm or a seat in local politics. The uncertainty was killing her. But at that moment she was sure of only one thing; that somewhere in D.C. or Cape Cod, or Yale, someone was deciding her future.

22

Hadley
Cincinnati, Ohio

It was a warm morning and the wind swirled Hadley's ponytail about her head as she walked. She didn't know where she was going but she knew she would know when she arrived. She'd woken that morning wondering about her father and about death and with a strong urge to go for a walk.

She'd snuck out early and set out with the rising sun, both ghost and angel behind her. She didn't know how long she'd been walking when a small brick Tudor caught her eye, a stream of morning sun shining on the front porch and a tabby cat licking its paws in the driveway. It was a well-kept house, the lawn neatly mown and edges trimmed, the flowers perfectly spaced along the path and the driveway freshly tarred and smooth. Mr. Ernest's ghost nudged her from behind and she moved toward the house, stooping to pick a bright peach-colored flower from a cluster at the edge of the drive. She'd never seen a flower like it before. It had thick rubbery petals and a long stem. She looked at it, contemplating its perfection, before continuing up the drive. She glanced in the car as she passed it, noting it was old but clean. The path to the door was made of small white stones, identical in shape and roundness. They seemed familiar to her. She gazed at them in the sunlight, noticing small engravings on them, some kind of foreign writing.

Thou wilt shew me the path of life: in thy presence is fulness of joy.

She approached the door and knocked. The door was heavy, the wood thick and old, so the sound from her knuckles was absorbed. She knocked again, using the palm of her hand.

The door opened quickly, and she jumped back and dropped the flower.

A man stood smiling at her. His skin was light brown and his hair black with loosely sprung curls darting in every direction. His eyes were bright and clear, a pale blue-green. They reminded her of the water in New Zealand.

"Let me get that for you," he said, stooping to pick up the fallen flower and handing it to her. His nose was sharp and steep above his white teeth and brown lips.

"Issa," he said, sticking out his hand.

"Hadley," she said, shaking it.

"I have been watching you."

Blessed is the man that heareth me, watching daily at my gates, waiting at the posts of my doors.

"Watching me?"

"From the window," he gestured toward his front window. "I saw you coming down the street and saw you pick the flower." His words were wrapped in a foreign lightness that made them dance.

"You have nice flowers," she said. "I hope you don't mind I picked one. Now that I think about it, it was quite rude of me, wasn't it?"

"Not at all. Would you like to come in?"

Hadley wanted to go inside but she stepped back, suddenly realizing she was speaking.

"Can you *hear* me?" she said slowly, placing a hand to her throat.

"Yes," he said solemnly, as if he understood the magnitude of her question.

She couldn't help but grin. "It has been a long time since I have spoken. I can't believe it." Her throat vibrated beneath her skin. She grinned wider.

And Jesus rebuked the devil; and he departed out of him: and the child was cured from that very hour.

"So, would you like to come in?" He asked again.

She hesitated, hand still on her throat. "Ummmm. I don't think so. I would like to, but I don't know you. How funny I'm talking!"

"How about the deck? Perhaps that would be more appropriate? It is around the side." He pointed to her left. "Follow the stone path and I will meet you there. Would you like a cold drink?"

"Yes, please."

Hadley knew it was dangerous to accept a drink from a stranger, but she knew the angel and the ghost would stop her if it was wrong, and she couldn't, after all, ignore the extraordinary fact she could speak to this man.

He shut the door and she walked around the house, following the funny little white stones to the deck. There was a picnic table and she sat at the end of one of the benches. He came out with a tray and handed her an iced tea, a fluffy white cat at his heels.

They sat and she laid the flower between them.

"What kind of flower is this?"

"It is an orchid."

"Oh." She looked at the flower. "I have heard of an orchid, but I don't think I've ever seen one before."

"Orchids don't usually grow in Ohio."

She nodded as if this explained things. Then she looked straight into his water-blue eyes and said, "I don't know why I'm here."

He laughed and then hastily apologized. "I am sorry. I am just pleased to have a visitor as frank as yourself."

"Well, I like being frank and I like it here on your porch a lot. I think it's so strange I am talking though."

"Tell me about that."

"I was in an accident and I haven't spoken until now."

"Why not?"

"I don't know."

"Give it your best guess. You may surprise yourself."

"Because I don't want to be alive," Hadley blurted.

"Oh?"

"That was weird," Hadley said, embarrassed. "Sorry."

"Not at all, dear. Life is weird."

"What do you think about death then?" she asked, taking a sip of her tea.

"I don't think much about death at all."

"Why not?"

"I am too busy living."

Hadley contemplated this and decided he'd certainly never been dead before.

"My grandmother used to tell me the only way to the Kingdom of God was through accepting Jesus into my life."

"Why would one need to do that?"

"Jesus saith unto him, I am the way, the truth and the life: no man cometh unto the Father, but by me."

"John 14:6."

"Yes, that's right." Hadley was comforted by the fact he was familiar with the Bible. "My grandmother taught me the Truth lies in the Bible and to always keep it near. She said your soul moves on to the Kingdom of God when you die. Do you believe that?"

"Oh, goodness." His eyes shone with humor. "You ask vigorous questions. To answer that one, I would need to know what she meant by the Kingdom of God."

"The Kingdom of God is where you go if you ask Jesus into your life, I think. Jesus saves you. Have you asked Jesus into your life?"

"I am not sure I have. Where do I find him to ask him?"

Hadley frowned at him. He was surely teasing her. "Jesus is all around you. All you have to do is ask with your heart."

"And where did you learn this?"

"It's all in the Bible."

"And you are sure the Bible is correct?"

His tongue lingered at the roof of his mouth when he spoke, causing his words to roll in small, rhythmical waves. It was a pretty accent. Where was it from?

"If you can't trust God, who can you trust?" she asked.

"You are taking it for granted that God wrote the Bible."

"Of course he wrote the Bible."

"What if I told you I know he did not?"

Should she explain to him about the misinterpretations of the other religions and the narrow path to heaven? The idea of her telling this man anything seemed ridiculous, like turning the light on in a sunny room. His calmness dazzled her. She'd never met anyone so *peaceful*.

"Are you a Buddhist?" She didn't know what a Buddhist was but somewhere she'd heard they were peaceful.

He lit up at this question, uncrossing his legs and leaning his elbows on the table. "What a remarkable man, Buddha! Have you studied his teachings?"

"So, you *are* a Buddhist?"

"No."

"So, what are you then?"

"I am me. I am part of the universe. I am a visitor. I understand."

"You understand what?"

"Everything."

There was nothing patronizing about his tone of voice, nothing condescending in his gaze. "No one can know everything."

Seest thou a man wise in his own conceit? There is more hope of a fool than of him.

"What a shame for such a bright girl to believe that."

"Grandma said we're imperfect and can't know the Truth without understanding the Bible."

"What do *you* think?"

"I think Grandma may have been confused."

"You are wise to question the Bible."

"I don't question it," Hadley said boldly. "I'm just unsure whether *all* Truth lies there."

"Where else do you think it might lie?" he asked.

"In death," she said.

"You have seen death?"

She nodded.

"What do you remember of it?" His face was kind and patient.

"It was easy. Clear and light."

He reached across the table and touched her arm. "Life, too, can be thus," he said. His touch was much like the spirits', light and misty, but also warm and tingly, like static.

"My grandmother said life is misery and providence exists only upon death."

His seawater eyes softened with sadness. "Do not believe that, child. Don't lose faith."

How strange he should imply her thinking was losing faith when it was faith she was practicing. Before she had time to question this paradox, she said, "Teach me. Please?" For she knew this was why she'd come.

"I cannot deny she who searches for the Truth."

She waited for him to say something else, but he only looked up at the sky and closed his eyes to the sun.

She waited.

He remained with his face basking in the morning warmth. "It is difficult to break through the holds and rigidness of religion. Are you sure you are ready?"

"Yes."

"How do you know?" He barely moved his lips, his voice soft. Was he falling asleep?

"Because the Old Testament confuses me," Hadley said. "It scares me. I feel something is wrong when I read it."

He opened his eyes and looked at her. "That is because the Old Testament is full of fear and with fear, we can do nothing. Except Genesis, of course. Genesis is brilliant and beautiful."

"Yes," Hadley agreed. "Yes, it is."

"I will teach you, if you will agree to learn."

Hadley contemplated her situation. She'd gone for a walk and seen a house that called to her, and she'd met a man who was gentle and wise and whom she could speak to. They hadn't talked about menial things but had spoken of God, of life and of death. He'd challenged her on the things she found most precious and she hadn't felt threatened. He'd agreed to teach her, without burden or enthusiasm, but with a humble sense of duty. It was the most comfortable and natural encounter she'd experienced since death.

Who comforteth us in all our tribulation, that we may be able to comfort them which are in any trouble, by the comfort wherewith we ourselves are comforted of God.

She looked at the orchid lying on the table. Was she being naive trusting this man? Was she being led by loneliness and not by God at all? She touched the orchid, fingering its rubbery petal.

"Do you know what you must do in order to learn?" he asked.

A fool hath no delight in understanding, but that his heart may discover itself.

"No," she said.

"You must quit dreaming of death."

"And when I do, you'll tell me the truth about life?"

"Exactly." His eyes sparkled.

She had so many questions. Why'd he put such strange intonations on his words? How old was he? What were those funny, white stones on his path? Why had he been watching her? How many cats did he have? But she was tired and meeting him was enough for now.

"I should go then," she said, pushing the bench away from the table and standing.

He stood with her. "I will walk you out."

She stared at the stones as they walked around the house, studying their tiny engravings.

At the front door she hesitated, tracing a stone with the toe of her shoe. "Why did I come here?" she asked.

"Because you wanted to see me again."

She looked up at him. "But I have never seen you before."

"Are you sure?"

"I've never seen you before, but I feel like I've known you forever."

"I suppose you are right," he said. "On both accounts."

She was so tired she wanted to lie down on the stones and sleep in the warmth of the sunshine. "I don't understand."

"It will become clearer."

"What will?"

"Everything."

"When? How soon?"

"I do not know for sure. But I think it will be soon."

A light breeze brushed against her face. "Okay," she said, stepping off the path and starting down the driveway, knowing she wouldn't speak again until she returned.

23

Renee
Cincinnati, Ohio

Renee had a headache. She would have stayed home if she thought it would help but she knew she'd only feel worse in the house. Hadley's silence was unnerving. Brett was disgusted with everything, not the least her mother. And Sara was determined to push the boundaries, relentless with her questioning and accusations. So, even though it was Saturday, Renee had decided work was the better place for a headache.

"Dr. Morgan?"

She looked up, the hall light silhouetting Jonas Powell in the door frame.

Oh God.

"Hi," he said, dipping his head to enter her office.

"Hello, Jonas," she said.

He took a seat on the other side of her desk, folding his arms over his books. "I'm sorry I haven't been to class in a while. I've been on the road."

"Yes, I know."

"It's nice you noticed I was missing," he said.

"I notice when all my students are absent."

"Of course."

Renee could smell aftershave, soap, and the musty wet smell of well-worn shoes.

"So, what do you want Jonas?"

"I'm here to make up class like you said. It's Saturday."

"You were supposed to *schedule* it. I'm not here every Saturday."

"Oh right, sorry." He stood to leave.

"But I suppose since we're both here," she said, opening the top drawer to her desk and pulling out the index card he'd left the first day of class. "We might as well discuss a few things." She placed the note card on the desk between them. "Last Tuesday when you rattled off your favorite authors, you forgot to mention John Irving."

He smiled. "*The World According to Garp* is one of my favorite books," he said. "But it's true, Dr. Morgan. I want to be your lover."

"Really, Jonas."

"But I do. It's not a joke."

"Do you know how old I am?"

"Mid-fifties?"

She'd expected him to flatter her by guessing younger. She liked that he hadn't.

"And how old are you?"

"Much older than you would have been when you met Ernest. And he would have been, what, sixty?"

Renee leaned back in her chair. It was common knowledge that she'd known Ernest before he died. But it had been years since anyone had questioned her about it. "And what do you know about me and Ernest?"

"Enough to guess you were probably more than friends."

More than friends! As if being friends was something typical and boring. It was a hell of a lot more difficult to find a good friend than a good lover.

"We were more than lovers," Renee said.

"I would like to be more than lovers too," he said calmly, confidently.

"Jesus, Jonas," Renee said, adjusting herself in her seat, warm blood rising to her cheeks.

"Tell me about Ernest, about how you met him."

A memory of Ernest appeared. He sat across from her, telling her about a trip to Spain and the bullfights, and beautiful matadors.

"Tell me?"

"No. We're here to discuss class," she said, suddenly aware how short his shirt was and how it was exposing the fuzzy, black hairs beneath his navel.

"I'm not flattering you for a good grade. I'm taking this class *because* of you."

"And if I refuse your advances, are you going to drop my class?"

"Are you refusing me?"

Renee laughed nervously. "Did you think I'd let you wander in here and bend me over my desk just because of a clever little note card?"

Oh my God, I didn't just say that.

He smiled. "That's not what I had in mind. I don't like smut."

"Well I don't like overconfident college boys who like to play games."

"The only game I play, Dr. Morgan, is basketball."

He picked the card up and replaced it with tickets, which he fanned out across the desk. "For me, it's all about beauty. I'd like you to come see me play. You'll understand when you do. Take these tickets and think about it, will you?"

She looked at the tickets. There were four of them.

Beauty? There he goes again with that word. And why four tickets?

"So, what did I miss in class?"

She continued staring at the tickets.

"Dr. Morgan?" he said. "Class?"

"Writing exercises," she said, looking back up at him. "You need to catch up on the writing exercises."

"But this is a class on theory not writing."

"Before we begin interpreting and analyzing the classics, we are going to interpret and analyze our own writing. So, pick an object in this room and write about it for twenty minutes."

He opened his notebook. "Anything in the room?"

"Anything but me."

He frowned.

"You're going to have to find something else to inspire you, Jonas."

"You can refuse me, Dr. Morgan, but you can't change the fact you're my muse."

"Just write, Jonas. I'll be back in a minute."

Closing the door behind her, she raised her eyes and arms to the ceiling. "Dear God," she said under her breath. "Is this your idea of a joke?"

She didn't like Jonas's advances, but she couldn't help noticing the size of his hands and the smoothness of his skin. It had been a long time since someone had talked to her like he was. In fact, she wasn't sure anyone had ever talked to her like he was. She didn't want to go back in the office. The room was small with him in it, the ceiling crushing down on her, pushing her closer to him.

Surely I'm not enjoying this flattery? It must be the way he talks about beauty. It's so like Ernest!

When she felt enough time had passed, she straightened her skirt and opened the door, half expecting him to be naked and spread across her desk, but he was still sitting in the chair, his long back curved over the table, his muscled arm moving the pen across the paper. He was beautiful, this huge young man, but she didn't want him. She wanted Tahoe. She wanted snow-covered mountains and antlers on a plaque.

She looked at the tickets fanned out on the desk.

How good is he?

He pushed the chair out and handed her his paper. "All done," he said, moving toward the door. "The other tickets, they're for your daughters. I was thinking you'd want to be spending time with them, with the death of their father and all."

He left with his head down, whether it was to miss the door or to show respect, she didn't know.

24

Sara
Cincinnati, Ohio

It was getting dark earlier each night. Sara watched out the
window, the moonlight shining on the flowerless lattice,
brightening the corner of each slat against the darkness of the
next. She smelled of patchouli and incense, her hair wet against
her scalp.

She chewed on her nails and spat the splinters onto the porch
roof, turning to look at herself in the mirror. She frowned; her hips
were too wide for her thin legs, her nose too small, her lips too
straight. She reached for her eyeliner and drew a black line under
each eye.

There was a light knock on the door and Hadley's face poked
through the opening.

"Hi, kid," Sara said.

Hadley swung the door open.

"What's up?"

Hadley shrugged.

"You know the doctor says there's nothing wrong with your
voice."

Hadley entered and picked up a notepad and pen off Sarah's
desk and began to write.

WHERE ARE YOU GOING?

"To meet a friend."

DON'T GO.

"Why not?"

I HAVE A BAD FEELING.

"*Savage*," Sara said. "Then it'll be a fun night."

Hadley glared at her.

"Don't tell Mom, okay, kid? *Low key.*"

IT WILL BE THE BEGINNING OF SOMETHING BAD.

"What, you read that in the Bible or something?"

Hadley crossed her arms and frowned.

"I have to go. It's important."

PROMISE TO BE CAREFUL?

Sara nodded.

Hadley stretched herself onto the tips of her toes and kissed Sara on the cheek. She wrote *BE CAREFUL* once more, waved goodbye, and left.

The Warehouse was typical with its blue lights, cages, and bubbles that smelled like Palmolive. Sara had been sneaking into clubs since she was sixteen.

"You made it."

She turned to see Penny, her hair wild and loose and gathered atop her bare, freckled shoulders. She wore a purple and green striped tank scooped low across her chest and a silver necklace that dipped into her cleavage.

"Hi," Sara said.

Penny took her hand and pulled her through the mob of pulsating people, past two bars and a room full of low-set yellow couches and through a hallway of single-stalled bathrooms. At the end of the hall was a metal door with a STAFF ONLY sign. Penny pushed through the door.

Inside was a stockroom, the ceiling open and revealing heating vents and plumbing. It had been sprayed with a plaster mix that hung in blue globules in the fluorescent light. Behind a table stood a man wearing a SECURITY T-shirt. On the table were small wooden boxes like the kind Sara used to store her movie tickets and special photos. One box was full of cash and the others contained blue, pink and orange pills.

"What color?" the man asked.

"What's the difference?" Penny asked.

"Pink's the cheapest but not so strong. The blue's stronger and the orange is like POW," the guy said, bringing his fingertips together and kissing them. "You'll still be singing tomorrow night and it's not even twice the price of the pink."

"The pink will be fine," Penny said, pulling her wallet from her back pocket and flipping it open.

"Sure you don't want to supersize?" He smiled, showing three gold teeth.

"No interest in peaking while I'm taking a midterm, but thanks." She turned to Sara. "How about you? Pink okay for you?"

"Pink'll do." Sara didn't know what it was. Speed? Ecstasy?

Penny paid cash and pressed a pink pill into Sara's palm and back out they went through the metal door, past the toilet stalls and the yellow couches to the first bar. Penny ordered them two Red Bulls and they toasted, a quick tap of aluminum, before chasing down their pills.

Penny's eyes darted back and forth as she scanned the room, her head nodding lightly to the music.

"Do you remember the day of the funeral?" Sara asked, relaxing her elbows against the bar. She could feel the music pounding up through the legs of the stool.

"Sure," Penny said, raising her eyebrows. "I remember it all."

"Me too," Sara said.

"Oh God," Penny looked at her, slightly horrified. "You didn't fall in love with me or something stupid like that did you?"

"Totally, *hundo P*," Sara said, slumping onto the bar.

"Really?"

"I think so." Sara paused. "Maybe."

"Christ," Penny said, annoyed.

"But don't worry. I'm over it."

"You sure?"

"Yes, definitely," Sara lied.

"Okay, good," Penny said, getting off the stool. "Don't expect any of that to happen again. That was just me being weird. Should we dance?"

"What're we doing here exactly?"

"We're having fun. Aren't you feeling your pill yet?"

"What was it anyway?"

"Ex."

How was she supposed to *not* be in love with Penny on Ex? "I thought we were going to do research or something."

"This is a cover-up. The more fun we have, the more drugs we do, the less serious anyone will take our friendship. Now, let's dance."

"Who are we hiding from?"

"From the Order."

"Who's the Order again?"

"A secret society. *The* secret society."

"Are they watching us?" Sara asked, looking around her.

"Maybe. I don't know."

"Why would they watch us?"

"Our fathers found something, and they were going to expose it. The two of us together is suspicious. We have to give the Order a reason not to watch us."

"And that is?"

"By acting like lowlifes."

"I don't have to act."

Penny laughed. "And in between, we have to retrace their steps and recover whatever they found."

"What? Go to Iraq?"

"If that's what it takes."

"How the hell will we afford that?"

"My father's dead and my mother's institutionalized." She stood and did a twirl in front of Sara and then leaned in close. "I'm officially a trust fund baby," she said with a wink.

"That's *lit*."

"That my parents are dead and crazy?"

"No, not that. I meant the money."

Penny laughed again. "Come on, let's dance."

Sara followed her to the dance floor, acutely aware of the warmth of Penny's hand. The lights were bright, the green especially vibrant. She looked into a green bulb. It was so *green*. She wondered if it might drip green. The square panels behind the light were a darker shade of green and as she stared, she could feel the back of her head turning green.

The music was green too, growing like vines up Sarah's legs, a pounding, monotonous beat overtaking the guitar. Raising her arms above her head, she began to move to the music, the vines twisting around her arms. Penny moved beside her. Their hips bumped and Penny's leg brushed Sara's thigh, the feeling like cotton and static. The dark shadows of Penny's hair were purple, a fine lime-green glow outlining her curls. Her skin was fuzzy and pale, her lips dark pink. Sara closed her eyes, swaying and twirling as the music slowed, the vines dropping away. When she opened her eyes, she was in front of a mirror.

She stared at her pale skin, her blue-black eyes and her spiky purple hair. She touched the glass, her finger meeting her finger's image. She pondered her beauty. Why hadn't she seen it before?

Penny appeared behind her in the mirror, wild orange hair sprouting from Sara's head. Sara giggled and pulled her phone out, posing for a selfie.

"We look *savage*," Sara said.

Penny's image grinned in the mirror, purple teeth.

Sara turned around, her lips an inch from Penny's.

Penny stepped back. "Tonight, we dance. Only dance."

"And tomorrow?" Sara asked hopefully.

"Tomorrow we avenge."

"Avenge who?"

Sara couldn't remember. Maybe the Green Arrow would help them. Maybe Penny would paint Sara and the Green Arrow rolling in the hay.

"Come to my apartment next Sunday," Penny whispered in her ear. "2A ½ West Fifth Avenue. Don't write it down, just memorize it. 2A ½ West Fifth Avenue."

"Don't you like live at the sorority house?" Sara said loudly.

"Shhhh," Penny said. "Now dance."

25

Brett
Cincinnati, Ohio

The letter arrived on a Sunday. Brett had been home for almost a week and was wondering how much longer she would have to withstand the drudgery of her family, when she noticed the mailbox was ajar. She hesitated before walking out to check it. Would the invitation to her future, her triumphant trophy, be left in a mailbox?

On the front path, she noticed a stick of eyeliner in the grass and a crumpled tissue and broken plastic bar bracelet. She'd heard the back door open early that morning and Sara stumbling and giggling to her room. She picked up the bracelet and turned it over in her hand. What would it be like to be unambitious, to seek pleasure instead of purpose? She shivered at the thought, carried the bracelet to the trash can and dropped it in.

She approached the mailbox with caution, for if ever there was a letter that could bite, it would be this one. She pulled the door back carefully and looked inside. Propped neatly at an angle was a single, square, gray envelope.

She pulled it out, noticing her name printed in courier type across the front and beneath it the familiar black wax seal. She sat on the curb and looked up and down the quiet street, half expecting a man in a hooded jacket to be hurrying away from her or a pair of eyes watching her from the bushes. But she saw no one.

She slid her forefinger beneath the paper slit and broke the wax, slowly pulling out a stiff, gray card.

PLEASE REPORT TO THE GREATER CINCINNATI AIRPORT

TUESDAY OCTOBER 5TH 1600 HOURS

IT IS SUGGESTED YOU PREPARE YOURSELF FOR NO IMMINENT

RETURN TO YOUR PRESENT PREMISES

She closed her eyes and clutched the letter to her chest, resisting the urge to stamp her feet in excitement. Nothing compared with the victory of obtaining something she'd worked hard for, and she'd been working toward this letter her whole life. Didn't she deserve a moment of celebration? Should she not allow herself to jump up and down and wave the letter in the air?

No, she would remain poised.

She tucked the letter in her pocket and stood on the footpath, looking up at the house. A flight meant she was going to Jekyll Island and that she may never return to Rosalind Drive. If her father was still alive, would he be proud of her? Or would he be jealous she was going where he'd never been invited? She longed for him to look down at her with the pride he'd shown her during her childhood.

But she was responsible for his absence and she would not pretend she wasn't.

At least now she knew her sacrifice had not been in vain.

26

Hadley
Cincinnati, Ohio

For the second time, Hadley stepped across the white stones and stood in front of the solid, rough-wood door. It was a sunny day and she was glad to be there again. Life had been tense at home. Sara was sneaking out at night, Brett was preparing to leave on a mysterious trip, and her mother was anxious.

There was a lemon tree by the front door Hadley hadn't noticed before. The sun shone brightly on the yellow fruit.

And for the precious fruits brought forth by the sun.

She knocked on the door, puzzled by the quietness behind it. She'd expected he would be home. She knocked again, harder this time, and turned to see that his car wasn't in the driveway. She looked at the ghost of Mr. Ernest, but he just shrugged, disinterested. Her father's angel, perched on a branch of the lemon tree, winked at her.

A cat appeared at her feet, lifting its orange chin and rubbing its whiskers against her jeans. She stooped to pet it.

"Where's your daddy? I was looking forward to having a chat with him."

She smiled at the sound of her voice. She'd spoken! And to a cat!

The curtains in the window moved and a pink, feline nose poked out. "Do *you* know where your daddy is?" she asked through the pane.

"Hello, Hadley!"

She turned to see Issa coming around the side of the house with garden gloves and a pair of clippers. She was overcome with familiarity. The corner of the house, the gloves, Issa's smiling face. It was all so familiar. But the house, the house was wrong, and the gloves were too clean. An image came to her of muddy green gloves and the sound of horses neighing from a nearby building. But it had not been a house, it had been stables and Issa had not been holding clippers but farriers' tools.

"Just trimming the hedge," he said. "Have you been waiting long?"

She shook her head, confused. "Trimming horses' hooves, you mean."

"No, quite sure it is a hedge." He smiled. "I am so glad to see you. Let me wash up and fix us some tea. I will meet you on the deck."

The vision left Hadley, and she saw clearly his gloves were yellow and the hedge trimmers were shiny and new with red handles. The smell of horse dung lingered in her nostrils. She shook her head again.

"Are you okay?" Issa asked.

"I'm okay, yes. I'll meet you around the back."

She made her way to the deck and took a seat at the picnic table, running her hands along the warm, splintered wood. She placed her hand on her throat. It was so peaceful to be back, so wonderful to be talking again. The vision already seemed insignificant.

The works of the Lord are great, sought out of all them that have pleasure therein.

"So, how has your week been?" Issa asked as he came out with the tea on a tray.

"I have read a bit of the Old Testament but I'm not sure I have found any piece of the puzzle."

Issa smiled and placed the tray on the table.

"There's a verse in Genesis that confuses me. It's chapter six, verse four."

"Oh, yes, the Nephilim," he said. "A peculiar verse. And one worth looking at. Let us look at it now. I will be right back."

He returned to the house and came back with a large leather Bible. He thumbed through the first few chapters, licking his fingers and running one down the pages, searching with fast, darting eyes.

When he found the page, he turned the Bible around so it was facing her, and tapped his finger on the verse. She noticed it was a New American Standard. She preferred King James. She liked the formality of the old English. Though she didn't always understand it, she found it beautiful.

"Should we read it?" he asked.

Hadley nodded.

He recited the verse. "The Nephilim were on the Earth in those days, and also afterward, when the sons of God came in to the daughters of men, and they bore children to them. Those were the mighty men who were of old, men of renown."

"See, it's so strange!" Hadley said.

"Tell me what you think it is saying," he said, sniffing the lemon on the rim of his glass.

She read it again slowly to herself. "I really don't know. It's so odd."

He winked at her. "You must dive in and discover the Truth, word by word. Tell me what is clear. Even if it is only one thing."

Hadley studied it again. "It's clear there was something called Nephilim on the Earth a long time ago and the sons of God had children with daughters of men. But it's not clear if the Nephilim are also sons of God, and if they're also the men of renown. The men of renown could be the children born. The Nephilim could have been on Earth during the time these children were born. It's confusing."

"Wonderful," he said, his eyes like water, catching the sun and throwing it to her in flecks of blue and green. "But there is something else you can gather from this verse. The sons are of *God* and the daughters are of *men*. Would it be correct to infer they are therefore different in ancestry?"

"I don't know. It could be the result of using too many words, couldn't it? I mean if men are children of God then being a child of God and a child of man could be the same thing."

"Then calling Jesus the son of God wouldn't really imply he was any more an immaculate conception than we are?"

"Is that why you've chosen this verse?" Hadley asked. "To prove Jesus was just a man?"

"Not at all."

Her exasperation must have shown on her face because he reached across the table and touched her arm.

"Don't get frustrated. Just think about it. What could be the opposite of what you just said?"

His touch relaxed her. "Well," she said. "If Jesus was a son of God while we're children of men then perhaps there were men like Jesus on Earth back then, men who were conceived by God."

He smiled.

"Does your smile mean this is true?"

He shrugged. "It could be Jesus was just a man. It could be, like you said, that they used too many words in the verse."

"So, what's your point? I don't get it."

He folded his hands and leaned into her, his breath sweet from the tea. "My point is that the Bible can be interpreted a number of ways and should not be a sole basis for the Truth. It should only be regarded as a piece of the puzzle."

"What puzzle?"

"The puzzle of why we are here and how we should spend our time. That is the Truth you are looking for, is it not?"

He was right. That was what she'd come for. Although she hadn't realized it until now. "So, do you know why we're here and how we should spend our time?"

"Yes, I do."

She stared at him for a long time before she asked, "How do you know?"

"That is for later."

"Why?"

"Like I explained last time, you must learn at a safe pace."

Hadley frowned.

"Listen, you cannot go on the journey if you already know the Truth, and the Truth will mean nothing to you if you don't go on the journey. All I can do is steer you in the right direction. There is no easy answer." He pulled back from her and snapped his fingers. "One thing I *can* tell you is that you cannot just pick what you like from the Bible, ask Jesus into your life and be off. It is not that simple."

He paused and she waited for him to continue.

"I think you knew that and that is why you are here."

A tabby cat rubbed against her leg, and she leaned to scratch the top of its head. "So how has *your* week been? What did *you* do?" she asked.

"I did some gardening and reading. Had some visitors."

"Don't you work?" she asked.

"Work?"

"In a job at an office or something."

"No," he said.

"Why not?"

"Well, if I worked then I would not be here when curious people like you stopped by, would I?"

"How many people like me stop by?" She didn't like the idea of other people stopping by.

"Many some months. Other times, not so many."

"What do you mean by curious people like me?"

"I mean there are other people who also search for the Truth." Hadley frowned.

"Although I stand corrected," he said quickly. "None are like you."

This comforted her.

"Do you think I could use your bathroom?" she asked.

"Sure. I will show you where it is."

They entered through the kitchen. The countertop was bright orange and the curtains were yellow and pulled back with a piece of lace. On the wall there was a black clock shaped like a cat, with eyes that rolled back and forth with each tick.

"The bathroom's through here," he said, and she followed him out of the kitchen and into a library.

The walls were lined to the ceiling with bookcases made of the same thick, dark wood as the front door. In the middle of the room was a wide backless bench like the ones in museums. Other than a peace lily in a pot and a photo propped on a small table, there was nothing else in the room.

She glanced at the photo as she stepped out of the room and continued a few steps into the hallway before stopping and turning around. She walked back into the library and stood in front of the photo, her heart racing.

It was an old-fashioned photo taken in black and white and yellowed for effect. It was of four men, their arms draped casually around each other. They were wearing top hats. Issa was on the far left, his head turned away from the other men, his long nose silhouetted against a fuzzy background of trees. The two men in the middle seemed vaguely familiar. One was tall and handsome, his eyes downcast. The other was tan and young with light hair. And on the far right was the man in the suit from the side of the road. The man from the accident. Sober and gray, he stared at her from the photo.

Issa came up behind her.

"The man on the right, in the photo. Is he your friend?" Hadley asked.

"A long time ago, he was, yes."

Beloved, believe not every spirit, but try the spirits whether they are of God: because many false prophets are gone out into the world.

She headed to the front door, forgetting about the bathroom. She wanted to get out of the house, to find her way home and make her way to the third floor. She wanted to feel the familiar orange light against her face and wait for her mother to come home.

"What is it?" Issa asked.

"I want to go home." She opened the front door, then realized her backpack was still on the porch. "I need to get my backpack."

She hurried through the library and kitchen and onto the deck.

He followed. "Tell me what's wrong."

"No. No. I've got to go." She picked up her backpack.

"Please," he said. "Please stay."

He looked sad, as if her leaving caused him pain. "I can't. I don't even know why I came. And we're going to a basketball game tonight. I can't be late."

"You mustn't run away from your fear."

She started around the front of the house.

"Facing your fear is the only way to the Truth," he continued.

She walked quickly over the little white stones.

As she stepped onto the driveway, he said, "Listen to your feelings, learn to understand them. They are the guide you are hoping the Bible can be. They are God within you."

Hadley wanted to say goodbye, but her voice had gone. She ran down the driveway toward home, her desire for death whispering in her ear.

27

Renee
Cincinnati, Ohio

The air in the arena was humid with sweat and sharp with the scent of new rubber. Above the murmur of fans and the shifting of bleachers was the squeak of shoes on polished wood.

Renee kept her hand on Hadley's shoulder as they followed Sara down the steps to the front section. She often had the urge to ground Hadley, to hold her tiny, thin frame down so she didn't blow away.

A referee stood at the bottom of the bleachers. "Tickets please."

She handed them to him.

"Front row. Right here behind the bench. Best seats in the house."

It was a preliminary game. The season didn't get into full swing until November, but regardless, the stadium was nearly full.

They sat down and Renee immediately felt small. The boys in front of them, even seated, were taller than Hadley standing up. She worried about her decision to attend the game.

Why am I here?

Because she was interested in a boy who spoke of beauty like no twenty-one-year-old should.

It was his feet she saw first. She glanced down at the blur of sneakers and noticed one pair, bouncing lightly side to side and moving to the rhythm of the ball, dribbling in sync, it seemed, with the breath of the audience. She watched his feet dance softly in their red-leather shoes, her eyes finally moving up the legs to the swishing white shorts, the red and black shirt, the vein-lined arms.

She was drawn again to his feet and followed them about the court. They'd been large in her classroom, huge like his hands. But all the large feet on the court caused his to seem average and brought to her the startling image of many large, thick penises concealed behind shorts. She shook her head, embarrassed at the vision.

"Which one is he?" Sara asked.

"Number eleven."

"Eleven," Sara said, following the jerseys until she found him. "Shit, *really*? He's hot. Is he in your class?"

"Every now and then, when he shows up."

"I thought you were strict about that."

"I am."

"If I were you, I'd make him sleep with you to pass."

"Don't be rude, Sara."

"I'm just saying."

Renee couldn't keep her eyes off Jonas. He glided and skirted at the same time, his movements so light and quick it was as if his feet were whispering. His legs bent at the knee, just enough to bounce, while his arms moved magnetically toward the ball, effortlessly; and with them went his eyes, simultaneously relaxed and alert. The other players seemed tight next to him, their brows drawn together, their shoulders held close to their necks in anticipation, their feet jumpy and anxious.

The bell sounded and Jonas ran across the court toward them, slapping a teammate on the back and stopping short of the bench in front of Renee. He rested his hands above his knees, his breaths quick and fast. He looked up, as if he suddenly remembered she

163

might be there. He met her eyes and waved before he was surrounded by red jerseys and they huddled around the coach, who began spitting and yelling and looking on the verge of a stroke. Renee looked at the scoreboard. They were losing by fifteen points.

The bell sounded again, and they were back on the court. The other team tapped the ball and drove it to Cincinnati's basket. They shot and missed, and Jonas sprang high off the court, knocking the ball with one hand and catching it swiftly with the other. Before either team had time to adjust, he was dribbling toward the other basket, the ball drumming smoothly between the court and his wide, sprawling fingers. The crowd became violent behind Renee, stomping their feet and screaming.

A good ten feet ahead of the rest of the players, Jonas widened his stride and closed in on the basket, taking three leaps and slamming the ball in the hoop. He let himself swing by one hand from the rim before he dropped to the court. The cheerleaders went wild, their pom-poms shedding red and white plastic strips onto the court, their breasts bouncing between. Sara whistled and tugged on Renee's arm.

"Oh my God, Mom, he's *so* hot."

The atmosphere was changed, and the points accumulated quickly, the other team's confidence broken. Jonas's teammates orbited about him, looking to his lead, and Renee didn't know how many points they scored before the game ended, but she was sure he scored most of them.

The coach and benched players rushed the court at the final whistle. Two cheerleaders wrapped their arms around Jonas and kissed his cheeks.

Look at them swoon.

"Why'd this guy give you tickets?" Sara asked.

Renee stood, her seat springing closed behind her. "To witness his poetry."

"His *poetry*?"

Renee began to move down the row.

"Where are you going?" Sara asked.

"To talk to him. You coming?"

"Fuck, yes."

"*Please* stop using that word, Sara."

"Do you think he'll like me?"

They waited for Jonas at the sidelines. He would expect her to be impressed and this made her uncomfortable. But she appreciated the opportunity to watch him play and she wanted him to know that.

Sooner than she expected, he broke from the crowd and moved toward them, less graceful than when he played, but still light and sturdy.

"Dr. Morgan," he said, breathless. "Glad you made it." He wiped a bead of sweat from his forehead with the back of his hand. "Are these your daughters?"

"Yes. This is Sara and Hadley." She watched as he nodded toward them and waited for him to take in the cleavage Sara had worked hard to reveal, but he didn't notice it.

"It was an exciting game for you to see. We don't usually get behind that much."

"Thank you for inviting us."

"Would you like to get something to eat?" he asked. "I'll be done and showered in half an hour."

"We have dinner waiting at home, but thank you."

"Why don't you come to our place for dinner?" Sara asked.

Jonas smiled. "What a nice idea. Thanks, Sara."

"No," Renee said quickly.

He looked at her, a flicker of challenge in his eyes.

"You can't, sorry."

"Okay, then."

"Thanks again for the tickets," Renee said. "It was inspiring to watch you."

"I'm glad you enjoyed it."

"It was, in fact, very beautiful, Jonas."

He smiled.

There. I have given him what he wanted and what he deserves and now that can be the end of it.

28

Sara
Cincinnati, Ohio

Sara preferred the roof to the stairs. It made her feel risky when there was, in fact, nothing to risk at home and everything to risk where she was going. She crawled out the window and onto the rough shingles, dropping the stub of her cigarette in the gutter. She swung her legs over the side of the roof and twisted onto her stomach. Then she gave a quick swing of her legs and jumped into her mother's petunias.

2A ½ West Fifth Avenue. She hoped she was remembering the address right.

"And about this apartment," Penny had said before they'd parted. "It's a bit of a dive and it's essential you dress like a tart and show up late, okay?"

It was almost one in the morning. Sara guessed it would be late enough for Penny and still give herself enough time to get her mother's car back before the sun came up.

It was a basement apartment and Sara descended the cracked steps in her skirt and blouse, her cheap bracelets clanking as she walked. She gave the door a quick tap and when no one came, knocked louder. She waited, shivering. She turned her back to the door and used her heel to pound on it. Finally, she heard footsteps and the sound of a chain being unlatched. Penny cracked the door and peeked through.

"I thought you'd never come." she said through the gap.

"Let me in. I'm fucking freezing."

"Promise you won't use that foul word and I'll let you in."

"Can't promise that. It just slips out."

Penny pushed the door open and Sara slid into the warmth of the apartment.

Candles were burning on bookshelves and wrought iron stands. The bedroom door was open, leaking green light into the main room. It flickered blue and then purple.

"I'm painting," Penny said. "Come on, I'll show you."

Penny had stopped painting action figures and now owned an old projector and collected episodes of 1970s TV shows that she played on a giant cement wall. "I paint over them and then I take a photograph of what I've painted and wash the wall and start on a new one."

There were framed photographs of these paintings littering the walls of the apartment.

"It's my gallery."

An episode of *Green Acres* played as they talked. It crackled as it went around the reel. A man was feeding pigs or sheep. It was hard to tell with all the paint on the wall.

"What time is it?" Penny asked.

"A little after one."

"You didn't have to make it *that* late. Good outfit, by the way."

She switched off *Green Acres* and pulled out a laptop. "Sit down."

Sara pulled up her skirt and took a seat on the rug.

"You know the folders I told you about, the ones my father taped under the pool table?"

Sara nodded.

"Well, I went through them and tried to make sense of them. There were lots of notes and references to historical events and groups of people and geographic places. I can't use the internet, of course, so it's taken forever to look into it all. I've had to go to the library and use books."

"What did you find out?"

"When I put the pieces together, I found three themes. The first one is here." Penny opened a file on the screen and said, "Genetics. They had a lot of articles on genetics, specifically autosomal recessive type inheritances. I have no idea what they were looking for, but I have no doubt it's important."

She clicked the screen again. "The second thing they spent a lot of time looking into was modern day secret societies, particularly the Calderbergers. Now, I've made headway with this. I'll get to that later. The third thing they were looking into was Iraq. They believed there was something important in Iraq *besides* oil." Her brown eyes were bright with excitement. "I found an email my dad sent to your dad saying he'd found proof the oil was nothing more than a decoy."

"I don't know what auto-whatever obsessive means," Sara said. "Genes? Iraq? No idea what you're talking about and definitely never heard of call-a-burgers. Are they a hamburger joint or something?"

"*Calder*bergers. They're an elitist group, members of the Calderberger Club. It originated in Germany."

"Oh," Sara said, disappointed.

"They also refer several times to two Truths." Penny handed Sara a stack of papers marked with highlighters. "All of these notes refer to two secret Truths. The First Truth seems to evolve around the secret of our origin. And I think the Second Truth is about a kind of superhuman power that existed a long time ago."

"Right," Sara said. "So, we're back to superheroes again. Speaking of which, I liked your superhero paintings more than these wall photo thingies."

"Stay focused," Penny said, going to a filing cabinet and fishing through it. "This will sound crazy, but ..." She pulled out a stack of folders and brought them over and dropped them on the floor. "I think the facts about our origin lie here."

"What do you mean our origin?"

"I mean where we come from."

"Who's we?"

"Us! All of us! Mankind! It's all here! Our fathers were looking into it. They found proof of something and they were going to expose it. We just have to put it back in order and retrace their steps." She opened the folders and spread their contents on the floor.

Sara stared at the cluttered papers, magazine articles, flash drives and CDs. "I thought we were going to figure out who killed them, not what they were up to."

"What they found out is *why* they got killed. It's all linked."

"I guess so."

"Don't you want to know what they found?"

"It sounds a bit *extra*."

"Even if what they found was important?"

"Important how?"

"Important to society! Important to life!"

"Sounds totally *extra*," Sara said. "But, saying all this is for real, how are we going to keep ourselves from getting killed if we *do* figure it out?"

"Keep up the front, stay off the internet and our phones, and don't get involved."

"Involved in what?"

"Politics."

"Well that's a shame because I was about to run for mayor."

"Seriously," Penny said. "No one's going to be watching us until we start making noise, and two pill-taking sluts in a basement apartment on Fifth Avenue won't be making the kind of noise they're worried about. It'll look like we're doing what they expect us to do."

"Which is?"

"Wasting our lives."

"I'd like to think of it as having fun."

"Well, whatever. It's an act anyway."

"Is it?"

"Of course it's an act." She paused. "Don't tell me you're doing this because you think it'll be fun?"

"No, of course not," Sara said quickly.

"Or because you think something is going to happen between us? I told you, it's not."

"I was just making a joke."

"You sure?"

"Chill, all right. Just tell me what you want me to do and I'll get started."

"I've spent months gathering information based on their notes and I've put it all in piles," she said. "One for genetics. Two for secret societies and three for stuff on Iraq."

Sara stared at the stack of folders.

"This looks like more than a few folders worth of stuff. How did they tape all of this under the pool table?"

"They didn't. I've been collecting information from their notes, trying to re-create the files they had. I think everything else was confiscated or destroyed." Penny pulled out a stack of photos. "These photos were in the folders."

She handed Sara four photos, all showing different views of the library. On every surface there were stacks of papers and files.

"See," she said. "None of this was here when we went in the library."

"Why would our fathers take photos of the library?"

"As evidence."

"Evidence of what?"

"I think they *expected* someone to ransack it."

"It was totally wrecked when we went in there," Sara said. "Someone definitely looted it."

"And then they killed my dad."

"And then they killed *my* dad."

"And now we have to make sense of all this."

"Why didn't the police look at this? Why aren't they putting all this together?"

"I don't think the break-in was ever reported. My mother rarely went in the library."

"So, we were the first people to enter it after?"

Penny nodded. "I think so."

"What I don't understand is that the newspaper said your dad died of cancer. How do you murder a guy with cancer?"

"Check this out." Penny sifted through the files and pulled one out, holding it up. "It had the letters JFK scrawled across the front of it. "There's all this stuff on Kennedy's assassination. But of particular interest is this." She pulled out a copied bit of paper from a book and pointed to a paragraph circled in red. "You know Ruby, the man who shot Oswald?"

"Not really."

"Well, he died of the same cancer as my dad. He didn't have a trace of it a month before, and then a month after a meeting in his cell with a couple guys from the CIA, he's dead from cancer." She sifted through the file and came out with another piece of paper.

It was a list of names.

"Who are all these people?" Sara asked.

"All had something to do with the shooting in Dallas and all died of cancer. And these," she handed her another list of names, "are all deaths from unexplained cancers over the past sixty years. All people related to a political incident."

"So, if your dad had all of this info, do you think he knew he was going to be killed by cancer?"

Penny shrugged. "Who knows."

"You still haven't told me where we start."

She grabbed a hardbound book and slapped it on Sara's lap. "You start with a history lesson."

Sara stared at the thick book.

"I've already read it," Penny said. "It's invaluable in making sense of all this. It's a history of secret societies."

"Should I take it home?"

"No, you read it here. I've got a great reading chair in the other room. The lighting's perfect. If you're fast, you'll have it read by the end of the week."

"I'm not much of a reader."

"Well, you better get used to it. There's a whole lot more to read after that."

"Like what?"

"A lot of their notes involve the Bible actually."

"I'm not going to read any Bible," Sara said. "Anything you want to know you can ask my little sister. She'd be able to tell you."

"We'll worry about the Bible later. Tonight, you start with the secret societies. Come on, I'll show you the chair."

29

Hadley
Cincinnati, Ohio

Hadley stood in the back yard, smelling the freshly mown grass. The air was crisp and cold on her warm skin, the sun bright and hot. She was trying not to think of Issa or the photo. She sung Psalms in her head.

Blessed is the man that walketh not in the counsel of the ungodly, nor standeth in the way of sinners, nor sitteth in the seat of the scornful. But his delight is in the law of the Lord; and in his law doth he meditate day and night.

She remembered there were clothes in the washing machine and decided she would hang them to keep her mind still.

She entered the laundry room through the back door and closed her eyes to better smell the perfumed powder. She pulled the damp clothes from the machine and lumped them into a basket, noticing items from that morning and remembering their spots and stains from the previous week: a ketchup smear from when her mother had squeezed her hotdog too tightly and the black smudges on the washcloth from Sara's eyeliner. Now these imperfections were gone and the clothes and linens, like herself and her mother and sisters and the grass outside, were born again.

She carried the basket through the sunroom and out the back deck into the autumn's sweet juxtaposition of warm sun and cold air. The empty clothesline rippled with the breeze. Her father, his wings partially spread, perched on the line, his weightlessness causing no bend or sway. She fingered a wooden clothes pin, the warm sense of appreciation replacing the fear that was burdening her.

There was something satisfying about the ritual of turning the dark clothes inside out and joining one item to the next with a shared pin. Later, when the line was full, she would glance out the window and notice the transition of darks to white, colors to grays, as the different loads met each other on the line.

It was New Zealand where she'd learned to use a clothesline. People there didn't use dryers unless it rained for days on end, and even then, sometimes they would wait. A long time ago, when she'd lived at a homestead in Austria, she'd hung laundry in the cold wind. She could remember the way it would whip about her hands as she pinned it to the wire, the wet fabric cold against her knuckles. That had been three lives ago, before the great wars, when it was still okay for women to take pleasure in domestics.

She wished her sisters and mother could find joy in the simple things. She wished they could let go of their desire to hurry ordinary tasks along in haste for what they thought were better things. She was thankful she was able to appreciate the mundane, thankful for the peace it brought.

30

Brett
Atlanta, Georgia

When Brett landed in Atlanta, there was a man in a suit staring stone-faced at her from across the terminal. With a small gesture of his head, he indicated for her to follow and they made their way through the corridors of gates, down two flights of stairs and out a set of glass doors onto the runway, where they were met by the warm southern air.

Three Lear jets sat idling in the late evening light, a woman in sunglasses standing at the bottom of the closest one.

"Brett. Welcome. How was your flight?"

It was De Payen.

"Unremarkable," Brett said.

"I suppose that's all we can ask from a commercial airline. I think you'll find the remainder of your trip improved." She offered her hand to Brett and circled Brett's palm. Brett promptly performed the secret handshake, catching the matriarch's eye briefly in acknowledgment.

"The plane on the far left is yours. You'll take off shortly. We're just waiting for the co-pilot."

Brett had to duck her head to enter the jet. The walls were lined with camel-colored leather. Two matching swivel chairs sat on either side of a table spread with fruit and meats and a bottle of white wine.

"Please, have a seat," a voice said from behind her.

She jumped, not realizing someone had followed her up the ramp.

"Well, you didn't think I'd tend to the stairs all day, did you?" His voice was light and nasally.

Brett took a seat in the far chair.

"I hear you are to have an accelerated initiation," he said, stooping to enter. "And, it appears, the nicest jet."

Unsure how to respond, Brett simply smiled.

"They have high hopes, very high hopes, for you, my dear."

"What else do you know?" Brett asked, finding her voice. "Tell me."

"Oh, that is it, nothing more."

"Don't be vague, please," Brett said. "It seems that's all anyone has to offer." She plucked a strawberry from the table and rolled it between her fingers. "Surely there's an entire file on me, including my bra size."

"Surely," he said, placing himself in the other seat. "But I can't say I've had the pleasure of reading it. De Payen did mention something about you being a spitfire, though."

Brett tilted her head to consider the comment, then asked, "And what would *your* file say, Mr.—?"

"Emulius," he said, reaching his long arm across the refreshments. "Mr. Japeth Emulius."

He looked to be in his early fifties, a plain man, with watery eyes and dull, flat hair. His lips were thin and straight, his chin undefined. She feared there wasn't one feature to remember him by, except that he was slightly effeminate. She shook his hand, waited briefly for a finger twirl and when it didn't happen, removed her hand from his grasp.

"And my file would say I don't have a bit of spitfire in me, and certainly no bra size. But I'm quite sure it would say I'm loyal, as true as they come."

"Loyal to whom?"

"To the cause."

"You mean the Order."

"Yes, I suppose we cannot separate the two."

"Why don't you use the handshake then?"

"Oh, the handshake, yes, that." He stuck out his hand in an effort to revisit their greeting.

Brett didn't move to extend her hand to him. "The rituals aren't important then?"

"They are and they aren't," he said, letting his hand drop back to his lap.

"Why is it those who are loyal are also so tediously vague?"

"You must earn the details, Ms. Morgan. This plane is but a prologue. Wine?"

"No thank you. If you had read my file, it would have told you I don't drink."

He reached in his breast pocket and removed a small, brass box. He flipped it open and presented her a row of hand-rolled cigarettes. His fingers were slender and smooth, the nails perfectly manicured and glossy.

When she shook her head at his offer, he removed a cigarette, snapped the lid shut and placed the box back in his jacket.

"You're nothing like your father," he said, lighting his cigarette from a port in the wall.

"What do you know of my father?"

"He was a good man, a handsome man. I liked him very much." He placed the cigarette in the corner of his mouth. "You have neither his attitude nor his looks." He inhaled, the cigarette standing erect and sparking orange-red. He closed his eyes, the smoke slowly escaping through his nose. It rose to the ceiling and gathered in wavy rings around the dim lights. As Brett opened her mouth to eat the strawberry the smoke floated to her tongue and through her nostrils and she was surprised to smell the sweet and sticky burn of cannabis.

"You were expecting tobacco."

"Wouldn't anyone?"

"I wouldn't subject my lungs to the perils of smoke unless there was a benefit beyond a simple addiction to manmade additives."

"Of course not," Brett said.

"Your father would have agreed."

There was a good chance this man had mistaken her father altogether. "My father is dead."

"Yes. And I understand you had a part in that?"

Brett ignored the comment. "Tell me how you knew my father."

The engine rumbled to life, her chair vibrating beneath her. The pilot pulled the curtain aside and stuck his head into the cabin. "Seat belts."

"I met him on the trip to Jekyll Island, just as I'm meeting you."

Brett was pretty sure her father had never been to Jekyll Island.

"That would have been a long time ago," she said, putting on her seatbelt.

"Ah yes, long ago indeed." He rolled the joint playfully between his fingers. "He was young like you, and handsome. Did I say that already? That your father was handsome? He wasn't as well treated as you though. I don't think their hopes were so high for him. He certainly didn't get his own plane."

"No?"

"There were five of them on the flight. It was a military cargo plane. There were no refreshments and, at that time, no women." She was sure he'd added this last bit to show his disapproval. "Your father was the only one of them from Yale. One young man had graduated from Cornell and the others from Harvard. I remember all the neophytes."

The cabin was enveloped with smoke and Brett felt light-headed. She wondered, briefly, about the pilot.

"What I remember the most about your father was his eloquence and talent for flattery. He moved with ease among the best of them, regardless of his low rank."

The plane released its brakes and started down the runway.

"Low rank?"

"Yes. In the end, he didn't make the cut. As I have inferred, he wasn't the best of them. All that etiquette and obsequiousness could not make up for the wrong blood."

"I'm not sure I follow," Brett said.

"I am getting ahead of myself; or ahead of you, at any rate. You'll learn all about it in due time."

Blood? What did he mean by blood? She came from the same blood!

She was pulled into her seat as the plane lifted and the weight shifted to the wings.

"Keep an eye out your window there, dear. It's a short flight. We should clear the mainland in about twenty minutes and the island will be in view."

She knew her father had fallen short of something somewhere along the line and that he'd hoped she, the eldest and most capable of his daughters, would make up for this. But she was sure he'd never been to Jekyll Island and the mention of blood eluded her.

"You look about the same age as my father. Surely you weren't escorting neophytes to Jekyll Island thirty years ago?"

"Some of us are initiated much younger, my dear. I have been in the Order since I was a child. But I have already said too much and would like to get a nap in before we arrive. I suggest you do the same. Jekyll Island is full of surprises."

31

Renee
Cincinnati, Ohio

"Mom!"

Sara's voice was getting closer as she ascended the stairs.

"Mom!"

She was at the door now, yelling as if she was still downstairs.

Renee opened the door. "What *is* it?"

"At the door ..." She said, breathless. "Mom, it's *him*. Downstairs at the front door."

"The reporter again?"

"No, Mom. *Him*—the guy from your class."

"What class?"

Sara stomped her foot in frustration. "The basketball player!"

"Jonas?"

"Yeah."

"What's he doing here?"

"I don't know. Are you coming down or what?"

"Right. Okay. Tell him I'll be down in a minute."

She closed the door and leaned against it, sliding down the length of it and cradling her knees. She didn't want to acknowledge her desire for the boy, but she couldn't disregard him. Since watching him play basketball, she'd been reading and working vigorously. His affection and beauty had restored her passion. She felt she owed him something for that.

Sara had let him in. He was standing on the tile of the entryway, his feet set wide as if trying to balance his height. He smiled at her and tilted his head. She saw uneasiness, shyness in his eyes. Then it was gone, and he was taking off his hat and moving toward her. "Dr. Morgan, how are you?"

"Renee," she said, correcting him before thinking.

"Renee," he smiled. "I was wondering if you'd like to take a walk."

"A walk?"

"Have you seen the sky?"

"The sky?" She'd been in a room full of windows, but she hadn't noticed the sky. "Jonas, how do you know where I live?"

"I looked it up in the phone book."

"Right," she said. "Of course you did."

"It's a beautiful night, and I was walking home from practice and I could tell by the redness of the clouds it was going to be a beautiful sunset. So, I was wondering ..." He put his hat back on. "Would you like to take a walk?"

Renee glanced at Hadley on the couch with her King James Bible and Sara, standing close to the coat rack, gawking at her.

I will go with him and end this. I will make him understand.

"Okay," she said.

He beamed. "You'll want a warm jacket, it's getting cold. But hurry, while the colors are still good."

Renee pulled her coat from the rack and followed him out the door.

She looked over her shoulder. "I'll be back shortly. Can you keep an eye on the meatloaf?"

It had rained earlier that day, and beneath the woodsy scent of living room fires, the air smelled of wet asphalt and damp leaves. The sky was dark orange with a thick layer of pink clouds.

"It's great, huh?" he asked, his hat back in his hands and the sound of his voice more relaxed than it had been in the house.

"I can't believe I didn't notice it."

"I can," he said.

"Why's that?"

"You always seem to be waiting for something else instead of noticing what's in front of you."

"Tell me, Jonas. What is this you're doing?"

"What do you mean?"

"*This*," she said, stopping and looking him in the eye.

"I thought I told you already. I want you."

She stepped off the driveway and onto the sidewalk. "You don't have to be so forward."

"It's the only way I know how to be. It's my position."

"Your position?"

"In basketball. I'm a forward."

"Oh, right," Renee said, fighting a smile.

"Why not laugh? You're beautiful when you laugh."

She quickened her pace. *This is not working.*

"Do you know when I first saw you?" he asked. "You were hosting a reading in the auditorium. Last year, remember?"

"Maybe. Which one?"

"Creative writing and politics. You read from *Atlas Shrugged.*"

"Oh, yes. I remember."

"I was there with my girlfriend at the time. She was an English major. She asked me to go and I felt drawn to accompany her. I didn't know why I should be interested. But I knew I was meant to go. When you walked on stage and began to speak, your voice soft and heavy and full of passion, I knew why I was there."

"That was last November."

"The next semester you were in New Zealand. Then I had to wait through the summer, and now, finally, I'm taking your class."

"Yes, you are."

"And you're just as stubborn as I expected you to be."

"Would you still want me if I wasn't?"

God, did I just ask that?

"What do you mean?"

"Well an easy older woman is hardly attractive."

"I would definitely prefer it if you weren't stubborn."

"That might be what you're really looking for."

"Stubbornness?"

"I'm sure when you're handsome and popular, it's nice to have a challenge."

"So, I'm handsome, am I?"

"You know you are," Renee said. "But being handsome isn't impressive." She turned her eyes toward the orange sky. The clouds had turned purple. "It's a beautiful night. Thank you for getting me outside."

"Why do you think there has to be an ulterior motive for my attraction to you?"

"Because things are never simple."

"Sometimes they are."

A car pulled onto the street, and Renee moved quickly into the shadow of a maple tree.

Jonas's face softened in the colored light. "Would you rather walk somewhere else?"

"There's a cemetery," she said. "We can cut between these houses and enter through the back gate."

Inside the cemetery, shadows from the gravestones stretched long black lines through the spotted orange light.

"My mother is buried over there," Renee said, pointing.

He leaned into her, looking down the length of her arm, his breath fogging in the air. She watched it dissipate, smelling a hint of spearmint.

"How long ago did she die?" he asked.

"Just over two years ago."

"Was it hard for you?"

"My mother was extremely religious. We didn't have a lot in common."

"And your father? Was he religious?"

"He was a politician, as was his father and his father before that. For him, religion was part of the role. For my mother religion was real. She believed it through and through."

"I don't think a person should have to choose."

"Choose?"

"Religion is about God being good and Man bad. I refuse to believe either is better than the other. It's like choosing between the country and the city. I mean there's no question the country is God's world with its bending wheat and worm-laden soil. But the city, oh the city, is *Man's* world. It's here we cry out with our rising buildings, 'Oh Father, look at us!'" He opened his arms wide as a gesture to the city around them. "It's as if we say with our sculptures, 'We can do it too!' The city is where we praise God as Men. How can that be bad? How can either be bad?"

Renee stared at him, less interested in his point than his prose.

"Don't you agree?"

"You aren't a typical young man, are you?"

"No," he said. "I've always been different."

An old sensation tickled beneath her shoulders. She shivered against it.

"I see a difference in you too," he said. "I saw it when you were reading on stage."

Renee allowed herself to look at him and saw his nose was narrow and his eyebrows thin. She noticed both of his ears were pierced, although unadorned. She saw stubble poking through the smooth skin of his chin. She had an urge to touch his face, knew somehow that if she did the sensation beneath her shoulders would grow.

"I knew that day I had to meet you, to *know* you," he said. "This knowing, it came from somewhere outside of myself and at the same time *through* me."

As he spoke, the lightening extended forward to her chest.

How long has it been since I have felt this?

She hadn't thought she would ever feel the feeling again. She'd thought she'd forgotten it entirely.

They began to walk again, the whites of his eyes glowing fluorescent blue in the rising moon, his steps the same graceful strides he used in basketball.

32

Sara
Cincinnati, Ohio

Sara liked it at Penny's. The dark windowless rooms, the flickering candles, and the weirdness of Penny's paintings comforted her. As the days passed, she not only wanted to be around Penny more, but found the vast amount of information before them exciting. From scraps of paper and random notes, they'd pieced together a skeleton of information.

Sara looked up at the timeline drawn on the wall. Fifty-four moments in history that spanned from 500,000 BC to today, all people or events their fathers had deemed important. Some of the things Sara had never heard of, like the five eras they kept finding references to. But a lot of it was the same history she'd learned in school. What had bored her then, interested her now. She wasn't sure if it was the link to her father's fate that appealed to her, or the way Penny came alive with each new discovery.

"Are you going to sleep here again tonight?" Penny asked. She was sifting through papers and didn't look up.

"Don't see any point in going home."

"No. Are you finding any more references to these guys Germain and Rhodes?"

"Yep, still finding them. Just a few more to go through. Is all this information really going to help us figure out why our fathers were killed? And if so, what do we do then?"

Penny looked up. "What we do about it is secondary. It's about knowing the Truth. Do you want to live your life in the dark?"

"Don't go all *salty* on me," Sara said. "And isn't it two Truths, not one?"

"Yes, two Truths. And we'll know what to do with the information when the time comes. Don't worry."

"What do you think the Truths are?" Sara asked.

"I think they're the answer to the ultimate question."

"Which is?"

"*Why are we here?*"

"That's only one question."

"But there are two aspects to that question. The first involves the past. *Where do we come from?* The second involves the future. *What're we capable of?* These, I think, are the two Truths."

"I don't know," Sara said. "I think it's all about money. It'll just turn out to be a load of political bullshit."

"And these five eras," Penny said, ignoring her. "Our fathers keep referring to them. I've never heard of them before, have you?"

She liked it when Penny looked at her as if she could help. "No, but I'm sure we can figure it out."

"They're important, like these two names Germain and Rhodes. They're everywhere. It's like our father's talked to them, knew them. Let's see if we can find a correlation between these guys and the eras."

A half hour later Penny tossed her last file onto the floor. "Okay," she said. "I think I'm getting somewhere. By looking at the dates, we know this man Germain has some valuable information about the first three eras, and Rhodes has valuable information on the last era. I think our fathers went to see these guys, trying to learn about the eras. Have you had any luck finding an address?"

"I've been through them all and there's no mention of Germain's address. But Rhodes looks like he's in Provincetown." Sara handed Penny a clip from the Provincetown newspaper. "An advertisement for yoga classes with Shane Rhodes."

"A yoga instructor?" Penny asked, taking the clipping.

Sara shrugged.

"Hey, it's something," she said. "It'll make sense later. The eras are clear to me now." She grabbed a marker and moved to the timeline on the wall.

"There are four. The first era, which our fathers simply called the Beginning, we know nothing about. But according to their notes, the Beginning ran from 500,000 BC to about 10,000 BC." She drew a large black bracket on the timeline beside these dates. "The second era is the Restoration, which I think involved an ancient civilization called the Sumerians. Then we have the Era of the Sages." She drew a smaller bracket from 2,000 BC to the birth of Jesus. "It seems the Egyptians, the Hebrews, the Greek philosophers, and Buddha all knew both Truths and practiced them during this era. Then there was the last era, the Corruption, running from AD 30 to present time." She drew another bracket. "This era apparently started over a feud between the secret societies and the Catholic church. Their notes imply a kind of split between the followers of the Great Sages." She drew a final giant bracket around these dates and started shuffling through some papers. "I think there might be a fifth era. I can't find any info on it, just one note that says ... the fifth era with a question mark after it."

A candle was flickering on the table next to Penny, making her face change colors. Sara wondered if Penny had any marijuana in the apartment.

"Are you listening?" Penny asked.

"Yes," Sara said. "A fifth era."

"*Maybe* a fifth era. I don't know."

"Why do we need to know about these eras?"

"I think each era represents a shift in the understanding and dealings of the Two Truths," Penny said, circling the whole timeline with a sweep of her arm. "But the details lie with two men—Germain and Rhodes." She wrote their names huge and sprawling across the wall. "I think our fathers visited both these men six months before they went to Iraq. Their credit card statements show a flight to Boston and then, a few days later, a flight to Paris. I'm guessing this Germain guy lives in France somewhere. But I can't find any address for either of them."

"So, let's go see this Rhodes guy in Provincetown. Can't be that many yoga studios."

Penny nodded. "We need to do it without being obvious. We need a reason to go."

"Maybe there's an event or something we can get tickets to."

"Good thinking. I'll track down Rhodes's address. You find an event. Find something popular, something we'd have heard about without looking."

Sara stared at a mark on the timeline. "Penny, what about *Saint* Germain? What if this Germain guy has something to do with Saint Germain? Our fathers marked him as significant on the timeline."

"Saint Germain lived in the 1700s."

"Well, it seems a bit weird our fathers thought Saint Germain was important enough to put him on the map, and they visited a guy named Germain as well. What if there's a connection? Shouldn't we at least look into this Saint Germain?"

"Okay. Let's get the file out on him."

Sara shuffled through the files until she found it. Inside were scraps of paper, articles, and a few pages torn from an old history book. She handed them to Penny.

"I wish we could just google this stuff."

"Well, we can't." Penny began flicking through the articles. "Okay, here we go. 'Saint Germain first showed in London in 1743,' " Penny read. " 'And was known as Wonderman. He spoke every language, and was a painter, writer, and violinist. His writing was published under lots of different names. No one really knows where he came from. He claimed to have lived for centuries after discovering the elixir of life and apparently staged his death numerous times.' "

"Is this guy for real?" Sara asked.

"It says here he knew Cleopatra, was alive when Jesus turned water into wine, put Catherine the Great on the throne in Russia, and was the grand master of freemasonry sometime in the late 1760s." She stopped and flipped through the scraps of papers. "The names he published his writings under: Christopher Marlowe, Valentine Andreas, Cervantes, Edmund Spencer ..."

Penny stood and hurried to a pile of files stacked against the back wall. She sifted through them, tossing them here and there. Finding one, she flipped it open and scanned her finger down the page. "Here! Edmund Spencer. Your dad has a note here about an Edmund Spencer in Paris. What if Edmund Spencer *is* Germain?"

"Wonderman himself, still alive?"

"I don't know about that," Penny said. "But I'm willing to bet it's the man our fathers visited, the man they called Germain."

"So, I was right. There *was* a connection," Sara said.

"I think so. Maybe Rhodes will be able to confirm it. And, Sara," she said.

Sara liked it when Penny said her name.

"Yeah?"

"Don't be so sure this isn't going to be *the* Saint Germain. Because whatever these Truths are, when we find them, I think they're going to blow us away."

33
Hadley
Cincinnati, Ohio

Hadley stood in front of Issa's door once again, her feet shuffling nervously on the white stones. She had wanted to return for days but had been unable to muster up the courage. Now that she was here, she couldn't find the strength to knock. Where were the cats? Was their absence a sign she shouldn't have come?

And he gave a sign the same day, saying this is the sign which the Lord hath spoken.

The door opened and Issa stood in the doorway.

"Hello," he said.

Hadley parted her lips but found she was unable to speak.

"It is very good to see you. Would you like to come in?"

She offered a slight nod.

"Would you prefer the deck?"

She shook her head, a tear working its way down her cheek. She wiped it off with the back of her hand.

"You can come in. It is okay," he said. "You are safe here."

She knew what he said was true, but she was afraid of what the photo meant. Who was the man? Why was he with Issa? There were so many questions she wanted to ask him, but her voice wasn't working.

"I can answer your questions without you talking. Come in and have a warm drink." He stepped back to allow her to enter.

She stepped in hesitantly, a cat rubbing against her leg and another hopping from the windowsill and darting out the door.

"How many cats do you *have*?"

"Ah, now there is your voice."

She placed her hand at her throat in surprise.

"Six cats live here," he said. "Four come inside and two prefer under the deck."

She leaned down and rubbed one under the chin. It purred warmly against her leg.

"Please come have a cup of hot tea. Let us talk about your last visit."

She looked up but didn't move.

"You know we must."

Be of good courage, and he shall strengthen your heart, all ye that hope in the Lord.

"A cup of tea would be nice."

"Come," he said, and she followed him into the kitchen.

Once the tea was made and they were sitting opposite each other at the kitchen table, Issa said, "Now, let us talk about Japeth."

"Is he the man in the photo?"

"He is."

"How do you know him?"

"We were friends. A long time ago."

"How did you meet him?"

"We used to work together," he said, sipping his tea.

"I met this man. He was very strange, and I kept wanting to ask him the same question I want to ask you."

"And what is that?"

"Who *are* you? That's what I keep wondering as I talk to you, and it's what I wondered when I was talking to him. And now there's a photo of you two together in there." She gestured toward the library. "It scares me because that man was at my father's death."

194

"Why don't you tell me what happened."

Hadley wrapped her hands around the warm mug. Should she tell him? Logic told her not to. Logic told her to leave. But her heart said she could trust him. "We were in a car accident, and just before the crash I saw a man on the side of the road. He was moving his hands around and around and they were glowing. My father died in the accident. I think this man *caused* it."

"And you spoke to him?"

"After the accident I followed him. He knew my dad had died and told me God's ways are mysterious. He said he was a servant of God."

And he shall spread forth his hands in the midst of them ... and he shall bring down their pride together with the spoils of their hands.

"Tell me again about his hands. You said they were glowing?"

"Well, it looked like it to me. Maybe that wasn't important. You think it was a different man, don't you? You don't think it was your friend Japeth?"

"Oh, I am quite sure it was him."

"You are?"

"Sounds like just the kind of thing he would be involved in."

"Do *you* think he caused the accident?"

"Maybe."

"Will you tell me who you are? Who this man is?"

A shadow came over his seawater eyes. "If I tell you too much, too soon, you will not believe me."

Hadley put her mug down and laid her head on her arm against the table. Her father's wispy hand caressed her hair and softly touched her cheek. He hadn't entered Issa's house last time and she was glad he was there.

"Please tell me what you can then," she said. "Anything."

He set his mug down and studied her, then said, "The Truth goes back to the beginning of time. Not just the fact of who Japeth is, or who I am, but who you are too. Perhaps that is what you really want to know? Who *you* are?"

"Yes," Hadley said softly, aware of her father and Mr. Ernest hovering above her. "I want to know why I see and feel things others don't. How did I know to come here and why can I talk to you but not to others?"

"We must start at the beginning. Go home and read Genesis," he said. "Read it thoroughly and with great curiosity."

She nodded, staring out the window, marveling at the strength of the orchids, at how they stood tall in the breeze, unbending.

"And patience, Hadley. Return to me with patience."

They sat together in silence; she, Issa, the ghost and the angel. She suspected Issa could see the spirits. Could he feel Mr. Ernest's restlessness? Could he feel her father's peace?

When she finally got up to go, Issa said, "Those who experience death in life always have a duty."

Hadley left without responding and made her way down the driveway. She stooped to feel the petals of the orchids, savoring their rubbery sturdiness between her fingers.

He hath made everything beautiful in his time: also he hath set the world in their heart, so that no man can find out the work that God maketh from the beginning to the end.

34

Renee
Cincinnati, Ohio

Jonas was sitting at the back of the classroom when Renee arrived. This was the first time she'd seen him since their walk through the cemetery. And the only place, she was acutely aware, where she should see him.

It was early and only two other students were there, on their phones by the window.

He smiled at her. "Good morning."

She withdrew her eyes, glanced to see if either of the other students were watching, then braved a look his way. "Good morning."

He stood and came toward her, turning sideways to fit down the narrow row between the desks.

She opened her bag, pretending to look for her phone.

He approached the desk and whispered, "It's good to see you."

"And you," Renee said, rummaging through her bag. "I think I forgot my phone."

"The only thing you've forgotten," he said, placing his hand on the desk beside her, "is to call me."

She stopped her fumbling and looked at him.

"Ten days is a long time," he said.

The door opened and more students came in.

Renee moved out from beneath the arch of his body. "Veronica," she said. "I'm glad you're early. I wanted to talk to you about your last assignment. Do you have a minute?"

Throughout the lecture he watched her. And despite her best efforts, she bloomed in the spotlight of his attention, her posture straighter, her enthusiasm heightened. The familiar, but nearly forgotten, lightness that came with feeling attractive rushed upon her. It had been so long since she'd felt wanted! What was it that Ernest had said once? That men desire women and women desire the desire of men. Or was that Madame de Staël who said that?

Quickly, shame set in. *How pathetic I am, falling for this boy's game!* And the fear of being made a fool turned her to the window, wishing for Tahoe, wishing to be anywhere but the front of the classroom, vulnerable with unexpected longing.

Then he caught her eye again and she found herself lost in the performance of her teaching, momentarily aware of her brilliance and beauty, only to cringe a minute later.

By the time the class was finished, she was exhausted.

As he was leaving, he brushed against her, making her skin tingle, and she knew he was a lover now, whether she let him touch her one day or not.

35

Brett
Jekyll Island, Georgia

Brett stood on the veranda watching the sun set over the Atlantic, the warm salty breeze tossing her hair about her brow. Her forearms were propped on the railing, and she held a glass of untouched Pinot Gris in her hand.

Below her, people were dancing. She gazed at the tops of their heads: amber bangs, gray parts, black curls, blonde buns. She enjoyed watching them from above, meditating on the fact they were the most powerful people in the world.

The brass instruments of the band played a light Caribbean tune, their bells and keys reflecting the pinks and oranges of the sunset. The ocean crashed against the beach, white caps meeting the sand every few seconds. Seagulls flirted on the horizon.

Eleven of the fifteen Claw and Bones initiates had been invited to the island. They'd all arrived on private jets twelve days ago. There was no mention of the four who were missing, but Eli was one of them, and this brought an emptiness Brett couldn't shake. Was he still a member of Claw and Bones? Had he received a rejection letter explaining the importance of the sacrifice or was he just ignored? And on top of this was an unease. What did it mean if you couldn't question customs or stand strong in a belief? What if the Order was nothing more than a tyranny? And for what? Extravagant rooms and parties?

Behind Brett, white linen curtains billowed from her room. Beneath her feet were slick ivory tiles, and a potted fig tree hovered above her. Her suite had its own spa. The shower was made of tinted aqua glass and had four shower heads and a seat with heat ducts that dried her before she got out. There was a bidet and gold enameled toothbrushes with bristles from exotic animals in Madagascar. The four-poster bed was covered with silk sheets, and sheer fabric scented with frangipani hung from its sides. The kitchen had a small window that opened from the hallway behind the counter. Fresh cuisine, appropriate for the time of day, was presented every four hours.

Jekyll Island was extravagant, the scenery divine and the entertainment constant. But nothing important seemed to be happening. Brett hadn't learned any new information. She hadn't been further inducted into anything. She hadn't even heard the name Calderberger spoken once.

She swirled the wine in her glass, watching it change colors from the sunset.

Was it her destiny to be perpetually waiting for something important that would never arrive?

The day she'd received the letter, she thought she'd finally gotten further than her father. He'd always implied the Truth lay on the island and claimed he didn't know the Truth. But everyone on the island spoke as if he'd been there. What did this mean? Had he come here but never learned the Truth? If so, what did that mean for her? What if there was no Truth? What if there was only money and pleasure?

This was her biggest fear: that there was nothing to be had but the power money bought. Her father had believed there was a deeper Truth, an answer hidden within. But an answer to what?

"Brett?"

She turned to see Noel standing behind the curtains, appearing intermittently as they blew in the breeze.

"Hi," she said.

He stepped onto the veranda. He was wearing a white linen suit, his tie loose, a glimpse of chest hair visible.

"What're you doing?" he asked.

"Watching the party."

He came and leaned on the rail beside her and looked out over the view.

"What is it with you?"

"What do you mean?"

"Why do you always hang back?"

"Because I'm not *in* yet."

"Supposedly it's tomorrow night."

She turned to him. "What is?"

"Initiation into the society that rules the world." He lifted his glass to the sea.

She could smell whiskey on his breath.

"The Calderbergers," she said, looking at the heads below her. So vulnerable. So human. She laughed at herself. Did she think they would wear armor?

"Yes, the Calderbergers," he said.

"I don't think so, Noel. Not yet."

"What do you mean?"

"There's something else still. There's another test to pass first."

"Oh, come on." Noel spread his arms wide. "You don't think they'd let us this close if we weren't in, do you?"

"That's the thing, Noel," Brett leaned into him. "There's in and then there's *in*. This is still outside."

"So that's what you're doing up here then, trying to figure it all out?"

"Partly. Mostly I just don't like people."

"No, Brett, you don't like the masses. These people here aren't the masses. Talk to them. They'll inspire you. Listen to them. Sometimes you won't even know what they're talking about because their thinking is so advanced. You're right. We're still on the outside. But this is the *door,* and these people you aren't giving a chance to are *it.*"

He was right. She'd spent so long waiting to be part of "the group", she'd forgotten the group was still made up of people.

"My God. I've been a snob for so long I've forgotten how to be interested in anyone."

"Come." He stood, offering his arm. "Join me?"

The sun was gone. Noel's thick black hair shone in the outdoor lamp, his eyes bright beneath his heavy eyebrows, challenging her to accept his company. She set her wine glass on the edge of the fig tree and placed her arm through his. He pulled her to him, the linen of his jacket cool, his arm firm and warm beneath it.

The fires had been lit, giant copper drums of burning driftwood casting an orange glow across the crowd. She sipped her wine and listened to conversations about the economy, the war in the Middle East, a scandal in Hollywood. None seemed particularly different than what she might hear off the island.

There was a tap on her shoulder, and she turned around to find a man standing next to her with an envelope. He handed it to her, bowed and left.

She walked toward the shadows of the building where a thin beam of light came from an upstairs room and opened the envelope.

MEETING HOUSE.

GROUND FLOOR

ROOM 26

2100 HOURS

She looked at her watch. It was already after 8:30, and the meeting house was on the other side of the island. She would have to be fast.

The building was dark except for a door glowing yellow at the end of the hall. It was open and she entered. A figure sat in an armchair in the shadows.

"Come in, Brett. Have a seat."

The voice was deep, strong and gritty. Arousing.

She approached the couch and sat down, the lighting so dim she couldn't make out his features.

"Have you enjoyed Jekyll Island?"

"I'm tired of the party. I want more."

"Good."

"There's another test, isn't there?"

"You've already passed it, of course. That's why I have summoned you."

The man brought his hand into the light. It was a lean hand, brown and beginning to age. She guessed he was probably in his forties. He flipped a switch and Brett heard the fan of a projector whir to life. A light shined against the wall and he withdrew his hand back into the shadows.

An image of a cluster of cells appeared on the wall.

"Do you know what this is?"

"Blood," Brett said.

"More specifically. Your blood."

The screen advanced to the next slide. More cells, but longer and paler. "Your saliva," he said and clicked to the next photo.

An image of capsule sized cells appeared.

"My hair," Brett said.

"Yes."

"This was the final test?"

"Yes."

"And you've collected these samples over the past twelve days?"

"Yes."

"From my apartment?"

"Here, there and everywhere. We took over two hundred samples."

"And if you hadn't found what you were looking for?"

"You would have gone home after the party and become a senator or a judge, something respectable."

"Like my father."

He didn't respond, a square-toed brown Rockport the only part of him visible.

She remembered what Noel had said about these people being a different caliber than she was used to.

"So, who am I related to?" she asked.

"An ancient bloodline runs through your veins." The Rockport withdrew into the dark. "You are one in a hundred thousand."

Brett was disappointed at the odds and was about to say so when he continued.

"You grew up in Cincinnati. By calculation, there are only ten people in the city with this blood."

"And in every other city too, I presume."

"Yes. But a person must be cultivated from a young age and then make their way here, and only about one in ten do."

"So, then I'm one in a million."

"That's more accurate."

His voice was disturbingly arousing. She thought about the mud pit, about how she'd stripped before stepping in. Had he been there? Had he seen her?

"And what of this ancient bloodline?" she asked.

"You'll learn about it later. First you must tell me about your sisters."

"My sisters?"

"We think one of them might be a prophet."

"A prophet?"

"There are some in which the blood runs thicker. We call them Prophets. There are considerably fewer of them than there are of you."

"And what're my kind called?"

"We refer to you as a Talent."

"And what makes you think one of my sisters would be a Prophet?"

"The ancient gene is passed down through the generations, carrying with it the ability to create a unique blood cell, called an Omega cell. It's similar to a basic red blood cell only a different shape, which causes it to move quicker throughout the bloodstream. We think this has something to do with why it can't be identified through regular blood tests. But the truth is, we don't understand much about it. We don't know how it works. We only know it correlates with heightened abilities and talents. And, like other autosomal recessive inheritances, there must be two genes present, one from the mother and one from the father."

"And my parents?"

"Your mother is a Talent, like you. And your father was a carrier. The correct term is Carrier Clone. A Talent and a Carrier Clone's combination of the ancient gene offers a twenty-five percent chance of creating a Prophet."

"Theoretically then, both my sisters could be Prophets."

"Or neither of them."

"Being a Carrier Clone wasn't enough to make my father a Calderberger?

"I'm afraid not. Although Carrier Clones have some Omega cells present and will show talents and abilities beyond Masses, their blood is still dominated by normal red blood cells. This is where he failed."

Masses? That was the word Noel used.

"And a Talent's blood?" Brett asked.

"Equal red blood cells to Omega cells."

"And," Brett said, making sense of it all. "A Prophet has more Omega cells than normal cells."

"Yes. And Masses have none."

"So, does anyone have *all* Omega cells?"

"Someone with one hundred percent Omega cells is called an Anunnaki. But we'll get to that later, much later."

"So, you need samples from my sisters?"

"To get the right samples takes weeks of vigilance. You would have to bring them here, and it would have to be on their own terms. Force creates resistance and that's a risk we can't afford. We had hopes you would be a Prophet. You have the signs of high levels of Omegas."

"Which are?"

"Intelligence. Ambition. Creativity. Resilience. A hunger for Truth."

"Washington D.C. is full of people like that. Pakistan is full of people like that."

"Yes, but Prophets also have metaphysical gifts. They have such a high number of Omega cells their powers are what some might call paranormal. Outwardly, none of your sisters fits this description. But inwardly, they may. Your father made a mistake only cultivating *you*."

"I was the only one interested."

"It is common for a Prophet to resist. They're free spirits."

Eli resisted! Had she given up the chance of love with a Prophet?

"Brett?"

"So, you want to know if any of my sisters have supernatural powers?"

"Yes."

Brett smirked. "I don't believe in magic."

"Another sign of a Talent," he retorted.

"Even if I did, my sisters are the epitome of unremarkable. One is an introverted religious fanatic and the other is a gothic wannabe."

"Introverted and religious?"

"Shy and weird. Currently she's obsessed with death."

"This is the little one?"

"Yes."

"She's independently religious at a young age?"

"My grandmother brainwashed her. Hadley's no Prophet."

"Don't be upset I'm asking about your sisters. They pose no threat to you."

She listened to the whir of the projector. It had heated up. The smell reminded her of melting crayons.

"Do I sound threatened?"

"Yes."

"I'm just disappointed."

"About what?"

"That I'm not a Prophet. That there are people with greater potential than me. Either way, I'm certain there's no Prophet to be found in a goth or a mute."

"Did you say a mute?"

"Hadley hasn't spoken a word since my father's accident."

"Tell me more."

Brett wished he would show his face. She found it ridiculous talking to a shadow.

"The doctors can't find anything medically wrong with her, but she doesn't speak. They think it's PTSD."

His hand came out of the shadows, and he tapped his fingers on the arm of the chair.

"How old is she?"

"Thirteen."

"You must bring her to me at once."

"But you said it was a risk bringing her to the island."

"Not here. You'll take her to Deer Island, in New York."

"And if she isn't a Prophet?"

"Then she's free to return to her life of biblical silence."

"And if she is a Prophet, what will you do with her?"

"We must keep the bloodline alive. We must keep the Masses from diluting it."

"So, you're going to *breed* her?"

The door opened automatically on the other side of the room. "Bring us your sister and I'll explain more then." His voice was raspy and short.

Brett stood and walked toward the door, the weight of his watching heavy on her back.

She turned at the door and looked into the dark where he sat.

"And if I don't?"

"Remember Eli."

She spun toward his shadow in the back of the room. "*What* did you say?"

He chuckled. "You aren't dealing with Masses anymore, Brett. Be careful."

36

Hadley
Cincinnati, Ohio

When Mr. Ernest's ghost came into Hadley's room that night, she wasn't surprised. She'd been expecting him. It was her father, the angel, who alerted her to the ghost's presence, his hand slipping from her shoulder and his form turning gray and opaque with loathing.

It was always like this. Her father didn't like Mr. Ernest, and looking at Mr. Ernest now, large as the doorway he stood in and robust even in death, Hadley understood her father's animosity.

Mr. Ernest glided awkwardly into the room. Although dead for half a century, he seemed uncomfortable floating.

Athletes have the hardest time adjusting to ghostliness, he said, *having once been so adept to gravity.*

He placed his buoyant hand on the crown of her head, his fifth finger and thumb touching Hadley's ears while his palm covered her eyebrows. She loved the way the spirits felt when they touched her. The stillness, the lack of blood and breath.

There is a boy, he told her with a heaviness that had seeped into the room with him and now settled about the carpet around his feet, misty and condensed.

What boy?

A boy your mother will love. I always knew there would be a second love.

Hadley's father was perched lightly on the headboard, crouching as Mr. Ernest spoke. Hadley wanted to argue that her father had been her mother's second love. But Hadley knew he'd been no such thing.

Why are you so sure she will love this boy? She asked. *Is he the basketball player?*

Mr. Ernest nodded solemnly. *I am as sure as I was the day she glided over the horizon, her hair like tumbleweed and her eyes yellow-green like the grass beneath the snow, that I would love her like I once loved war.*

Mr. Ernest always answered questions like this. Hadley found it irritating.

I'm happy for her then, Hadley said. *Aren't you?*

Yes, Ernest, her father said from behind her. *Aren't you?*

No, he said. *I do not want to be replaced.*

You always were a coward, her father said to Mr. Ernest.

At the sound of these words, Hadley remembered the jealousy she'd experienced earlier that week when Issa had mentioned that other strangers also visited him. Such a strange feeling it was! It had been full of anger and desire and possessiveness and love all woven into a knot in her stomach.

You loved her differently than I, Mr. Ernest said wordlessly. *You think being selfless is noble but being in love and jealous is its own kind of beauty. Of course it doesn't make me happy, this talented boy. How could it? But because I know she will love him and it will be requited, there is nothing for me to do.*

He proceeded to cry, that strange living emotion he'd taken with him to death.

Hadley was tired and slid into the cool smoothness of the sheets. She thought of her mother in love, smelling of springtime and bouncing when she walked. She imagined the orange and pink flowers that would come to her door and the way her mother would tap her fingers on the roof of the car. She could feel the sheets growing warm from the heat of her body, the pillow taking on the form of her head and the ghost's crying fading with the day.

37

Sara
Cape Cod, Massachusetts

"Sorry it took so long," Penny said, coming up behind Sara, breathless and red in the face. "He's here. I found him."

Penny had left Sara by a tree on the outskirts of the concert over an hour ago. Squeals of laughter and singing were echoing through the park, the beat of the drums rising from the ground.

"Where?" Sara asked.

"He says if we want to talk, we have to do it in there." She pointed to the undulating mass of bodies.

Something was different about Penny. Was it the breathlessness?

"How are we going to talk in there?"

Penny shrugged and licked her lips, tucking a loose curl behind her ear.

"What's going on with you? You seem weird."

"Talking to him could get us killed."

"No, that's not it. It's something else."

"What're you talking about?" Penny rolled her eyes and flicked her hair from one shoulder to the other.

"That," Sara said. "That right there, flicking your hair. It's not like you."

"Who cares about what I do with my hair? This is dangerous stuff we're doing."

"If it's that dangerous, why would he bother talking to us?"

"He's not worried about himself," Penny said. "We're putting ourselves in danger talking to him."

"Great."

"We knew this before we came."

"Yeah, I guess."

"Well, what else can we do? Take our mothers' approach and turn our backs on the Truth?"

"Okay," Sara said, pulling herself off the tree. "Let's go."

He was waiting for them a few hundred feet from the stage. He wasn't old like Sara had expected but young and tan. He wore a brightly colored Hawaiian shirt and a baseball cap. He took off his sunglasses and smiled as he shook Sara's hand, his teeth broad and white against his bronze skin. His hair was light brown, the ends sun-bleached. His eyes were the same light brown, the whites around them clear and bright.

"You girls take a great risk meeting me," he said.

"Did you meet with our fathers too?" Sara asked.

"Yes."

"When?"

"About a year ago. They're dead now, I hear."

"Murdered," Sara said.

"As I mentioned, you're taking a big risk." He turned to the stage. "But I'll help you if I can."

Penny's eyes lingered on his face, then dropped to his shoulders and down the length of his arm. She was attracted to him, that was why she was acting strange. Sara went limp with the realization.

"Our fathers were studying the great secret societies throughout history," Penny said, twirling a curl of hair around a finger. "They referred to four distinct eras in their papers. They're nothing we've heard of before and they seem to be linked to two Truths. What do you know about the eras and the Truths?"

"Or," Sara said. "You could just tell us who killed them."

"I don't know who killed them," he said. "But I can help with the eras. What do you know already?"

"The first era we know is called the Beginning," Penny explained, blinking her long orange-yellow eyelashes. "But we know nothing about the significance of this time. According to their notes, it ran from 500,000 BC to about 10,000 BC and has something to do with Biblical Genesis. Is that right?"

He nodded. "That's correct."

"And the next era was the Restoration," she said. "We know even less about this time. All we know that is that it ended with the disappearance of the Sumerian civilization."

"Go on."

"After this was the Era of the Sages. This was the time when all the great religious leaders and philosophers thrived. Our fathers' notes infer the Great Sages knew and practiced Two Truths, but we don't know what they were, or are. And last is the era we called the Corruption, which apparently began with the formation of the Catholic church and continues today to the wars in the Middle East. The only thing I'm sure about," Penny added, "is that each era seems to represent a shift in the understanding or dealings of Two Truths."

"What else did their notes say about the Truths?"

"Nothing really. Just that they're kept secret by a group of people who stretch back before Christ."

He nodded.

"Well, what're the Truths?" Sara blurted.

"Just like that, you want me to tell you the secrets of our existence?"

"Do you know what the Truths are, Mr. Rhodes?" Penny asked.

214

"Shane," he said. "Call me Shane."

"Shane," she said, smiling at him.

Sara rolled her eyes at Penny. "Shane, do you know the Truths?"

"The First Truth involves facts about our creation. But I'm not the best person to talk to about that. I'm still learning myself."

"But our father's notes said you were a historian."

"I am a historian. But I specialize in the last few centuries. I'm afraid I'm not a BC man."

"So, you would know about the Corruption then, how it started?" Penny asked.

He shrugged, then nodded. "I don't know much about how it started. Like you said, it began with the formation of the Catholic church. And I know that the oppression of the Catholic church gave rise to a string of secret societies, the first of which was created around AD 1090 and was called the Priory of Sion. It was created by people who refused to let the church own the sacred Truths. The Priory grew and morphed and divided over the years. There were many societies that originated from it: the Knights Templar, the Rosicrucians, the Freemasons. They all knew the sacred Truths and tried to protect them. Today, remnants of these secret societies live on, but there's only one society that is still organized around the Truths." His foot tapped to the music as he spoke, his eyes watching the band. "It is commonly known as the Order."

"How big is the Order? How influential?" Penny asked.

"It encompasses our government, our whole political system. But the number of people who actually know anything are probably only a few hundred. Most politicians, although part of the Order, are just pawns. Within the Order there is only a small group of people who know the Truths. They're called the Calderbergers."

"So, most members of the Order don't know the Truths?"

"No. The Truths are the carrot within the Order. The higher up you are, the more you know. The Calderbergers are the top of the pyramid, the ones who pull the strings. The rest are puppets."

"But, there are people outside the Order who know them, like yourself, right?"

"There are other groups that know about the Truths, yes. But over the years all have become corrupt."

"Including the Order?"

"Oh yes, as corrupt as they come."

"And you? Where do you fit in?"

"It's a long story," he said, looking at Penny.

Penny held his eyes, her cheeks reddening.

"What're the other groups?" Sara asked.

"There are two main alliances besides the Order." Rhodes continued. "The Catholic church is one and the money launderers is the other."

"Who are they?"

"The men who own the banks."

"The Rothschilds and the Rockefellers," Penny said.

He tapped his hand against his leg and began to sway to the music. "Listen to this solo coming up. I love this band. They've got grit."

Penny watched him move to the music, her fingers unconsciously stroking her hair.

"But what about the word *federal*?" Sara asked. "Isn't the Federal Reserve Bank controlled by the government?"

"Once again, don't mistake alignment and control with matching motives and history. They're all terrifically intertwined, but they're separate. The government is in debt and always has been. Have you ever asked yourself who owns their debt? This is *good* music, isn't it?" He began to dance.

"So, what does any of this have to do with our fathers?" Sara asked. "Did one of these groups kill them?"

"It's the Truths lodged in these societies that our fathers were trying to understand," Penny said. "It's the Truths that got them killed, isn't it?"

"So, who was it?" Sara asked. "Was it the Order then? The Catholic church or some rich bastard? Tell us."

Rhodes flashed his bright teeth, still dancing. "It depends what your fathers found out and what they did with the information. If it was something small, it's unlikely it was the church or the money men. If it was a profound threat to the secrecy of the Truths, the Order probably killed them. But if they found something big and if their plans were big enough, it's probable all three groups were after them."

"Our fathers were part of the Order," Penny said. "Weren't they?"

"Yes," he said.

"If they were part of the Order, why would the Order kill them?"

"Your fathers most likely had low standing."

He closed his eyes, shoulders jigging slowly as he danced.

"And you," Sara said. "What about you? Isn't Rhodes a rich family name?"

Penny looked at Sara for the first time since they'd entered the crowd. "What do you know about that?"

"Some guy named Rhodes, can't remember his first name, was the creator of one of the secret societies. He owned a bunch of diamonds and was prime minister of something. South Africa maybe? I don't remember. I read it all in that book you made me read."

"You're referring to my great-great-great grandfather, Cecil," Rhodes said. "He was part of the Corruption. He founded the

Round Table society, which was one of the last societies formed at the turn of the twentieth century. Some say he was the founder of the money launderers. I, however, am not a member of any of these groups. I'm only interested in living the Second Truth."

"What does that mean?" Penny asked.

"It means political power doesn't inspire me."

"No, I mean living the Second Truth."

"It means I have grasped the essence of the Second Truth, the only Truth that matters." He turned his attention on them fully, his eyes darkening. "It is impossible to remain a member of any of the sects when you understand the Second Truth."

"Which is?" Penny asked.

"Omnipotent power, power that's independent of approval or status, power that comes only through submission and faith."

"So, you're part of the church group?" Sara asked.

"Oh my, no. The church is just as much about approval and status as the Order is. The Second Truth," he said, "is about a magical power, a power we display in our superheroes and wizards, unaware we're capable of it ourselves."

"Magic?" Penny asked.

"This isn't what you came for, is it?" Rhodes asked.

"I don't know," Penny said, toeing the grass with her shoe.

"We came to find out who killed our fathers," Sara reminded her.

"And when you find out who killed them, and realize they were killed to protect two ancient Truths, will you stop there? Or will you need to know the Truths?"

Neither responded.

"You've embarked on a long journey. The more you learn, the less you'll be able to turn back and bury your head in the sand like all these happy people." He turned his palm upward, extending it to the pulsating crowd.

"Happy? How do you know they're happy?" Penny asked.

"Don't they look happy? Dancing and drunk and not the least bit concerned with murder or the Truth?"

Sara wished she could be dancing and drunk with them. She could smell marijuana. The sweet burn was ripe around them.

"Sure, they look happy now," Penny said. "But ask them later when they're paying taxes for something they don't agree with or watching their child die of cancer. Then they'll want to know where they come from and why this is happening."

"Taxes and cancer won't make them search for the Truth," he said. "For most people, those things are only excuses for playing the victim, vehicles for getting attention. Few people really want to know *why* things happen."

The music grew louder as the band joined the guitarist and the crowd began to roar. Rhodes turned to the stage and began dancing again.

"I still don't understand how the money launderers play in all this," Penny yelled over the music. "What did they do?"

Rhodes beckoned them with a tilt of his head, moving backward out of the crowd. They followed him, the multitude thinning as they moved further from the stage. He stopped by an overflowing trash can.

"For years there had only been the church and the secret societies holding the knowledge of the Truths. But in the 1700s Mayer Rothschild, born of lowly ranks in the German ghetto, cleverly managed to embezzle a large amount of money from a number of wealthy men and set up his sons with bank branches across Europe. He then leveraged his wealth further through intermarriage, until eventually he accumulated so much money he started buying royalty and church debts. Not long after, the Rothschilds became their own group, known as the money launderers. They have expanded to include others, including the Rockefellers."

"And they knew the Truths too?"

"Rumor has it they bought them off the secret societies through blackmail and debt bribes."

"So," Penny said, touching his shoulder, "you're saying the church, the Order and the money launderers are the three main groups of power in the world today but that they all differ in their belief about the First Truth."

"No, they all *believe* the same thing. It's their motives and ways of handling it that differ. It's why the era is called the Corruption. The church distorts it, the secret societies hoard it, and the money launderers leverage it. And the rest of us ..." He lifted his arms, gesturing about the wide lawn, "we live in the corruption, most of us ignorant of it. Some, like yourselves, trying to figure it out, and a few, like me, are past being affected by it."

"You mean you don't care?" Sara asked. "I'm in that camp, hundo p!"

"I care. The corruption just can't touch me. It's a consequence of practicing the Second Truth."

"So, the First Truth is what our fathers discovered and were going to expose, and the Second Truth is something different, some kind of magic?"

"Completely different indeed. When one experiences the Second Truth, there is no need to expose it. It's not something that *can* be exposed. You can tell people about it, but they won't understand it until they've experienced it, and once they've experienced it, exposure is pointless. It's all very ironic." His eyes sparkled. "You see, these three groups, they only know *of* the Second Truth, they don't understand it. They don't know how to *live* it."

"And you do?"

"I'm learning how, yes."

"How? Who teaches you if none of these groups understand it?"

"Ah," he said. "Now you're asking the right questions."

"I don't understand," Penny said, deflating.

"We're moving into a new era, where more and more people will come to live the Second Truth."

"A fifth era?"

He nodded.

"Our fathers' notes said something about a fifth era. Do you know what it is, when it begins?"

He shook his head. "I only know it's imminent."

"How can we learn more about this Second Truth?"

"If you want to understand the Second Truth, you must go see Germain. I'm merely a Prophet, as they call people like me. But Germain, Germain is the Truth itself."

"Can you take us to him?" Penny asked.

"Or an address," Sara suggested. "An address would be good. No need for you to take us."

"He's in Paris, goes by the name Edmund Spencer. Address is 44 Rue de Saintonge in the Marais. No doubt, he'll be expecting you."

38

Renee
Memphis, Tennessee

Renee thought about Jonas often. She found her attraction to him, while definitely lustful, was also due to admiration. For when she thought of him, she thought of the way he quoted Ernest as much as she thought of his smooth skin. She thought of the way he spoke of beauty as much as the size of his large hands. And she thought of the way he played basketball, the swiftness of his movements, as if he'd been crafted for the court.

The classroom was becoming a prison, his adoration a tease within the confinement of the brick walls. And after two weeks had passed, she understood he wouldn't ask her on another walk or invite her to another game. He was waiting for her to requite his affection. He was calling her over mountains and she had to follow.

So she found herself in Memphis, nestled in his hotel bed, the silk of her lingerie and the cotton of the sheets cool against her skin. He was playing in the last pre-game before the season began. Twenty minutes earlier, she'd convinced the hotel receptionist she was part of the management team and been let into his room. She was anticipating his reaction, excited by her own daring, when she saw the girl.

She stood rigid behind the bathroom door, dark hair pulled back in a rubber band, a sweatshirt tight under her armpit, a backpack slung over her shoulder. She was staring at Renee, her mouth open.

Renee wanted to run, to disappear.

"Well," she said, trying to forget about the lingerie she was wearing. "This is a bit awkward."

The girl remained frozen behind the door.

"You may as well come out. You're going to have to eventually."

The girl didn't move.

"It's my fault," Renee said. "I should have checked to make sure no one was here before I let myself in. It was ignorant of me to not suspect it."

The girl stepped from behind the door, her eyes wide with disgust. Renee remained poised, adjusting the pillows behind her so she could sit up straight. She pulled the sheets higher over her. "Now, come, haven't you seen a senior citizen in silk before?"

Oh God, that wasn't funny.

"I know who you are, Dr. Morgan. Don't you remember me? I took your class last year."

Renee wasn't sure if she'd ever seen the girl before.

Have I slept through another student? They're so unremarkable now!

The door in the front room clicked open and slammed close. Footsteps padded across the carpet toward them and a long shadow came into the room. Jonas stopped in the doorway. He looked at Renee, glanced at the girl and back at Renee and sighed, simultaneously reaching his hands above his head and gripping the door jamb.

"Lizzy, you should leave," he said.

Lizzy gaped. "What?"

He closed his eyes and dropped his head. "Go on. You shouldn't be here."

"*I* shouldn't be here?"

"You need to go."

"This is crazy," the girl said.

"No. Just crowded."

"What is *she* doing here?" she asked, not budging.

"She's here to see me."

"In your bed ... in her underwear?"

This is a silk and lace Victoria's Secret teddy and it cost a hundred and eighty dollars. It isn't meant to be worn under anything.

"Look at me, Jonas," Lizzy demanded.

Jonas looked up at her. "Yes, she's in my bed and hopefully wearing nothing."

"That's disgusting."

He held up his hand to stop her saying any more. "Just go, Lizzy."

"Disgusting," the girl said again, her voice was deflated, edgeless.

Jonas took his hand off the door jamb and crossed his arms. "What exactly do you find disgusting, Lizzy? The fact Renee is older than me? Is that it? Because Renee has more character in one crow's foot than you have in both those fake breasts."

"You asshole!" She shook her head and started to the door, pushing her backpack further onto her shoulder. As she passed Jonas, she thrust her elbow into his stomach. "Pig."

She slammed the door behind her.

He remained in the doorway, grasping the door jamb. "I fear I have defended you weakly."

"I wanted to surprise you," she said.

"And you did."

Renee laughed. Her hands were shaking. "I wasn't expecting ..."

"You don't have to explain." He came and sat next to her on the bed. "I'm not worried about Lizzy. She wasn't invited. I'm thrilled you're here."

"I'm afraid the moment is lost."

"No," he said, moving closer to her. "It isn't."

"So, who is she?"

"She's one of the cheerleaders. We usually hook up on away games."

"Hook up?"

"We just sleep together sometimes. Nothing more. I've never pretended it was anything more than that and neither has she." He pulled back and looked at her with a straight face. "Didn't you once say a friend was harder to come by than a lover?"

"Would you have slept with her if I wasn't here?"

"I don't know," he said. "Probably. You haven't talked to me in two weeks."

Renee nodded. She liked his honesty. "Does she really have fake breasts?"

"Yes."

"Oh God," Renee groaned, wishing she hadn't chosen to breast feed. "How many others are there?"

"Fake breasts?" he asked. "More than you would think."

She laughed. "How many other *cheerleaders*."

"None now," he said and brought his lips to hers.

Lightness spread through her, not in the slow and undulating way it had some forty years ago, but in a sudden encompassing sensation that started nowhere and ended everywhere. His flesh on hers was a commotion of static, his hands aware and responsive, his eyes alert and conscious. When they joined bodies, the lightness erased Renee's mind. Her thoughts, for the first time in her life, ceased.

Afterward, Renee reflected on the lightness she'd experienced with Ernest. It had been in the absence of physical union where her years with Scott had been the opposite. There had been sex without lightness. She'd thought intercourse was a poor man's substitute for real connection. Now that she'd experienced both simultaneously, she realized how wrong she'd been.

"Let's go away together," Jonas said, his voice moving with his warm breath across her shoulder.

"Where would you like to go?" she asked. "If we could go anywhere?"

He kissed the soft skin at the inside bend of her arm. "I don't know. Somewhere in the Mediterranean maybe. On a sailboat."

Ernest had loved sailing. He'd had a boat. He'd told her about it one night. She remembered how he'd talked about the boat as if it was a woman, as if it was his mother. She wished she'd had a chance to stand next to Ernest as they approached home after a long day, his arm strong around her shoulder in the setting sun, the fishing lines trolling behind and the sharks surfacing as they scavenged the day's catch. She'd dreamed of this often.

Jonas laid his head on her stomach, his scalp rough with new hair. "You're thinking about Ernest."

"How did you know that?"

He closed his eyes. "Tell me about the two of you. It's such a mystery."

"Is it really?"

"Everyone knows you were his last lover. They found his writings. But you've never admitted it."

"No," Renee said. "We weren't lovers, not in the way people think. I was only fourteen. Let's order room service. Champagne?"

"I don't drink in season," he said. "And I want to hear about Ernest. Tell me in what sense you *were* lovers."

"I have never explained Ernest and myself to anyone."

226

"So, try me."

She propped herself against the headboard, Jonas shifting to lie by her side.

"We were lovers because there was love between us. It was highly sensual but we didn't *do* anything."

"I don't understand."

"I can't make it make sense."

Jonas moved up to the pillow and pulled her into the crook of his arm. "Okay," he said. "I get that."

"You do?"

"Yes," he nodded. "There's lots I can't explain."

"Like?"

"My mother, my basketball, the distance I feel from most people. The way I feel about you." He kissed her hair. "I always think life is full of possibility, that nothing is unknown, just untried. I think about these things. Thinking, I'm always thinking. I walk home at night and I wonder how many other people are thinking like I am. How many others are aware of the beauty life holds? And then I see the flickering blue and purple screens of televisions and I think, no one. No one thinks. It's only me."

She smiled at his soliloquy, remembering how he'd spoken this way when they'd walked together in the cemetery.

"I was once like that," Renee said. "Always thinking."

"Once?"

"I don't think as much as I used to. Maybe the questioning dies with age."

"No," he said. "It's not age. It's a choice. You haven't lost it. You still seek truth." He sounded tired, his arm growing loose around her.

She thought of the basketball game he'd played earlier, of the swiftness of his feet across the court, the energy it would have taken. "You're wrong. I don't seek the Truth."

"Yes, you do," he said sleepily.

"No, I run from it."

"Well, you know it's there then," he mumbled.

"Yes," she said. "I know it's there."

"Then you can only run for so long."

His words trailed off and his breathing slowed. Short spasms jerked his arms and legs as his breathing became louder and deeper. Then, like a great and powerful machine shutting down at the end of the day, he shuddered, and his head fell heavy against hers.

39

Hadley
Cincinnati, Ohio

For days, Hadley had been reading Genesis. She'd read it and reread it, scrutinized it, noted it, and endured the confusion created by the juxtaposition of what she'd been taught at church and what she saw in the words and chapters.

She was once more at Issa's doorstep. She would have visited sooner but her mother had become suspicious of her walks. How could she explain that she regularly visited a strange man at his house? Luckily, her mother had left town that morning, providing the perfect opportunity.

It was a beautiful Sunday morning and this time she found Issa's front door open. Two cats were sunning themselves on the white stones.

Behold, I have set before thee an open door, and no man can shut it: for thou hast a little strength, and hast kept my word, and hast not denied my name.

She knocked, and poked her head into the entryway. The windows were open, drapes blowing in the wind. She stepped inside, Mr. Ernest floating casually into the house ahead of her.

"Hello?"

She moved into the library and stood between the tall bookcases, reading the foreign titles. Many of the books were labeled with characters she didn't recognize. Mr. Ernest was touching the books with his see-through hand. He came to one and pulled it out, smiling and leafing through its pages. It was a small book and there was a photo on the front of an old man in a small sailing boat. She left him there and made her way to the kitchen. Finding the back door open, she stepped out onto the deck.

"I am out here," Issa's voice said from the backyard.

She crossed the deck and found him sitting on the ground among his flowers.

"Hi," she said. "I couldn't find you."

"Here I am." He smiled. "How are you?"

"I have lost my peace."

"That is because you have become afraid."

There is no fear in love; but perfect love casteth out fear.

"Don't worry. By understanding your fear, you will overcome it."

"I read Genesis and I made notes."

"Perfect. That is a start. But we must teach you to erase your mind. Let us not be so obsessed with the Bible." He motioned to the grass beside him. "Come, sit down."

"But you *told* me to the read the Bible."

"But it is not everything. Now, please, sit."

"In the grass?"

"Yes."

She set her backpack and Bible on the stoop of the deck and went and sat next to him. The grass was damp and immediately soaked through her jeans.

He placed the backs of his hands gently on his knees. "The key to good instincts is meditation. So, you shall learn to meditate."

"Like Buddha?"

"And like Jesus."

"Jesus didn't meditate, he prayed."

"Prayer in its highest form *is* meditation. Now get comfortable."

230

"Do I have to cross my legs?"

"When you get proficient, you will want to pay attention to your posture, but when you are beginning it does not matter. You can sit however you like."

She crossed her legs anyway.

"I do suggest you close your eyes. It limits the distractions."

She looked around her first.

The garden was alive with color. The hedges were trimmed square and rose bushes towered from their center showing off orange, yellow and pink. Red and black butterflies and large, fuzzy bumblebees hovered between the petals. Purple and yellow petunias grew in pots set routinely about the yard. A mosaic birdbath glistened in the afternoon sun, two robins flirting on its rim.

Awake, O north wind; and come, thou south; blow upon my garden, that the spices thereof may flow out. Let my beloved come into his garden and eat his pleasant fruits.

"Meditation is a state you find yourself in," Issa said. "It is not something you can force. It is important you are gentle with yourself and do not try too hard. You must not try to control anything. It is our mind that tries to control. That is what it is for and it has its place, but you must also know how to turn it off. I want you to sit here until your mind disappears."

He closed his eyes and Hadley watched him for a moment before she said, "I have no idea what you are talking about."

"You will," he said, eyes still shut. "The key is not to care one way or another. Attach no emotion to anything, especially not to your thoughts. Now close your eyes and try to be present."

She closed her eyes and sat still, trying not to do anything or think anything. She found herself thinking about how trying not to do anything was still trying to do something and exactly what she wasn't supposed to be doing. These thoughts made her restless. She wanted to move, to get up and run, to laugh.

"Breathe," Issa said. "Frustration and humor are feelings attached to thought. They are like birds you only need let fly away. Pay attention to your breath."

"How am I supposed to not think about the fact you know what I'm thinking?"

"Who cares if I know what you are thinking."

"Anyone would."

"Do you want to be anyone, or do you want to know the Truth? Now quit talking. It has only been forty seconds and we have all day."

There was a playfulness in his voice she hadn't heard before and it made her giggle. She didn't know what he meant by all day, but she didn't want to be just anyone, so she took a deep breath and held it until the itch to giggle went away.

She listened to the birds. At first, she heard random peeps and tweets that seemed to come from several birds. But the more she listened she noticed there were different patterns and soon detected four birds singing. As she listened, she noticed there was also a pattern between the chirps as they answered each other. She'd always known birds used their song to communicate, but she hadn't realized the birds were *talking*. A bird flew from one side of her to the other, chirping until a chirp came back. When it got the response it wanted, it gave a different chirp and flew in another direction.

How significant these details seemed when she paid attention! She smiled and opened her eyes.

Issa sat with his palms faced upward and his fingers curled in. His face was expressionless and soft.

How long had they been sitting there in silence?

"About fifteen minutes," he said.

She closed her eyes and focused on the wind. It was cool against her skin. She shivered at its touch, contemplating how it was always here, always moving. Where did it come from? What was its purpose? Maybe like the birds, it was part of the intricate process of life and didn't have to have a purpose beyond that.

The thought of there being no deeper purpose beyond existence scared her. Frustration welled again, bringing nervousness.

She soon realized she was giving meaning to her frustration. Her frustration, like the wind and the birds, simply existed. She didn't need to give it any attention if she didn't want to. Immediately, it disappeared.

Be still, and know that I am God.

She didn't know how much time had passed before Issa spoke, but it had been long enough for her frustration to return and disappear several times with the shifting of her emotions. It reminded her of waves coming in off the ocean.

"There is a place inside you," Issa said, "where earthly things don't matter, things like thoughts and feelings and reasoning. Meditation is about going there. It is here we tap into the Great Universal Energy that is existence. It is here we connect with our true power."

His eyes were open and he was looking at her.

"It's like death," she said.

"I have not experienced death, so I don't know."

"You haven't?"

"No."

Hadley was confused and disappointed. She was so sure he, like herself, had seen death.

"Those thoughts are for another time, Hadley."

How did he read her mind?

"That question is also for another time."

"I can't stop thinking and wondering!" she said, exasperated.

"You will learn."

"How long will it take?"

"As long as it takes."

She wanted to stop meditating and discuss the Bible. That's what she'd come to do. But she took a deep breath and dismissed the impatience. She closed her eyes and listened to the birds again, and the inaudible chatter of the neighbors. She listened to her breath, played with the depths of her lungs, inhaling and exhaling, noticing her breath vibrating her lips.

For a moment there was stillness, a void, a bright nothingness. She wasn't aware of it until it was gone and her emotions rushed in, excitement, elation. She'd been there, to the place he spoke of! She opened her eyes, acutely aware of her surroundings, the flowers, the wind, the fly on her knee.

Ye shall know that I am in my Father, and ye in me, and I in you.

Issa began to speak.

"They asked Buddha, 'Are you a God?' and Buddha said 'No.' They asked, 'Are you an angel?' and again Buddha said 'No.' 'A saint?' they asked. 'No,' Buddha said. 'Then what are you?' they asked, and Buddha answered, 'I am awake.' "

Hadley sat still, the birds chirping loudly, the wind crisp.

"You are awake now," Issa said. "However short the experience was, you are now aware of the place beyond your humanness. Each time you will find it easier to reach and you will stay longer."

She closed her eyes and straightened her spine, placing the back of her hands against her knees. She took a deep breath and observed herself as she analyzed the absurdity and simplicity of what she was doing, the thoughts no longer scaring her. They were waves off the ocean, rolling in and backing out without meaning.

Then they were gone, and there was only a buzz deep within her sternum, a warm generator humming, a purple-white ray of steady light.

When she opened her eyes, the garden was a brilliant sea of color.

"Over ten minutes," Issa said. "You tapped in for a good ten minutes that time."

"Is that a long time?"

"Eventually time is irrelevant. But, yes, it is a long time for your first try. We will continue until the sun sets and then you will go, and you will find life very different indeed."

The Lord of peace himself give you peace always by all means.

40

Brett
Jekyll Island, Georgia

The initiation into the Calderbergers, full of candles, robes, and rituals, had happened the night following Brett's meeting with the dark man. Only six of the original initiates had been accepted. The others, they were told, had been sent back to comfortable government positions where they would serve the Order through implementing decisions and influencing social focus. They were still brothers and sisters of the Order, but they wouldn't learn the Truths. They wouldn't make decisions. They were, Brett interpreted, puppets.

Fourteen had lined up behind her outside Weir Hall that first night at Yale. Ten had joined her on the island. And now only six of them remained. Noel was still among them, and she sat with him on the veranda contemplating the glory of becoming a Calderberger.

She didn't feel much more than a puppet herself. A week had passed and the only Truth that had been revealed had been an odd explanation about the power of sex between Talents. It seemed everyone was content to bask in the sun and copulate while she was churning over the dark man's request and waiting for a bigger Truth.

And still wondering about Eli. What had become of him?

"So, when are you going to go get Hadley?" Noel asked, sunning himself in his robe.

"I don't know if I'm going to yet."

"If they give you a mission, you do it. It'll all work out in the end," Noel said, eyes closed and tilted toward the sun.

"In the end!" she exclaimed, getting out of her deck chair and stepping inside. "What is the end? When does it come?"

"What is it you want exactly?"

She paced across the plush carpet. "Truth and power."

He sat up, his robe falling open and revealing his dark, furry chest. He ran his fingers over the shadow of his navel, the light catching the ripples of his stomach. "There are many kinds of power."

Sex with Noel *was* a kind of power. It had been one of the few things in life that had surprised her. But the pleasure it offered came with a vulnerability that appalled her.

She turned away. "I have to come up with a plan. I'm not giving up Hadley for free."

"Are you rejecting me?" he teased.

"Yes," she said. "We've been at it constantly. I need to talk this out, make a plan."

"At *it*?" He stood. "Maybe *it* is what we should talk about."

"What's there to discuss?"

"They promised it would be amazing. They promised it would be powerful. And it is. I mean we're experiencing what they said we would. Is that nothing to you?"

Brett shrugged.

"They've done everything they said they'd do. They told us we'd receive a letter and we did. They said they'd make us Calderbergers and they did. They explained to us how we passed the test. They told us about our blood and our importance and then, upon initiation to the Calderbergers, they explained power would be ours."

"What through *sex*? I thought we'd be able to leave that obsession to the Masses."

"It's just the first step. Didn't you listen?"

Brett shrugged again.

"They explained sex together would offer us a portal to what we'll be capable of later. There's still more to come. Something bigger than this. Why so impatient?"

She leaned against the back of the couch and crossed her arms.

He came and stood over her. "You know what I think it is? I think you're undervaluing the sex we have because you've never had sex with a Mass."

"Perhaps."

"I'm surprised you've never asked me if it's better."

"Better?"

"Better than what I experienced with others. You know, before."

"Hmmmmph," she laughed. "I'm sure it's better. How could it not be?"

Noel brought his lips close to hers. "You accept it so easily. But you can't appreciate it because you have nothing to compare it to."

"That's because I held out for something more, for something remarkable."

"And they've given us remarkable. You just can't see it. If you had experienced sex with a Mass, you wouldn't be feeling slighted." He began loosening her robe. "I wish you'd been with other men, so you'd know the difference."

An image of Eli flashed before her, stretched on the couch as he'd been the last time she'd seen him. What might sex have been like with him? He must be a Talent. It explained her draw to him. But Noel was a Talent and she hadn't been drawn to him initially. Or was Eli a Prophet? Something greater than she?

"So, how's it different then?" She asked.

He groped her breast through the robe. "With you, everything else disappears. It's like we go someplace else, some other dimension. I don't know how to explain it."

She knew what he meant. It was like they lost themselves and gained something else altogether, some kind of force.

"And with others?"

"It just felt good," he said. "Like a nice meal or a good shit."

"Lovely analogy, Noel." She pushed him away.

"Well, you asked."

"Surely it was more than that, the way Masses are so obsessed with it."

He looked away, silent for a moment, then said, "At times there was a glimpse of something more. I used to try and hang on to those moments. But I could never catch them." He pulled her back to him. "With you there's no frustration. I think it might be love."

"Oh, spare me." She rolled her eyes.

"Didn't they say the movies are depicting love between Talents and Prophets? Remember, they said the Masses spend their lives striving for this romantic, all-encompassing pleasure, but it always eludes them."

They had said that.

"That's probably why a lot of people give up on love and think it isn't possible," he said. "Masses can't experience it and most Talents and Prophets find themselves unmatched and unsatisfied with a Mass."

What would it be like then, to be with a Prophet? She thought of the dark man, pictured his lean hands, fingernails like pale almonds.

"The girls you were with," Brett said. "They would have felt it, that overwhelming infatuation. You would have given them that, being a Talent."

"Yes, and they always claimed love and never seemed to be able to get over me. Now I understand."

Her desire for Noel was more pleasurable than anything she'd experienced. But it wasn't pleasure she sought.

"If you're saying the girls you were with felt what we're feeling now, then the feeling is ordinary."

"Unrequited attraction is ordinary. Ours is reciprocated. Ours is high level passion and connection. Don't underestimate that."

A vision of her parents came to her, beside the fireplace at Rosalind Drive. They'd been having an argument and her mother had walked away, frustrated. Her father had watched her go with a love and admiration Brett had found pitiful. She'd thought her father weak and her mother uncompassionate.

"You may have just explained why my mother never loved my father the way he loved her. I always thought it was her ridiculous obsession with Ernest. But it's obvious now. My father was a Carrier Clone and she was a Talent."

"She couldn't feel for him how he felt for her," Noel said. "Because he had fewer Omegas."

"And Ernest," Brett said. "He was probably a Talent." She walked onto the veranda and looked out to the ocean. "She experienced this with Ernest."

Noel followed her out. "What did you say?"

"My mother must have experienced this," she pulled him to her. "When she was with Ernest."

He nibbled on her neck.

"Or what if Ernest was a Prophet," she murmured.

"That would explain her eternal obsession, wouldn't it?"

"And she was so young. It would have *rocked* her." She whispered.

"Can we make love now then?"

She wished he would just take her instead of asking.

He must have understood because with one hand he opened her robe and with the other he pushed her against the wall. Her head fell back, a tingling warmth spreading from her breasts to her thighs, her identity dissipating into a small purple dot behind her eyelids.

Bright, pure, nothingness.

Afterward, they lay on the tiles of the veranda, embracing each other in a thin layer of sweat. Noel's breathing was heavy. She could feel the quick beat of his heart beneath his chest.

"How can I help you bring Hadley here?" he asked.

Brett shrugged. She always found herself less ambitious in the wake of sex. And if sex created apathy, how was that power?

"Getting her isn't the problem."

"What is then?"

"Saving her."

"From what?"

"From the Order."

"They won't hurt her."

"They killed my father."

"Hadley's a child," he said. "She's a Prophet. Your father was a rebellious Carrier Clone."

"My father served the Order most of his life."

"I thought you agreed it had to be done."

"The fact is, they're capable of killing and I care if they kill Hadley. She's a little girl, Noel."

"The fact you care about her shows she's a Prophet like they suspect, and I don't think they'll kill a Prophet. I don't think they *can*."

"What makes you think that?"

"I don't think anyone has more power than a Prophet. If Hadley doesn't want to die, they won't be able to kill her."

"But that's exactly what Hadley wants."

"What?"

"To die."

41

Sara
Paris, France

Three days, one car, two planes and a taxi later, Sara and Penny stood on a narrow, dimly lit street in Le Marais.

"He lives there," Penny said, pointing to the top floor of the building across the street.

Sara looked up and saw wide French doors behind a small veranda glowing yellow in the dusk. The warmth of the glow would have been inviting in different circumstances.

He is the Truth.

What had Rhodes meant by that? Sara feared Germain would be even more handsome than Rhodes, pulling Penny further from her. More daunting was the fact that this was the last place their fathers had visited together before they'd both been killed.

Penny crossed the street.

Sara pulled her coat tightly about her and followed.

On the covered stoop, the wind whipped and whistled. Penny pushed a button next to an old, ornate mailbox and they heard a buzz from above. The wooden door in front of them creaked open.

The entryway was dark except for a single lamp casting shadows across an Oriental rug. They crossed to the stairs and began to ascend, stopping on a landing in front of a massive painting of men, horses, and tigers wrestling with swords and capes. It reminded Sara of Penny's superhero paintings.

"Rubens," Penny said under her breath, her fingers caressing the air above the painting. "I think this is an original Peter Paul Rubens."

Sara had never heard of him.

"He was a fabulous man, Rubens," a voice said from above. "We spent many a night pondering the choices a man can make, the delights he can experience, the traumas he can endure."

Sara turned toward the looming figure. There was a light behind him so she couldn't see his features, but she could see he was broad.

"Come on up," he said. "I have only had one visitor since your fathers, and he was just a wee frog who slipped in through the fire escape. I am sure you two will offer much better conversation."

Penny smiled up at him with curiosity and began to ascend the stairs.

Inside the apartment a fire gleamed in a marble hearth surrounded by books stretching from wall to ceiling, their spines flickering words and colors in an array of patterns. A table sat beside the fire with an open bottle of Scotch.

Germain was a large man, but not tall. Most of his weight was across his shoulders and chest, the rest of him tapering off below. His face was young, despite his thick silver hair and the deep lines around his eyes. He was closely shaven except for a thick white mustache. He caught Sara looking at the Scotch and gestured toward it. "Would you like a glass?"

"Yes, please," Sara said, calmed by the softness of his voice and the fact he wasn't, in the least bit, sexy.

He opened the Scotch and poured a glass. "You know what your father said about me, Sara?"

She shook her head.

"He said everything about me was a paradox."

She didn't know what to say and so she said nothing, swiping at her phone mindlessly.

"Penny?" he asked, holding up the bottle.

"Sure," she said, placing her bag on the leather sofa and moving toward a framed portrait on the far wall. "This is another Rubens, isn't it?"

"That's his daughter," Germain said. "She died not long after he painted it."

The painting was considerably smaller than the one on the landing, but Penny seemed equally impressed. "An original?"

"It certainly is."

"Look, Sara! There are fibers from his paintbrush dried in the paint."

"Is that exciting?" Sara dropped onto the couch, her face buried in her phone.

"That phone," he said. "Can you give it to me, please?"

"Why?" Sara asked.

"Because you will learn better without it. Both of you, please." He beckoned their phones with his fingers.

Penny handed him her phone and when Sara didn't, she glared her.

"Okay, okay, don't get all *salty*." She held the side button to switch it off and handed it to Germain. "For how long?"

"As long as you are here." He took her phone and handed her a glass of Scotch. "Penny, yours is here," he said, holding her glass up.

"Only two glasses?" Sara asked.

"I don't drink," he said. "It does not suit me."

He plucked a golden tin from his pocket and flipped it open with his thumb. "I prefer marijuana," he said, pulling a wafer of white paper from the tin.

Sara jerked her head toward him.

He laughed. "One of Earth's many miracles!" His chuckle was wide like his shoulders, his jaw jutting forward with enthusiasm. "It is not just the high, it is the ritual of the roll, the smell of the burn!" He placed the paper in his hand and pinched the green leaves between his forefingers.

Penny came and sat next to Sara on the couch. "Obviously, Shane told you we were coming?"

"Life told me you were coming."

"When our fathers arrived, were you expecting them too?"

"Yes."

"And did you expect their deaths?"

"Yes," he said again, rolling the joint between his finger and thumb. "I did."

"And what about us? Are we going to die?" Sara asked.

"Most likely, someday."

"I mean soon, over all this."

"It depends on what you decide to do when you leave here."

"You know what we'll do, don't you?"

"Yes, I do. But knowing one's future without earning it is dangerous."

"Well, we must live then, or you wouldn't worry about danger," Sara smirked.

Germain raised his eyebrows and pointed at her. "Only if you think death is the epitome of danger."

Sara sighed. It hadn't taken long for the clever conversation to start.

"Smoke?" he asked them, holding up the joint.

Penny shook her head. Sara reached for the joint.

"Are you sure?" he asked her.

"Hundo p. I don't know how else I'll get through this."

He recoiled his hand. "Then you shall not have it."

"Why not?"

"We are given these beautiful enhancers not to be used as crutches to our fears but as augmentations to the Truth. You must *earn* them."

Sara rolled her eyes. If he was wise enough to have known she wasn't ready, then why would he bother offering it to her at all?

"An opportunity to educate you!" He sat back and flicked his lighter open. "So how can I help? Why have you come?"

Sara was aware he'd read her mind but decided not to be impressed.

"We want to know who killed our fathers," Sara said.

"More importantly, why they were killed," Penny said. "And we want to know what the Two Truths are. Shane said that you *are* the Truth. What did he mean by that?"

"Let me guess," Sara said. "You can't tell us. We have to go on some bullshit journey first."

He chortled and blew smoke. "You are on the bullshit journey, dear." He leaned toward her and lowered his voice to a whisper, his silver hair glowing in the fire. "This is the part where you get to learn something big."

He wriggled back into his chair. "So, if you are ready and comfortable, I will start with my arrival in London in 1743." He gave them a mischievous wink. "The eighteenth century, although well into the story, is a great place for us to start, a safe place for new ears."

"Sorry," Penny said. "*What* story?"

"The story of the Two Truths, the story of me. I thought that was what you were after?"

"Yes, okay, sorry."

"You see, in the eighteenth century Europe was on the verge of big change. The population was growing, bringing different cultures together and many were searching for new inspirations, tired of tyrannies of the church and the government." he explained. "So, I decided to show up, to offer the world a bit of direction, to give it a shake up if you like."

"Show up from where?" Penny asked.

He held his finger up to stop her. "May I?"

"Sorry," she said. "Go on."

"I drew quite a bit of attention when I arrived. You see I was perfectly fluent in all the European languages and my accent was nothing they had heard before. No one was quite sure where I came from. And the stories that I shared caused great gossip. For you see I did not restrain from talking about the old days. I often let it slip how I had known Cleopatra and Muhammad and Aristotle. And this, coupled with my talents in alchemy, my amazing violin playing and my general charm, soon had people more than just talking. Many suspected I'd found the elixir of life." He paused and drew off his joint. "That is why they called me *Saint* Germain."

"Are you claiming to *be* Saint Germain?" Penny asked. "*The* Saint Germain from three hundred years ago."

"It is difficult to accept, I know. People struggled back then too. They thought I was a lunatic. But when a person is as powerful as I was, as I *am*," he said, "we must reevaluate the definition of crazy, must we not?"

He drew off his joint again, flicking the ashes into the fire.

"And for those who believed in the existential, for those who belonged to a longstanding society that knew what great things were possible, I became a novelty and my company was coveted. Powerful men came from all over to meet me. This, of course, was my plan all along. I was on a mission to steer the world back on the right track. But I must admit," he leaned toward them, grinning devilishly, "it was amusing as well. I was asked to join secret groups, to lead soldiers, to advise kings. It was great fun!" He chuckled, his eyes merry and flickering, his teeth shining. "You know it was me who put Catherine the Great on the throne in Russia?"

"I read about that," Sara said. "It said you were her lover too."

"Ah, yes. I must admit it was a move of passion, putting her on the throne." He sighed and glanced to the ceiling. "And my, what a lover she was."

"So how is all this possible? *Did* you find the elixir of life?" Penny asked. "Is that the Second Truth?

"Ahh, if it were that simple!"

Sara put her glass down on the side table and crossed her arms. "I think it's more likely you're crazy."

He laughed heartily. "A crazy person is not in touch with reality. Reality is the laws of nature and life. And, my dear, I am more aware of all of this than, possibly, anyone."

"Anyone?" Penny asked.

"There is one other who is equal. I have not seen him in a long time though." He looked to the ceiling again, smoke wafting from his nostrils, warping his features as it rose in front of his face.

"Is it Shane?" Penny asked, "Shane Rhodes?"

"Shane? No. I am referring to someone you have not met."

He looked back at Sara. "You are right to be cautious, dear. It means you are listening and weighing things up. But you must not let fear get in the way. Be smart and sometimes cautious, but never afraid."

Sara bowed her head and rubbed her temples. "For what? What am I doing all this for again?"

"To learn the truth about your father's death."

"Why don't you just tell me?"

"I am telling you. But the only way I will continue is if I am certain you will believe me."

Sara closed her eyes. She thought of her pillow at home and the way it formed to her head when she sunk into it. She was tired from the traveling.

"I will believe you," Penny said, "because I've studied my father's notes and I've read all the great books and there are too many mysteries and signs surrounding me to doubt there's something we don't know, something we aren't being told."

Sara opened her eyes to find Penny had stood up and gone to the fire, her hair glowing yellow from the flames. "If you really have been alive for centuries, then can you tie all these ancient mysteries together? Can you explain to me how you've lived so long? Can you tell me what my father knew? I need to know in order to decide how I will continue."

"Continue what?" he asked.

"Continue living," she said, moving back toward the small Rubens painting and standing squarely before it. "I want to know, to be aware, so I can live consciously."

"Good," he said. "That is good. What mysteries do you want to know about?"

"There are so many," she said, still staring at the painting. "Starting with the Sumerians and their cuneiform writings and ending with you sitting here reading our minds and casually referring to friends of yours who died hundreds of years ago. I want to know everything." She turned to him. "Will you start with the first era, which they call the Beginning? It all starts with the Sumerians doesn't it?"

"The beginning started long before the Sumerians," he said. "But the Sumerians are a good place for us to start. What do you know about them?"

"Sumer was in Mesopotamia," Penny said. "It was one of the first known great civilizations. Today it's known as Iraq." She came away from the painting. "The Sumerians were, obviously,

Sumer's people, and nothing was known about them until about a hundred and fifty years ago when an archeologist began to dig into the strange mounds dotting the countryside in southern Iraq." Her eyes grew bright. "Lots of amazing artifacts were found, the most important being the cuneiform writings, etched and preserved perfectly into stone."

Sara slouched in her chair. She had learned these things too, but they didn't excite her like they did Penny. What did all this have to do with their fathers anyway?

"These writings," Penny continued, "together with artifacts, have shown us they were the first civilization to have the wheel, schools, medicine, science, written proverbs, history, congress, taxation, laws, social reforms, coined money, and not to mention, an amazing knowledge of astronomy. They understood it all: the three-hundred-and-sixty-degree circle, the zenith, the horizon, the poles, the equinoxes ... everything!" She was pacing the room now, her hands flying in the air as she talked. "They created the world's first calendar, which was used for centuries afterward by the Egyptians and the Greeks."

"And why does this excite you so?" Germain asked.

"In their texts they claimed everything they knew and achieved had come from their gods. But not gods that directed them from a different dimension, not an untouchable god like we refer to. But gods that lived among them and ruled them from Earth; real, tangible gods."

"Yes," Germain nodded, his eyes lighting up, matching hers.

"Then," she said, "Two thousand years after the Sumerians appeared, they mysteriously vanished." Her voice had been rising as she spoke, but now she stopped and shook her head. "Where did they go?" she asked Germain softly. "Who were these gods and why have we been taught so little about them?"

"There are plenty of similar mysteries in history," he said. "The ancient Chinese 'seals' discovered all over Ireland during a time when there was no known commerce between China and the Emerald Isle; the life-sized crystal skulls, obviously made by a power cutter, that were found in South America dating thirty-six hundred years ago; the giant stone balls in Costa Rica made of granite, a rock not found in the area; the ancient stone forts throughout England, France, and Germany that could only have been made by a heat not possible from conventional fires; a computer-like device containing differential gears dating back to the sixteenth century found in Crete; a battery run from alkaline grape juice found in an Iraqi village dating 220 BC; Stonehenge; the huge heads of Easter Island; the Peruvian Nazca lines; the Great Serpent Mound of Ohio. Why does this mystery of the Sumerians interest you so much when so many mysteries abound?"

"I guess science has explained some of those mysteries, hasn't it?" Penny asked

Germain's eyes sparkled. "How they were done, I suppose, for some of them."

"More importantly than how they were done," Penny said, "is that all the mysteries you mention are linked. They're all signs that technologies and discoveries of the past few hundred years were already known a long time ago, and if you study them closely, they all trace back to Sumer. We knew more six thousand years ago than we know now because we were integrated with gods, not separate from them!"

Sara watched Penny, the facts and theories they'd read about over the past months flung forth in a package Sara hadn't put together.

Germain snuffed out the butt of his joint in an ashtray. "And," he asked, "what do you want to know?"

"Who were these gods?" Penny asked.

"They called them the Anunnaki," Germain said, scooting forward in his chair. "Or those who came to Earth from heaven."

"So, it's true?" Penny asked, stepping toward him. "These gods existed? They were real?"

"Very much so. But that is enough for tonight. There is a bed in that room." He nodded toward a door in the corridor. "It is big enough for both of you. I will answer the rest of your questions in seven days."

"Seven days!" Penny exclaimed.

"You girls are tired and anxious. That is not the way to the Truth. You must rest for six days, and on the seventh day, I will show you the Truth you are after."

"What do you mean rest for six days?" Penny asked.

"I mean sleep in, eat, lie around the apartment, sleep some more, eat again. Sleep again. Exhaustion is no way to the Truth."

"You must be kidding," Penny said.

"Not at all. Now, go and sleep."

"Thank you," Sara said, relieved.

He smiled at her. "Sleep well, child. You are going to need it."

42

Hadley
Cincinnati, Ohio

Life was different now for Hadley, although not in a tangible way. The furnace still clicked on in the morning and the sun still cast pink clouds across the sky in the evening. Her mother's Audi still idled when it was in first gear, and the raised cracks in the driveway still caught Hadley's toes and made her stumble. The change lay in the fact there was no longer a right or a wrong associated with these things. They just were, each object or situation existing in its own beauty and consequence. There was something beneath and beyond each of these things, something that held no moral judgment, and this gave her an odd peace like the purple-white fuzz she went to when she meditated. And she meditated constantly, eager for dinner to finish so she could find a spot in the backyard or in her room, where she could close her eyes and go to the timeless space.

Returning from a deep trance one day, it occurred to her she didn't have to wait to meditate until her mother stopped talking, or the TV was turned off, or they got home from the grocery store. There was no reason she couldn't meditate with her eyes open while she was standing in line with her mother at the bank or stuck in traffic on I-75. Because there was no wrong nor right anymore. There were also no more rules. There was only awareness, a powerful sense of consequences. She often knew what to do, or where to go, or how to respond to matters that would once have stumped her. This change brought joy and excitement and she thought less of death. How strange that learning to dismiss her feelings had, in fact, brought about more intense feelings than she'd ever experienced before.

Happy is the man that findeth wisdom, and the man that getteth understanding.

She sat with her mother in the back garden having a cup of tea. Her mother passed her a notepad and said, "I don't see you reading the Bible much lately."

Hadley took the notepad and wrote neatly across the top of the paper.

I'M NOT INTERESTED ANYMORE.

Her mother raised her eyebrows. "Really?"

She wrote, THERE WAS NO PEACE THERE.

"No peace? What do you mean?"

TOO MANY WORDS. NOT ENOUGH FEELINGS.

"When did this change?"

I'VE LEARNED TO MEDITATE! She made the exclamation mark large on the page, drawing the dot at the bottom with perfect roundness and coloring it with solid dark blue. She took pleasure in watching the ink take form on the paper.

Her mother raised her eyebrows again. "Where did you learn that?"

FROM ISSA.

"Who's Issa?"

MY FRIEND.

"What friend is this?" her mother asked. "Have I met her?"

Hadley giggled, shook her head and wrote, ISSA ISN'T A GIRL. HE'S A MAN I MET LAST MONTH.

"A *man*? Where does he live? How did you meet him?"

255

HE LIVES ON FAIRFIELD STREET. I WAS JUST OUT FOR A WALK AND I MET HIM.

"A walk?"

Hadley could feel her mother's fear brewing.

IT'S OKAY, MOM, she scribbled. HE'S A VERY NICE MAN.

"Hadley, you don't just make friends with strange men."

Hadley turned away.

Her mother's voice softened. "Could I meet him?"

Hadley smiled at this. MAYBE WE COULD HAVE HIM OVER TO DINNER. The thought of Issa at their dinner table pleased her. She hastily scribbled, MAYBE WE COULD HAVE JONAS OVER TOO?

"Maybe. I really don't like you visiting a man I don't know. Did you say you meditate with him?"

Hadley didn't want to talk anymore. Her mother's fear made her tired. She set the notepad down.

"Now don't clam up on me, Hadley. I'm your mother and I need to know if you're meeting a man at his house."

Hadley shrugged.

"Where does he live? Can you take me there?"

Hadley nodded.

"Can you write down his address?"

Hadley turned the pad of paper over and wrote, I DON'T KNOW THE NUMBER. IT'S A BROWN HOUSE ON THE CORNER OF FAIRFIELD STREET.

"Thank you," her mother said. "You need to tell me when you have a new friend, especially a man."

Hadley smiled and wrote, HE IS NICE. I PROMISE.

In the presence of her mother's questions, Hadley's peace had begun to slip from her, a faint desire to die filling the void.

Even in laughter the heart is sorrowful; and the end of that mirth is heaviness.

She hurried upstairs to her room and shut the door. In life, people didn't understand peace and love; everyone was so suspicious and afraid. But, somewhere behind her longing for death, she knew she'd chosen to return to life, that she'd come back for something. The feeling of an imminent purpose revealing itself was familiar to her. She'd experienced the sensation in other lives. But like always, the details were hazy, her breath and thoughts got in the way.

You must make yourself strong, Mr. Ernest whispered in his rough, ghostly voice. His misty form had been hovering about her more than usual lately.

Strong how? she asked, looking up.

Humanly strong, he said. *There is going to be much fear and confusion. You will need physical strength, human strength, to endure this. Your will to die has caused you to forget about your body.*

Know ye not that your body is the temple of the Holy Ghost which is in you, which ye have of God, and ye are not your own?

So, I must eat, she said through her thoughts.

You must do more than eat. You must eat good things and be active and get out in the sun and drink water. You must do the things that make you alive.

Alive she repeated

Well you are alive.

How soon will she come?

Will who come?

Hadley shrugged. *Someone is coming for me.*

There was a knock on her door.

"Hadley?" her mother said. "May I come in?"

Hadley opened the door and went and curled up on her bed, hugging her pillow.

Her mother looked worried. "Darling, what is it? Is it this man?" Her mother sat next to her and rubbed her hair. "I wish you would talk to me."

Even if Hadley could speak, she couldn't explain to her mother why she hated her mother's fear, how she sometimes wanted to die, how she talked to the ghost and the angel. It would scare her mother more. Hadley began to cry softly.

Her mother stroked her hair. "You've always been an intense child. Amid the garden of your innocence there have always been thorns of inconsolable sadness." Her mother continued to rub her hair. "And I've never been able to help."

Hadley looked up at her mother, surprised at the awareness in her mother's words.

Only by pride cometh contention: but with the well advised is wisdom.

"When you were a baby," her mother continued softly. "You would, with no warning, become overwhelmed with grief. You would cry and tremble, not from terror but from some kind of longing I couldn't understand. The only thing that would calm you was that funny little rock. Do you remember? You used to cuddle the rock like it was a stuffed toy. I never did know where it came from. I found you clutching it in your crib one day. I wonder whatever happened to it."

The rock! Hadley sat up.

"What darling?"

She went to her desk and wrote on a piece of scrap paper. WHERE'S THE ROCK?

"Gosh, I don't know. I haven't seen it in years."

"I want to see the rock," Hadley wrote.

"It'll probably be in the attic somewhere in a box. Do you want to look for it?"

Hadley nodded and grabbed her mother's hand, pulling her out the door.

They found it in a crate among kindergarten drawings and a pair of plaster hands from preschool. It was wrapped in faded green tissue paper. "I remember putting it in this now," her mother said.

Hadley reached for it and placed it, still wrapped in tissue, on her lap. She carefully folded back the layers of paper, letting the stone fall into her hand. It was smooth and white, its touch familiar.

She turned it over.

There they were, the dark intricate engravings she used to run her fingers over as a small child. The same characters etched in Issa's footpath.

43

Brett
Cincinnati, Ohio

Brett and Noel made their way through the airport parking lot.

"Where'd they say the car would be?" Noel asked.

"It's supposed to be here in short-term parking. Row J. Looks like it might be a truck," Brett pointed ahead of them at a black Dodge Ram, its tires too wide for the parking space.

"That'll do." Noel smiled. "That'll do just fine." He pressed the remote and the truck beeped twice, the headlights flashing. "You said you wanted power. Well, they're giving us power."

She was reminded of the boy he was before the island and how differently she'd felt about him then. Was this new relationship really a strength?

"Here, you drive," he said, tossing her the keys.

She caught them in mid-air and approached the truck.

It was huge and sleek, and as she climbed in, she was aroused by the size and smell of it. How was it possible that in the search for power she found herself attracted to boys and trucks?

They drove out of the airport and through the city in silence, the deep purr of the vehicle a distraction from contemplating how she would deal with her mother. She hadn't expected to see her again so soon. Did her mother know the truth, the truth of what she'd done to her father? Now that Brett knew her mother was a Talent, she couldn't underestimate her.

"So, what's the story again?" Noel asked as Brett veered the truck off the freeway and onto an exit ramp. "We're in town for a night and thought we'd take Hadley to the movies. Is that it?"

"Yes. Let's not make it complicated unless we have to."

"Won't it be weird if we don't stay for dinner?"

"It would be weird if we did. I don't like my mother and she knows it."

She steered the truck through the familiar streets of her childhood, passing the park where her father had first told her about her destiny. The swings they'd sat on that day were empty and swaying in the late afternoon breeze. She could remember the way a chain had hidden one of her father's eyes as he'd taken her hand and told her she was more special than her sisters, that she would one day be powerful and important.

As she turned onto Rosalind Drive, she was reminded of the lessons he'd taught her as they walked the chipped sidewalk to school in the mornings and how he'd told her that she would go to Yale one day, that she *must* go to Yale. She remembered how she'd avoided stepping on the cracks, afraid of breaking her mother's back if she did, a silly myth her school friends had told her. She'd only been, what? Seven? Eight?

She pulled the truck into the driveway, the house dark except for a purple-gray haze coming from the third-floor windows and shut off the engine.

"It doesn't look like anyone's home," Noel said.

"My mother's working upstairs. Hadley doesn't usually go anywhere without her. She'll be here somewhere."

They got out of the truck and approached the house, the bug zapper on the porch flashing blue and buzzing as they passed it.

Brett opened the door and stepped inside, turning on the entryway light. It cast a wide beam of yellow through the living room and over Hadley, who sat cross-legged on the Persian rug in front of them.

"Hadley?"

Hadley tilted her head and looked up at Brett.

"This is Noel," Brett said, gesturing toward him. "We're in town for work. Thought we'd stop by and say hi."

"Hi," Noel said.

Hadley nodded at him.

"We were going to go to a movie. Thought you might like to come?"

Hadley shook her head.

"It'll sure beat sitting here in the dark by yourself," Noel said with a friendly laugh.

"Hadley," Brett said. "This isn't healthy, you sitting around on your own. Where's Mom?"

Hadley pointed to the ceiling.

"Why don't you take a bit of a vacation, come with us for a while. We're working on a beautiful island, have our own private plane and can fly onto the island during sunrise. It's magnificent. You'll love it. Let's go talk to Mom and see if we can get you out of here for a few days. It'll be good for you."

Footsteps pattered upstairs.

"Hello?" The stair light came on and her mother appeared on the top step.

"Hello, Mother."

"Brett?" She came down quickly, her feet bare, her hair in a loose bun. "What's going on?"

"Mother, this is Noel, a friend of mine from Yale. We're in town for the night. Thought we'd stop by and say hi."

"Right."

"We thought we'd take Hadley to the movies, seeing as she's just sitting about in the dark doing nothing."

"Why didn't I know you were coming?"

"Last minute work thing," Noel said.

Her mother came over and extended her hand to Noel. "It's nice to meet you. Please, have a seat. I'll make some coffee."

"No, no coffee," Brett said. "We're not staying."

"Of course you're staying. Sit down. Hadley, darling, would you go put the coffee pot on?"

Hadley scurried into the kitchen.

"Just in town for the night, eh?" Her mother glanced at the gold ring on Brett's index finger. "So, you're a Calderberger."

"Yes."

"That would have made your father very proud."

Was that a dig? A sign she knew?

"This has had nothing to do with Dad for a long time now," Brett said.

Her mother looked at Noel. "Please tell me she has a warmer side. A mother hopes."

Noel smiled. "Yes, Dr. Morgan, she definitely does." He winked at her.

She turned back to Brett. "So, is it everything you hoped it would be? Are you happy?"

"A long time ago, you decided you didn't want to know. Don't start asking questions now."

"Oh, Brett, I don't care about the bloody secrets! I care about *you*. I want to know if you're happy."

"Happy?" She thought of Noel in the silk sheets on her four-poster bed, of his body reflected in the mirror above, of the nights they lay talking until the sun rose. "Yes," she said. "I think I am."

"Well, that's something then. I'm glad to hear it. Now, why are you really here?"

"I told you. We're in town for work. Thought we'd take Hadley to the movies."

"I think it's more likely you're here on a mission. Your father had missions too you know. Eventually one killed him."

Hadley came into the room with a tray.

"Hadley, darling, did they ask you to go to the movies?"

Hadley nodded.

"Do you want to go to the movies?"

She shook her head again.

"See. Look, she doesn't want to go. So why don't you have a cup of coffee and we'll watch a movie here, like a family."

Brett sighed. "I'm not here to be a family. I just wanted to see Hadley."

"Well, you can *see* her right here."

Brett smiled at Hadley. "Come on, little one. It'll be an adventure."

Hadley shook her head.

Noel reached for a coffee.

Brett stared her mother down, head lowered, eyes raised. She saw a knowingness in her mother's eyes. There was no accusation in it, only resolve, a determination not to be played. The room felt heavy and thick with inevitability.

"Hurry up and drink your coffee, Noel. We're leaving."

"What do you want with Hadley, Brett?" her mother asked.

Brett walked to the door and opened it.

"Leave Hadley out of this," Her mother said to her back. "You can do whatever you choose with your life. You can hate me and cut me off, but don't bring Hadley into it. She's too good for it."

Brett came back pulled Noel, coffee in hand, to the door. "I'm only leaving because Hadley wants me to. Your opinion means nothing."

"I wouldn't have flattered myself as much."

They left, leaving the door open to the cold, dark air.

"That was weird," Noel said.

"My mother's a Talent. She knew exactly why we were there. She might be a dissenter but she's clever. She's not going to let us walk Hadley out of there."

"Hadley knew we were up to something too," he said, swinging himself into the driver's seat. "She's older than I expected, but smaller."

Brett climbed in beside him. "She's changed. Something's different about her."

"Your mom's sexy," he said. "You look a lot like her."

Brett rolled her eyes as he started the truck and it rumbled into gear, drowning out the sound of the mosquitoes electrocuting themselves on the porch.

44

Renee
Cincinnati, Ohio

Renee hadn't slept for two nights.

She paced the room, different tones of orange light passing over her hands and arms. The phone was ringing. She hadn't answered it for days. She let the answering machine take the call.

"Renee. It's me, Jonas. Why aren't you answering the phone? Call me please."

She paced faster. She couldn't talk to him. Not until she cleared her head. She needed a plan.

What is Brett messed up in?

What does she want with Hadley?

Who is this man Hadley has met?

And where was Sara?

Sara had been gone for over week. She'd called to say she was fine but refused to tell Renee where she was.

I've lost touch with my daughters when they need me most.

Distracted by romance!

There was a time long ago when she would have known clearly what to do. She stopped pacing and sat on the floor, facing the orange light. She took a deep breath and raised her face to the warmth, focusing on the green-black blotches of light on the back of her eyelids.

Issa isn't a problem. Hadley is more content than she used to be so he can't be bad. Brett is the problem. She's up to something. Who do I talk to? Who can help me?

She focused on her breathing, turning off her mind so the answer could get through.

Clara.

She opened her eyes and stared at the wall in front of her.

"Clara," she said out loud. "Of course."

She found the address to the hospital in the phone book. It was only an hour and a half drive to Columbus. Her logic told her she should stay close to Hadley, that she shouldn't leave her home alone. But a gentle voice that had guided her many times before said Hadley would be fine, Brett wouldn't be back in a hurry and she must go now. She found her purse and car keys and left immediately.

The man at the desk was heavily wrinkled. "Mrs. Weishaup? Yes, she's here. Did you have an appointment?"

"No, sorry."

"What is your name please?"

"Renee Morgan."

The man looked at her. "Morgan did you say?"

He isn't going to let me see her. The Order has already had me cut me off.

"You wouldn't be related to Sara, would you?"

"Sara?"

"Yes. Sara Morgan. She was here last month."

"Sara was *here*?"

"I'm sure that was the name. Not many people visit Clara. Let me look." He fingered through the guest book. "Ah, yes. I was right. Sara Morgan. It was September 7th she was here."

"Sara's my daughter. I can't imagine why she would have been here."

"She came to see Mrs. Weishaup, like you."

"Are you sure you don't mean Brett? What did she look like?"

"Short black hair. A sarcastic little number. Did a handstand right here against the wall. Dressed a bit inappropriately if you don't mind me saying."

"Yes, that's Sara." Renee sighed. "And you say she was here to see Mrs. Weishaup?"

"Yes, she talked to Mrs. Weishaup and then tried to pry information out of me about Clara's daughter."

"What kind of information?"

"She wanted an address."

"Did you give it to her?"

"No. Now did you want to see Clara still?"

"Yes, please."

He pointed through a door into a lounge. "Please wait there. I'll see if she's in a position to see you."

Renee entered the lounge and sat down.

Why would Sara have come here?

The 7th September. Why is that day familiar?

That was the day Sara skipped school!

A door opened and a stocky man in a uniform entered with Clara and helped her into a high-backed chair where she looked away from Renee and out the window.

"Hi Clara."

She didn't respond.

"I know in the past you wanted to talk to me, and I ignored you. I'm sorry. But from one dissenter to another, can you forgive me?"

Clara gave no response and continued to look out the window.

"I wanted nothing to do with it back then. In many ways I thought Scott deserved what he got. I was so sick of the secrets and the snobbery."

She thought she saw Clara's eyes narrow.

"I think our daughters are in danger," Renee said. "I need your help."

Clara turned and looked at her.

"Brett is in the high ranks of the Order now, and I think they're after Hadley. I've reason to believe Sara and Penny are up to something too. I'm worried, Clara. I think our husbands were in over their heads and now our daughters are in trouble."

Clara turned to the security guard. "Can we be alone, please?"

He looked at Renee. "You'll have to sign a waiver, ma'am." He grabbed a form from the coffee table and pushed it toward her. "Clara can be unpredictable."

Renee signed the form without looking at it and turned back to Clara.

"I'll be right outside," the man said.

As he closed the door behind him, Clara spoke. "Our husbands discovered something they shouldn't have. They were going to expose it, so the Order got rid of George and then came snooping around our house. They questioned me and eventually decided I didn't know anything and gave up."

"And do you know anything?"

"No."

"But you came to me once," Renee said. "A few years ago. You asked me to help you."

"I was suspicious, thought they were up to something. That's old news now. Tell me about Penny."

"I think she's with Sara. They've gone away somewhere. I don't know how they're tangled up in this."

"They're in Europe. They've gone to find Saint Germain."

"Saint Germain?" Renee asked.

Clara nodded.

"*The* Saint Germain?"

"Yes."

"Surely he doesn't really exist?"

"They think he does. Our husbands thought he did."

"Well, if he does then he will protect them, won't he?" Renee asked, hopeful. She'd learned about him before she dissented. He was an anomaly the Order feared, a powerful man who had dissented years ago and eluded them.

"He didn't protect our husbands."

"How do you know they went to see him?"

"Penny came to see me. She wanted my support."

"Support for what?"

"To find out what her father had discovered and to see out his mission."

"Oh God," Renee said. "And Sara?"

"They were going together."

"And you supported it?"

Clara shrugged. "Penny is stronger than I am, smarter too. I can't expect her to sit around and ignore the Truth."

"Well, Sara isn't."

"What do you plan to do?" Clara asked.

"I suppose I have to get involved. I have to learn what they know."

"Why?" Clara asked. "What can you do? You can't stop Penny, trust me."

"I might be able to stop Sara."

"Why? So she can live in ignorance like you?"

"I suppose it's better than living in here, like you."

"You think I'm crazy because of what I know. But I'm crazy because of what I *don't* know. Half the Truth drove me crazy."

"You're not crazy, Clara."

"I am and I think that's why I was never shown the full Truth. Or maybe it's because I was a woman. Times were different then. I don't know. But I hope for more for Penny."

"If you can articulate why you're crazy then you're not crazy," Renee said. "You're just a coward."

"No different than you."

"No. No different than me."

"So, what're you going to do?"

"I'm going to face the Truth," Renee said.

"Why?"

"So I can connect with my daughters."

Clara looked back out the window. "I suppose that's as good a reason as any."

"Tell me where the girls are then."

"I don't know. They were following their fathers' trail. Some man in Cape Cod told them where Saint Germain lives."

"What man? Who?"

"I don't know."

"Well, can you find out?"

"I have no idea who he was. But there's a man in Cincinnati who knows how to find Germain."

"In Cincinnati?"

Clara nodded.

"Why didn't you tell Penny about him?"

"I couldn't remember his name. George mentioned him a few times. He visited him before he went to France."

"You must remember his name."

"I'm telling you, I don't."

"Surely you remember *something*."

"It was an odd name. Short and strange."

Issa.

"I think I would recognize it if I heard it."

"Was it Issa?"

"Yes, that was it. Issa. Do you know him?"

Renee stood. "I must go." She caught Clara's eyes. "Thank you. I'll let you know what I find out."

Clara shook her head. "Don't worry about me. Just take care of the girls."

45

Sara
Paris, France

Sara woke to the sound of a clanging cowbell and a flashlight in her eyes. She held up her hand against the brightness. Germain's head was poking from the half-open door. He shook the cowbell again.

"Rise!" he said. "Paris will soon be awake."

"Paris?" Penny said sleepily from beneath the covers.

"Yes, Paris!" He came fully into the room and raised the cow bell above his head, shaking it again. "You have rested for six days. The seventh is for living and learning!"

Sara pulled the duvet over her head and looked at the clock. It was six o'clock.

Penny sat up and rubbed her eyes. "Aren't we learning about the gods today?"

"The most fabulous city in the world is outside your door and you want to learn about gods!" He flipped on the overhead light.

"But that's why we came here, to learn the Truths. We've been waiting for a week."

"To understand the Second Truth, you must understand life, and there is no better place than the City of Light!"

Sara brought her head out from under the duvet. "Shouldn't we be avoiding public places?"

"Now, where did you get that idea?" Germain raised the bell again.

"Please," Sara said. She pulled herself from the sheets. "We're up. See?"

He lowered the bell. "Now, why should we avoid public places?"

"Won't we be watched?"

"If I don't want anyone to take notice of us, they won't. The Order has been looking for me for hundreds of years to no avail."

Penny rustled the sheets nervously next to her. "But we have so much to do," she said. "Surely we don't have time for sight-seeing."

"Don't be in such a rush. Your fathers are dead. You cannot save them. And history will always be there."

"But more people could be killed," Penny said.

"Oh right," Germain said. "I forgot you are trying to save the world."

"I'm not trying to save the world."

"Well, it seems that way to me. Why don't we go out and immerse ourselves in the world you are trying to save?"

"Those who create social change don't have time to play," Penny said.

This time it was Germain who put his hands over his ears. "It is much too early in the day," he shook his head between his hands with an impish smile, "to hear such nonsense. One must at least eat before listening to such claptrap! I am going to go have breakfast."

He winked at them and turned to leave, waving his arm with a wide sweep to invite them to follow. "Hurry now. We haven't much time!"

"Time for what?"

"And after he said not to rush!" Penny added.

Sara went to the bathroom and brushed her teeth. When she came back, Penny was still sitting in the bed.

"Aren't you getting up?" Sara asked.

"I'm not sure about this," she said. "Going into Paris?"

Sara picked her bra up off the floor. She pulled her nightshirt over her head and stood bare breasted in front of Penny. "We could stay here if you wanted?"

Penny rolled her eyes and threw a pillow at her. "We'll go."

"Shame," Sara said.

Penny got out of bed. "I'm sure there's a point to this diversion. Germain doesn't seem like someone who wouldn't have a point."

"No," Sara sighed. She preferred it if there was no point at all. She was tired of purpose. Even the days of rest had had purpose.

They found Germain in the kitchen with a cup of tea in one hand and toast in the other. His toast was dark and crumbling, most of it collected in his beard.

"Toast?" he asked, holding up the charred bread.

They shook their heads.

"Never mind, we haven't time anyway." He looked at his watch. "Let's go. We must not be late!"

"For what?" Penny asked.

"You shall see!" He grabbed his jacket from a hook by the door and hurried out onto the landing. "Come on. Come on."

They followed him down the steps and into the dark, early morning chill. It had rained in the night and the smell of fresh dampness rose from the street as they stepped onto the cobblestone.

The streets were lit by tall, black lamps that shone dim orange light on the sidewalk. Penny studied one, her face flickering.

"These are gas lamps," she said.

"Originals," Germain replied. "This is the historic district. Everywhere else they have been replaced, but here we are still true to the City of Light!" He clapped with enthusiasm. "Paris was the first city, you know, to have gas lamps, but that is not why it was nicknamed the "City of Light". It was because it was the hub of ideas during the Enlightenment. La Ville-Lumière! What a wonderful time to be alive. These, my dears, are the streets of Voltaire and Rousseau and Montesquieu."

Sara feared a day of history lessons and names she didn't recognize.

"This is the city of *Les Misérables*, the conurbation of Victor Hugo!" he continued, looking at them with glowing orange eyes. "Come, my dears. Before Paris wakes."

They followed him, the hard soles of his boots clapping against the street and splashing through puddles. It was dark and they made sure to stay close. He turned often and abruptly with little warning. Sara struggled to match his pace.

He took a sudden left around an old covered cart and they entered a wide street. He stopped and turned to them, not the least bit out of breath. "Here," he said, "we face precisely east. And that there, looming in the dark blue sky, is the rear of Notre-Dame. Now sit." And with that he promptly sat on a wrought iron bench, placing himself in the middle. He tapped each side and they both sat, grateful for the rest.

"It's so quiet," Penny said.

"Oh yes," Germain said. "There are few things as wonderful as walking through Paris in the cool autumn morning when it is still dark and quiet. Even better is when the sun is just up and the men begin to wash the pavement and you can hear the water from Montmartre gushing down through the city gutters, and the garbage trucks begin to grunt and add their gray fumes to the day, and the rich yeasty smells begin to waft from the bakeries. But first, oh first, we will watch the glow."

As he said this, a thin line of indigo drew low across the sky at the place where the sky and the city met. The line stopped at the black square of Notre-Dame and began again on the other side. The purple expanded and became lavender and then turned to a pink candy floss puffing itself over the city's edge. The profiles of dark, rounded trees appeared, and then a bridge, and finally the dual peaks of the cathedral. For a moment the sky stood still, the only colors in the world pink and black, the city one dimensional in its silhouette. Then a line of orange appeared along the top of the bridge and spread into pink and the cathedral came alive with gold and amber as the crest of the sun broke through the horizon. With the first rays of full light, the river was revealed, purple ripples on black glass. They were sitting on the edge of the Seine.

In an apartment above them, a shirtless man opened a window and stretched. A duck waddled down from the street and put a webbed foot in the river, the water rippling orange in answer. A man dressed in green coveralls appeared on the other side of the street with a broom. A light came on behind him, the letters of a shop sign appearing in the window.

"And with the dawn, Paris is awake!" Germain said, standing in ovation, his arms outstretched before him. He sighed deeply and turned around, placing a hand firmly on each of their heads and looking from one to the other. "That, my dears, was a feast for the eyes, a true vision extraordinaire!" He leaned in close. "No sound, no touch, no smell was necessary was it? The visual effects stood alone, provided satisfaction in isolation. Did they not?"

Penny was staring calmly at the Seine. "Yes," Penny said softly. "It was wonderful."

"This is the world I love, the world I see every day and that most people walk by without noticing. If you do not love what the world is in its simplest form, you will not be able to save it."

Penny blinked and looked away from the river and up at Germain.

"Today you will notice the world," he said. "Today you will remember your senses in a city of plentiful pleasures. You have seen her gloriously break into day. Now you will smell her, taste her, feel her. You will hear her sing and you will find you do not want to ask me about gods."

His playfulness was gone, his face revealing only passion and respect.

Neither of them said a word.

"Come then," he said, his humor returning. "Let us indulge!"

To Sara's delight, the day became one of the senses and nothing of the mind.

Germain began by leading them with a long stride to the square in front of Notre-Dame.

"*Parvis Notre-Dame!*" he said as they stopped in front of the sacred building, the statue of Charlemagne rising on its pedestal before them. The horse and men stood aqua blue in the morning light, behind them the rays of the sun creating an eternity of shapes and shadows on the stone surfaces of the cathedral.

They sat for a while before Germain walked them to a gate and through a park beneath flying buttresses flanking the roofline of the cathedral, then over a pedestrian bridge that dumped them on a busy street on the other side of the river. The street was narrow and lined with parked cars, the windows of old restored hotels and restaurants glowing yellow in the morning sun and throwing pale squares of light on the sidewalk.

"Our eyes have feasted. Now let our tongues lap at the concoctions created from the spices and fodder of the earth!"

Germain led them to a small red door set in an entryway of brown brick. "Enter, my children and prepare your palates!"

Inside, Sara was accosted by the smells of baking, a blanket of warm yeast and cinnamon enveloping her. "Sit," he said, pointing to two wrought iron chairs beside a glass-top table. When they sat, he placed a small, round iced bun in front of each of them.

Powdered sugar fell to the plate as Sara lifted the warm bun to her mouth. The baked shell was crisp and flaked as she bit into it, the icing coating her upper lip with sweetness. The dough beneath the shell was soft and hot. She could taste vanilla and tart apple. Another bite was followed by a cool rush of sweetened cream and salty caramel. As she bit again, the flaky coating added texture to the dough and cream and fruit so it crunched while the rest melted and oozed in her mouth.

She ate the last bite with her eyes closed, breathing in the aroma while she chewed. When she opened her eyes, there was a croissant on a fresh plate in front of her. She picked it up and bit into one end, warm raspberry spilling into her mouth as the hot dough collapsed around it. There was a hint of coconut, or was that almond? She bit again, closing her eyes and not opening them until her fingers were empty.

When she opened her eyes, Penny was licking her fingers and Germain sat between them, smiling.

"One word," he said holding up his finger. "You are only allowed to say one word."

"Yum?" Sara said.

"Yes, I suppose that sums it up."

"Enchanting," Penny said.

Sara expected Germain to smile at Penny like her father used to smile at Brett when he was impressed with her. Instead Germain said, "Equally as worthy a word!"

After their patisserie extravagance, they followed Germain back onto the street and passed three blocks of cafes and bakeries, rounded a corner and hurried across the lawn of a huge palace, until they finally stopped in front of an unremarkable gray townhouse with wide concrete steps rising to tall black doors.

He pointed to the steps. "Take a seat."

"On the ground?" Sara asked.

"On the steps. Now do hurry. He will begin soon."

Penny brushed some gravel from the third step and they both sat. Germain remained standing, one arm bent so he could look at his watch. He examined it for a few seconds and then lifted both hands like a conductor and said, "In the flat behind you lives a man of not only exquisite talent, but also of finite punctuality. In less than a minute he will open the lip of his grand piano and expose the keys. And then for an hour he will play the most passionate Debussy and Stravinsky you have ever heard!"

"An *hour*?" Sara asked.

Lifting his arms higher, Germain said, "Now close your eyes." And with a flick of his wrist, a single note resonated out the window behind him.

For an hour, which seemed like a minute, Sara listened to music that felt as if it was coming from the stone beneath her and from the street in front of her and from the sky above. She was propelled by the speed of the sound, her heart racing with it. Her thoughts calmed with the low, mellow notes and invigorated with staccatos. There was a dissonance in the changing notes, a subtlety in the length each was held, an intensity in the combination. There was despair and jealousy, fear and rebellion in the music, too. As it ebbed and changed, she sensed the stone beneath her sinking away, her body floating upward, and she watched herself from a distance, her shoulders and fingers pulsating to the beat. She didn't think of Penny or Germain or of the public street they lounged on. Nor did she notice the faint aftertaste of raspberry from earlier. She did not think at all. And with a final crescendo of empathy, the music stopped and the cement beneath her became solid and her shoulders grew heavy, and she opened her eyes to find Germain lying on the footpath in front of them.

A man with a dog strolled down the street, not the least bit curious about a large man lying on the ground. Ah, the joys of a large city!

Germain sat up. "Well, that was a surprise. He did not play Stravinsky at all today. He played Massenet instead. A beautiful surprise for a beautiful day! And so, my dears, let us see what else the city has to offer."

He sprung to his feet and the girls rose trance-like from the warm stone and followed him.

For the next few hours, he led them down main streets, through bus stations, past ornate churches, through leafy squares, beside mounted statues of kings, and under stone archways. They passed elaborate shops, old canals, and harbors of private boats with weekenders gathered along the edges.

"Come," he said. "Just one more place before we arrive at our final destination."

They passed through a sculpture garden and across a bridge, Notre-Dame rising in the distance. The sun was high, and its full glare bleached the building so it appeared flat instead of the dynamic structure it had been at dawn. Sara thought of how Germain had rushed them that morning and understood his haste.

"We are coming into a special part of Paris here," Germain said as they entered a square of posh galleries and boutique hotels.

He stopped in the middle of the square and said, "This, my dears, is Saint-Germain."

"After you?" Penny asked.

"After me," he said, smiling.

"It's grand. You should be pleased."

"It is not only an area of splendid quality and wealth, but it leads to the green oasis of the Luxembourg Gardens. Come, for it is nearly two o'clock and Mother Nature bids!"

The palace was framed behind the gardens, the sun low and shining on the large square of water in front of it. A fountain flashed silver, blue, and white sparkles against the sky as children sailed model boats in the metallic water. White ducks splashed droplets of silver onto the stone feet of ancient kings carved in turquoise stone. A blanket of green lawn striped with gravel paths stretched to meet their feet.

"Enter," Germain said. "The end of our day. The finale! A sensual symphony!"

It was indeed exactly that. A symphony made of sunlight on the water and flowers of pink and purple planted so close together Sara couldn't see leaves or stems, only boundless color. The music of birds and the low buzz of bees and the laughter of children were joined occasionally by a barking dog. Intermittently, there was the sound of a fiddle and the clanking of wine glasses. There was the smell of fresh cut grass and lilies and chrysanthemums.

Sara wandered alone, finding herself at a puppet show and then beside a busker strumming a guitar. She knelt between the thorns of two rose bushes and watched a fuzzy bumblebee extract sap from the inner side of a petal. She ate lemon sherbet and lay in the grass watching the white cotton clouds spread and change shape in the fragrant breeze. She rested against an apple tree, its leaves pale and rustling against dried, un-bloomed fruit. She ran her hand along a sculpture, its marble like ice, and stood against the golden stone of the palace, feeling the warmth of the rock against her back.

Eventually the breeze grew cool and the sun lowered in the sky and the trees stretched long black lines across the lawn. The children pulled in their boats and their mothers draped jackets across their shoulders. The music from the gazebo changed to the slow strum of a harp, and the sound of meat sizzling on a grill traveled from beyond the hedge with the smell of blackened grease. The carousel lights came on, red, green and gold sparkling against the dimness of dusk.

Sara found a last slice of sunshine on the lawn and sat down, pulling her jacket around her shoulders, and watched as the sun disappeared behind the palace.

She didn't know how long she'd been there before she heard Germain say, "Come."

She turned to see him standing in the near-dark light, Penny at his side.

"Let us go home," he said.

She put her hand in his warm, fat palm and he pulled her to her feet.

They walked home in silence, the natural gas lights they'd passed that morning lighting the way.

46

Renee
Covington, Kentucky

Renee found Jonas's leanness odd, his strength so close to the surface it reminded her of his mortality. Perhaps that was why people put on weight, as a subconscious desire to cover up their mortality?

His leanness wasn't the only thing that was strange to her. He also used the back of his hands to caress her body.

"The basketball," Jonas explained, "has dulled my fingers. I can feel you better this way."

She didn't need an explanation. She liked his knuckles against her breasts, the tight tendons against her thighs.

"Where are we?" he asked.

"You'll see in the morning," she said, "when the sun comes up."

They'd left earlier that night and driven to Red River Gorge in the dark. It was a place Renee had come to often as a child. They were in a rented cabin by a slow burning fire, drinking tea while Hadley slept in the other room.

"I have missed you," he said. "Are you going to tell me why you stayed away for so long?"

"It's complicated."

He smiled, his teeth glowing in the dim light. "I just want to understand what's going on. You've been uptight since you picked me up, looking over your shoulder every few minutes, nervous and weird. I'm worried about you."

"Can we wait until morning? I promise we'll talk about it then."

"Okay," he said, nestling his head into her neck.

The next morning, she lay cupped in his body as she watched the sun come up over the hills.

"It's as if an inevitable war is coming and you're the only one who knows about it," Jonas said.

"I thought you were asleep."

"It's hard to sleep when you're sighing and fidgeting."

"Am I? Sorry."

He kissed her on her shoulder and rose onto his elbow. "So, are you going to talk to me about whatever it is?"

"I decided a long time ago I didn't want to know about it."

"Well, you know enough to worry about it."

Suddenly she couldn't breathe, panic welling in her . She sat up.

"What's wrong?"

"How do you know it's a war?" she asked.

"What're you talking about?"

"Why did you choose the word *war*? Why'd you ask me that way?"

"I don't know."

"I've been stupid, haven't I?"

"About what?"

"This is what you've been after the whole time, isn't it?"

"What?" he asked again.

"The story. That's why you wanted to be my lover, for the story."

"What story?"

"You know what I'm talking about."

"The story about you and Ernest?"

"No, not about me and Ernest, about Scott and the Order."

"What's the Order?"

"Really? You don't know?"

"I only want to know what makes you tense, why you are so worried about Hadley. I don't know anything about a story or the Order."

"It's strange I didn't think of it before."

"Think about what?"

"Think you were chasing me for information. Usually it would have been the first thing that crossed my mind."

"Maybe it's because I'm not."

She laid her hand on his shoulder. She believed him.

"Have you heard about the mystery surrounding my husband's death?"

"A bit. Any politician dies and it attracts attention."

"I never cared before."

"About his death?"

"About the whole damn mystery. My family. The secrets. The politics. All of it."

"So, what's changed?"

"My daughters. It was always to come to this for Brett. But now Hadley and Sara are involved too."

"Involved in what?"

"I don't know how to talk to you about it. I'm not sure I should."

Jonas swung his legs over the side of the bed. "I'm going to make us some coffee."

He moved to the kitchen in three long strides.

She looked out the window. She'd forgotten how colorful the trees were in autumn, how steep the slope of the gorge.

"I only want to know so I can help," he said from the kitchen.

She glanced through the half-opened door to the other bedroom where Hadley was sleeping.

It's better not to know.

Jonas came back in the room, the coffee pot gurgling behind him. "My mother always used to tell me to keep it simple and come up with the first step, that everything after that would fall in place."

"You've never talked about your mother before."

"No?"

"Tell me about her. I need to ease into this."

He sat down next to her. "She was the kind of person you could feel approaching before you saw her. It was like her happiness reached you first. She used to play basketball with me, taught me to dance on the court. She made me play with my eyes closed, taught me to smell and hear the ball, to use my senses to play and not my mind. 'Let your feet decide when to move,' she used to say, 'not your head.' She never saw me play college basketball. She died before I graduated from high school."

"I wish I could have met her."

"You wouldn't have wanted to meet her. You would have worried about your age."

"How old was she?"

"She would be thirty-nine if she were still alive."

"Wow," Renee said. "She must have had you very young."

"So, are you going to tell me about this so-called war?"

Renee sighed. "It's an ancient game of power that has been passed down for centuries. If you are born into it, the secret of this power enshrines your world and you either follow the path to the secret or you ignore it and try to live a normal life."

"And you were born into this?"

She nodded. "I chose to ignore it. I wasn't interested. But to do that, to be let off, you must give them what they want first."

"And what's that?"

"You breed for them."

"*Breed* for them?"

"It's no different than many cultures. You allow yourself to be married to another who comes from the same ancient society."

"So, you have to buy your freedom from them?"

"It's not freedom because eventually your children grow up and choose the other path, and if you love them then you must walk it with them." She placed her hand on his thigh. "And that, my dear Jonas, is the predicament."

Jonas glanced through the door at Hadley sleeping.

"A dissenter is someone who has chosen not to pursue the Truth," Renee continued. "I dissented so long ago that I don't know how to become involved now."

"Involved in what?"

"The ridiculous game of secrets, of Truth."

"Truth?"

She shrugged.

"What will you have to do?"

"I might have to go away. I might have to fight something. I might even get killed. Somebody will probably get killed anyway. Death seems to fall in the wake of the Order."

"Killed?"

"It's possible."

"I don't know what to say," he said.

"It's crazy. That's why I didn't know how to tell you."

"Who's the Order?"

Renee shook her head. "I can't tell you any more, and you mustn't ask anymore. I only wanted to tell you enough that you would understand I have no choice."

"No choice about what?"

"About ending this. We must stop seeing each other."

"*What?*"

"We haven't spent much time together. If we end this now there's a good chance you'll be left alone."

"You can't be serious." He stood and began pacing the room.

"If I'd had any idea this was going to happen, I never would have let you in my house, much less my bed. You've chased the wrong old bird, I'm afraid."

He stopped pacing and looked at her. "I'm not going anywhere."

"Not today. Not tonight," she smiled. "But tomorrow we'll stop this."

"And you get to make that decision without me?"

"I'm doing it to *protect* you. If you're close to me and I cause any kind of a stir, they'll use you to get to me."

"I don't want to be protected. I'm not interested in living a narrow life."

"You could be killed, Jonas."

"Death isn't my greatest fear."

"Life as you know it will change."

"Good! That's what I've been waiting for." He kneeled in front of the bed and pulled her to the edge of it, taking her hands in his. "I'm meant for whatever this is, Renee. I can *feel* it. You know it's true. I'm different. You said it yourself."

"I'm not going to be responsible for your suffering."

"I will suffer far more if you cut me off."

I shouldn't have told him anything.

"Tell me about the Order," he said. "I'm not afraid."

"You should be."

He stared at her, unflinching. "Fear will get us nowhere."

He won't go. He will be relentless in his questioning.

289

She took a deep breath and exhaled, looking out the window at the rusty orange hills.

"The Order is a society with great influence throughout the world," she said, bringing her eyes back to him. "Apparently this influence comes from some kind of ancient knowledge or power retained throughout the years. I don't know much. It seemed to me, as a child, that no one did. But I didn't choose the path that answers these questions, and I think there are some who have chosen the path and do understand. Both my mother and father were members of this group and their parents before them. I grew up on the fringes of this society, raised to believe I was special and groomed to move up the ranks as my parents had. It was understood I would know great secrets one day, perhaps even secrets my parents didn't know. But you see, being part of the Order, part of the society, doesn't guarantee you'll learn the Truth. It only meant you have a chance, and you'll be protected."

"A chance at what? Protected from what?"

"A chance to know the Truth and be protected from ignorance. They chastise the Masses by holding back knowledge and creating fear. They believe withholding the Truth from common people is the ultimate torture. Without the joys of the Truth, the Masses flounder and suffer."

"When you say the Truth, do you mean the facts of this power?"

Renee shrugged. "It's the secret to their power, I guess. I don't know what the Truth is. My parents didn't know either. I do, however, believe it exists."

"Go on."

"So, I was groomed by elite schools and driven to excellence. It was expected I would get into an Ivy League school, preferably Yale. I feigned interest, until I was fourteen."

"Until you met Ernest," Jonas said.

What do I say about Ernest?

She'd never admitted to herself Ernest could be connected to all of it.

"Should I get that coffee?" he asked.

She'd forgotten about the coffee. The thought of a warm cup in her hand was comforting. "Yes, please."

She watched him through the door as he poured the coffee.

How has my life come to this? An unlikely lover, three vulnerable daughters, and a fate I can no longer run from.

She remembered Ernest's words.

You will have three daughters. They will be important.

Jonas brought her cup of coffee, and she cradled the steaming mug in her palms.

"Ernest and I met on a mountain," she said. "He'd been waiting for me. When I reached him, he led me to a cabin where we lay together by the fire for hours talking. He knew about my parents, and he warned me against the path they had planned for me."

"You lay together?"

"We *talked*."

"People believe Ernest had affairs with young women."

"And they believe I was one of them."

"So, were you?"

"I think he was probably capable of what they suggest. But what Ernest and I exchanged was something different. At the time, in my innocence, I wondered if it was sex. But I learned later, in disappointment, that it wasn't."

"Throughout that winter, Ernest and I met frequently at the cabin. Sometimes we didn't talk at all, just sat and watched the woods. Sometimes I asked questions. Sometimes he talked endlessly about his life. In early May, when the ski season was over and it was time for my family to leave, I saw him for the last time.

I can still remember him standing beneath the mounted antlers, rising like huge extensions from his hair. 'I am old,' he said. 'I have met death before and we have shared many a drink. Next time she comes, I will go with her.' Then he kissed me on my forehead and pushed me toward the door, and I left him there in the woods. He died the following July."

"When I heard of his death, I was inconsolable. I decided, in some kind of youthful tribute, I wanted nothing of the world I was being brought up in. I told my parents I was no longer interested in any of it. I changed schools and began reading furiously. Everything Ernest had written I read. I began critiquing his books in school papers. My parents were disappointed, kept telling me I was capable of so much more, that there was this Truth that was my birthright and that I could only get to through specific schooling and special selection. I assured them I wasn't interested in the Truth, and eventually they accepted my indifference. But only under one condition: that I marry someone ascending into the Order and keep the bloodline strong. I agreed."

"So, you just quit?" Jonas asked.

"It's called dissenting, and as long as you agree to pass on your genes, they don't argue. They believe a person will never make it to the Truth if they don't want to and apparently there are very few of the bloodline left."

"What is this bloodline? How do they know who has it?"

"Like any line of royalty, by lineage and DNA testing, I guess. But there's something else. There's a test to pass. I don't know what it is. Scott was tested and failed. I think Brett might have passed recently."

"She's a prodigy," Renee continued. "Scott groomed her well. She got into Yale. She got into the Order. And she's learned to hate me and her sisters like she hates the Masses. Last week she came for Hadley. The Order will have sent her."

He lowered his head and looked toward Hadley's room. "Are you sure we should talk about this here?"

"Hadley knows more than I do. She senses it, I think, instead of knows it. That's probably why they're after her."

He shook his head. "Is all this for real?"

"*They* believe it's real, and I suppose that's enough to make it so. My father used to tell me the saga of secrets goes back to the Kennedys, the Rockefellers, even the Catholic church."

"But what will they do with Hadley?"

"I don't know, but their methods are obsessive and righteous. They're capable of terrible things. They killed my husband."

Jonas nodded. "I wondered."

"I'm afraid it's probably true," Renee said. "Scott turned against them when he failed the test. He was angry and I'm guessing he got close to exposing something, some big secret, so they got rid of him. He knew it was coming. After his friend died, he became overrun with fear and begged me to take the girls and leave the country. I took sabbatical and we moved to New Zealand. But it was all in vain. You can't run from the Order. They aren't contained within a continent."

"So, what do you think they want with Hadley?" He asked again.

"They want her to join them. I think Brett has alerted them to her uniqueness. She's too special for them to ignore. If I stand in the way, they won't hesitate to get rid of me. I'm a dissenter who has already passed on my blood and no longer fertile. I'm worth nothing to them."

"But wouldn't it be suspicious if you died too?"

"I will die of something unsuspicious. They have many tricks."

He put his coffee mug on the table. "So how do we keep Hadley away from them? It sounds hopeless."

"It's not just Hadley. Sara's involved too. She's in Europe, following Scott's trail. I never thought Sara would get involved. Never." She stared out the window again. "It's funny, you know. I don't think there's anything I can do to protect any of them. But I still have to try because I'm their mother."

Jonas took her hands in his.

"There's a man Hadley visits. His name is Issa. I believe he can tell me what I need to know."

"So, we must go see him," Jonas said.

"Really, Jonas, this isn't something you jump into lightly."

"If there is a secret of significance in this life, I want to know it."

"You can't just *want* to know. You must commit to dealing with whatever you find out. It's a big decision. It's why I've been so distant recently. I've needed time and space to decide."

"And have you decided?"

Renee nodded.

"From the day I met you," he said. "I've been committed to you. So, if you decide to take this path, then I'm going with you."

Renee stared at him. Despite all the far-fetched facts of the conspiracy of power, it was his love she found the most unbelievable.

PART III

Remembrance

47

Sara
Paris, France

The morning after their day in Paris, Sara and Penny sat in front of Germain's hearth, the fire raging. Outside, rain spat against the windows and the wind whistled and stretched the walls.

"We had fun yesterday, did we not?" Germain asked from his chair.

Penny held a socked foot up to the flames. "It was a wonderful day," she said, twisting her foot in the heat. Sara was pleased to see her face was still soft from the spirit of the previous day. How long would it last before Penny became hard and focused again?

"But you still want to know about the Anunnaki," he said.

She brought her foot away from the fire. "Yes. I want to know even more about them now. I want to know everything I can know about everything. I want to know about their powers. I want to know how many of them there were. And where did they come from? Where are they now?"

"That would about cover it," he said, smiling.

He sat forward and looked each of them in the eye. "We will get to the gods, I promise. But first I want you to understand Earth and humans. That is why I took you into the streets of Paris. You see, everything human, everything beautiful, everything ugly is what it is because of its vibrations. You must first understand this."

"Vibrations?"

"Yes, vibrations. Earth is a small particle of a massive universe of bouncing molecules that create energy," he said. "And energy is *life*. Like blood runs through a body, energy soars through the universe and through everything that exists within the universe. Energy *is* existence. It has always existed and always will. The illusion of time passing is only energy changing form. And as energy accumulates, it becomes powerful. That is what people are, you see. We are an accumulation of a complex form of energy. But we all come in different degrees of energy and are therefore capable of different degrees of power."

"What makes a person differ in energy from another?" Penny asked.

"Those who vibrate at a higher level, have a greater amount of energy. Many things can affect the level of your vibrations. Physical exercise and learning can raise your vibrations to a moderate degree, and love and appreciation can raise them to a higher degree. The higher your vibrations are, the more you connect with the Great Universal Energy. And it works the other way around too. The more you connect with the great energy of the universe, the higher your vibrations."

Sara decided she must not vibrate at all.

"I, for example, vibrate at a higher level than you two." He pointed at them as he said this. "Hence my connection is greater, and I can see and sense things you two cannot. Everything is energy. Thoughts are energy and feelings are energy too. And objects are just forms of bouncing molecules, which, if seen, can be manipulated."

"Manipulated?" Sara asked.

"Moved," Penny said. "He's talking about moving matter."

"Yes," he said. "That is exactly what I mean."

"What, with your mind?"

"Not with my mind, but with my *energy*. Would you like me to demonstrate? I mean, if you think you are ready for the bullshit journey that is." He winked at her.

"Okay, then." Sara pulled her feet up beneath her and nodded at him. "Go on."

He looked across the room, his eyes gathering as he concentrated, his head bowing forward. A dim light formed at his brow, and before Sara had time to wonder about the fact he was beginning to glow, something moved in her peripheral vision. She turned to see the small Rubens painting come unattached from the wall and float toward them, hovering in the air until it settled softly on Penny's lap.

Penny stroked the frame, seemingly more impressed with the painting than the magic.

He continued as if he hadn't just sent a painting flying through the air. "When one's vibrations are at a higher level, or as I prefer to call it, when one is *enlightened*, one is not vulnerable to the things that vibrate at a lower level, things like disease and danger. An enlightened one does not come into the path of things that vibrate on a lower level unless one chooses to."

"Why would someone choose to lower their vibrations?"

"I have lowered my vibrations purposefully for your visit. Otherwise you would not be able to see or hear me. In fact, if one lets one's vibrations get too high, one will cease to exist." His eyebrows rose. "And get your vibrations just high enough and you can live forever."

"The elixir of life," Penny said.

He clapped his hands together. "Yes, my dear. The secret to immortality is to increase your vibrations."

Sara wasn't feeling enlightened. She was feeling frightened, and it wasn't the floating painting that had startled her. It was something else, something she couldn't place. She crossed her arms and sank into the couch.

"Once you understand energy," Germain continued. "Once you can see it, you have control over your future. You can decide what you want to happen in your life. You can even make decisions about death."

"And that's enlightenment?" Penny asked.

Germain nodded. "Yes."

"You make it sound like it's a beautiful thing," Sara said.

"Enlightenment is always beautiful," Germain said. "What makes you think it is not?"

"I don't know," Sara said.

"Manipulating matter can be learned superficially, and when this happens, it can be ugly. You are wise to be aware of this. What is it that is scaring you?"

Sara shrugged.

"My moving matter has reminded you of something, has it?" He reached out and placed his hand on her knee.

A vision came to Sara, of a man standing beside a road with glowing hands.

She sat up and moved to the edge of the couch. "I saw a man standing beside a road doing something with his hands, and they glowed. It was the same way your brow glowed, but it was his hands. I don't know where I saw him, but I remember him."

"An un-enlightened," Germain said.

An image of the truck flashed before Sara, and she remembered the great squeal and crunch that followed. She gasped and opened her eyes.

"What is it?" Penny asked,

"It was you," Sara said, standing and pointing at Germain. "This power is what killed my father. You made the truck hit us. You used this power to kill my father!"

Germain sat back in his chair and opened his golden box. "Yes, this power was the weapon behind your father's death." He sifted through the green and orange buds with his finger. "But I can assure you it had nothing to do with me."

The man on the side of the road looked nothing like Germain, but blaming him sent a rush, a thrill, through Sara's body.

"How can someone enlightened do something so awful?"

"Having power hardly guarantees good will. And you said it was his hands that were glowing, not his brow. So, he is clearly *not* enlightened. His power is learned. He knows how to find it and use it, but he does not know how to tap into it and *become* it."

"Is this how my father died too?" Penny asked.

Germain shook his head. Then nodded. "Yes and no."

"The autopsy said he died of cancer," Penny said. "But he'd never even been sick."

"Cancer is our cells' response to very low vibrations, or bad energy. Anxiety, hatred, fear, these emotions create low vibrations that distort our cells. When we are exposed to them for a long time, they mutate and cancer forms. The Order has learned how to create a concentrated cloud of low vibrations, so that when a person is exposed to them, their body reacts to the low vibrations and matches them. Because it is concentrated, the cancer forms quickly. It can appear within hours. An autopsy will reveal a tumor that is only days old but as lethal as one that has been festering for five years."

"You mentioned you can tap in and become it," Penny said. "What did you mean?"

"Whoever killed your fathers was connecting to power outside himself, probably through a tool of some kind, instead of raising his vibrations and tapping into a power *inside* himself. Only through love can you become the power itself."

"Love?" Sara rolled her eyes.

"I understand the physics you're describing," Penny said. "But how does this tie into the Sumerians and the Anunnaki? And what're the Truths?"

"I was about to talk about love, and you rush me on," he said, chuckling. "This energy concept you are so keen to dismiss *is* the Second Truth, and high vibrating energy in its purest and simplest form is love."

Penny looked, disappointedly, at the painting in her hands. "So, love is the Second Truth?"

"Whatever you want to call it," Germain said. "The fact there is a Great Universal Energy, a stream of boundless power that can be tapped into at any time, by anyone, is the Second Truth. It is more beautiful than the First Truth. The Second Truth is beauty itself. It is the sunrise you watched yesterday. It is the pastries and the piano and the park. Do not make the common mistake of obsessing about the less important First Truth."

"The Second Truth can be tapped into by anyone?" Penny asked.

He sighed and began rolling a joint. "I fear you have not heard me."

"I understand. I felt it yesterday. I see how gratitude and appreciation are a portal to the Second Truth. But I fail to see how *anyone* can tap into it. If it was that easy, everyone would."

"Anyone lucky enough to be aware of it, encouraged to pay attention to it and keen enough to learn, that is. It is inside us all." He placed the joint in his mouth, his lips grasping it as he spoke. "For some people it comes easier though. Some are born at a higher vibration and learn quickly."

"How?"

"It is part of their genetic makeup."

"Genetic how? Random or inherited?" Penny asked, excited.

"Inherited."

"Autosomal recessive?"

"Yes," Germain said smiling. "Are your pieces fitting together now?"

Sara stopped listening, overwhelmed by the memory of the man by the roadside. Who cared about genetics?

She stood and walked to the window, pulling the curtain aside and watching the rain hit the pavement below. A headache was coming on and she rested her head on the cool pane. "I don't want to hear any more stories," she said. "I want to find this man and make him pay for what he's done."

"Don't be ridiculous," Penny said. "Going after one man isn't going to accomplish anything."

"Maybe I don't want what you want. Maybe I don't care about the Truth!"

"How many times have we been through this?" Penny asked. "This is about finding out the Truth. That's all it's ever been about."

"Careful, Penny," Germain said. "You are making one of the greatest human mistakes, assuming everyone else is like you. People's differences are far greater and more predetermined than you realize. Sara has never wanted anything but to be close to you and to appease her grief. She is not interested in being enlightened. She was not born that way."

"Not born that way?" Sara asked, pulling her forehead off the glass. She watched the circle of her breath shrink and disappear.

"Penny is what they call a Talent, born with a special blood. And you," he said, looking at Sara. "Are pure human, one of the Masses. You can learn to be enlightened, but for the most part you are not interested in it. You are driven mostly by fear and desire and rarely ever by faith and knowledge. You are, and will be forever, attracted to those who are more enlightened. That is why you love Penny, and why she does not feel so strongly about you.

And even as I speak, instead of gaining perspective as Penny is, you grow more afraid, and this will lead to more anger and if you are not careful, you will end up like your father."

"Who killed my father?" Sara asked. "Tell me his name."

Germain sighed. "His name is Japeth."

"Will you help me find him?"

"No."

"Do you know where he is?"

"I am not going to help you find him."

Sara stomped her foot and crossed her arms.

Germain flipped his lighter open.

"Brett!" Sara said. "Brett will know, won't she?"

Germain lit his joint and looked at her, his face revealing nothing.

"Hadley," Sara said. "Yes, Hadley saw the man too!"

"Please can we continue about the Anunnaki," Penny said. "About these genetics?"

Germain snapped his lighter closed, shut his eyes and inhaled. "Can I continue, Sara? Can we stop this revenge nonsense?"

"Just tell me where I can find him."

"If you follow your anger you will see your demise."

"Whatever."

"Set aside your anger for now, at least, and see how you feel tomorrow."

Sara turned back to the window.

"If you are smart, you will listen."

"I'm not smart." The glass fogged with her breath.

"You *can* be smart. I believe in you."

Sara stared into the rain. For as long as she could remember, she'd wanted someone to speak those words to her. Now that someone was, she was too angry to care.

"I will continue, then," he said. "We were talking about the biology of the Second Truth, the fact you are a particle of the Great Universal Energy and because of this you are capable of creating whatever you want. And you can only do this by accepting you are part of something greater than yourself and through that concept learn to need nothing, fear nothing."

"But how does that give you power?" Penny asked.

"Because when you feel complete and utter love, high vibrations will allow the Great Universal Energy to flow freely through you, creating the ability to manipulate and morph."

"Morph?" Penny asked.

Sara turned around in time to see his image become wavy and the edges of his form shrink and warp until what sat in his chair was a small frog.

Sara leaned into the sill behind her and closed her eyes, a sharp pain pulsating between them.

Penny looked at the frog of Germain and said, "I thought the frog was supposed to turn into a prince."

And suddenly, before them sat a prince, dressed in white and adorned with gold tassels. A grin of perfect white teeth spread across the prince's face and in Germain's voice, the prince said, "You must give up your greed in Order to have what you want, and as this happens, you become more and more full of the high vibrations of the Great Universal Energy and in turn can become anything you want. This is immortality."

"Stop!" Sara said. "Please stop."

The prince immediately turned back into Germain. "I am sorry. That was probably too much. But you did say that you were sick of the journey and wanted the facts."

"I didn't want to see you turn into a frog."

He stood and went to her, placing his hand on her shoulders. "The magic you just saw is not only what killed your fathers, but also what they wanted to expose."

He pulled her toward him and embraced her. His touch was soft and light. It reminded her of her father. "It is okay," he said.

"So, are you going to tell us the First Truth?" Penny asked from her chair.

Germain loosened his embrace so he could look Sara in the eye. "I promise I will not morph again. We can stop talking about these Truths for now."

Sara looked at Penny.

"Don't worry about her," Germain said, touching Sara's face softly and pulling her gaze back to him. "Penny needs to learn compassion. Let her wait."

He led Sara back to the fire and sat her down. She noticed her headache was gone.

"Your headache is gone because by treating you with kindness, by slowing down and being in the moment, I raised your vibrations and healed you. These are the powers of the Second Truth."

He moved to Penny and knelt in front of her. "This is something you will struggle with. But what is the hurry, child? Remember yesterday?" He placed his large hand on her crown of orange curls. "Sit and watch the fire and contemplate the Second Truth. You are not yet ready for the first."

48

Hadley
Cincinnati, Ohio

Hadley had been patient about taking the stone to Issa, but after Brett's intrusion and a trip to Kentucky with her mother, she didn't want to delay her questions any further.

His door was open, and she went inside, pulling her feet from her shoes and leaving them in the entryway before hurrying into the back bedroom where she could hear the steady knock of a hammer.

Issa stood on a ladder, hanging a picture over the bureau.

"Hello, Hadley," he said through a mouthful of nails.

"I need to show you something," she said, holding the stone out to him.

He straightened the frame and came down from the ladder, taking the stone from her.

"They're the same ones you have outside, aren't they?"

"Similar, yes. But this writing is much older."

"My mother used to put this stone in my crib when I was a baby. She said it would calm me. She doesn't know where it came from. She says she just found it with me one day. What do you know about this stone?"

Surely you remember where it came from? Mr. Ernest asked from behind her.

Hadley jumped. She hadn't realized Mr. Ernest had followed her into the house.

"And you have just found it again?" Issa asked.

He must not see the ghost.

"Yes, my mother and I found it in the attic."

Issa sat on the end of the bed and moved the stone lightly between his fingers.

Mr. Ernest glided toward him and peered down at the stone. *I brought this to your crib when you were a tiny baby. Don't you remember?*

Issa swatted in Mr. Ernest's direction as though he were a fly. "This stone was once your ancestors'," he said to Hadley. "It represents who you are and who you can become."

"So, it's my grandmother's?"

"No. It belonged to ancestors from a very long time ago."

"Why'd I have it as a baby? How did I get it if my mother can't remember it?"

I told you, I gave it to you, Mr. Ernest said.

Hadley ignored him. "Was it my father's? If so, why didn't my mother know that? And how do you know it's my ancestors' if I've only just met you?"

"That is for you to remember."

"A ghost is telling me *he* gave it to me," Hadley said boldly.

Issa sighed and looked in Mr. Ernest's direction. "Ghosts are often self-absorbed. Do not give them too much attention."

Mr. Ernest chuckled and shook his head, then surprised Hadley by holding up his middle finger to Issa before he floated out of the room.

Hadley giggled and turned back to Issa. "Tell me about the Bible, about how it all fits together. I'm beginning to understand truth and love come from something outside a book. I won't be disappointed or scared with what you tell me now."

He handed her back the stone and she put it in the front pocket of her jeans.

He stood and brushed his hands together, flakes of drywall floating to the carpet, and started for the library, motioning for her to follow.

"The Bible is one of many books that combine ancient facts and current politics. It is no more holy or astute than the Talmud, the Torah, the Tipitaka, or the Quran. They are all holy books, and all have great truths hidden amid a maze of jumbled stories, stories that can confuse you if you have not experienced spirit."

"What's the use of a book that isn't needed by those who understand it and is used in vain by those who don't?"

"For reference," he said, reaching the library and sitting on the bench. "You see, what you are beginning to understand is that there is no world, no universe, no substance, separate from anything else. There is only energy forming and reshaping and Earth is simply a concentration of this energy, and you, too, are a small part of it. And these sacred books are here for reference, to remind and inspire those who understand and plant a seed for those who don't."

Hadley nodded that she understood. "I see Truth in the New Testament where I didn't before. It's the history of the Old Testament that confuses me."

"That's because God is completely misunderstood," he said, his eyes like running water in sunlight. "Do you remember how we talked about the Nephilim?"

She nodded and sat on the carpet in front of him, crossing her legs.

"Before Jesus," he said. "Before Moses, there were gods that ruled over humans. The God of the Old Testament was much like the Bible represents him: ruthless, selfish, and angry. As you may have noticed, this is very incongruent with the loving God portrayed by Jesus. But the first thing you must understand is that originally there was more than one God. Genesis clearly refers to

311

plural Gods. Genesis 1:26, '*Let us make Man in our image ...*' and Genesis 3:22, '*the man has become like one of us,*' and Genesis 11:7, '*let us go down and there confuse their language.*'"

"I noticed that last week when I was reading. Funny, I hadn't noticed it before."

"Seeing only what one is looking for is normal. With your new-found knowledge and spiritual growth, you will notice many things you missed before."

"So, what's the Truth then, about these gods?"

"On one hand there *is* a monotheistic God, the God that Jesus loved and taught the world to honor. This God is the Great Universal Energy. It is the ever-abundant flow in you and me and the sun and the moon. It is love and joy and passion. It is beauty and faith and playfulness. It is this God you have been learning to connect with, to become one with through meditation. But it is not a *being*. It is spirit that is everywhere."

"It's not a man on a cloud in the sky."

"No," he said, smiling. "It is not. But personifying something makes it easier to believe. It is understandable people portray God in this way."

"And the plural gods, the wrathful ones in the Old Testament?"

"The gods of the Old Testament were vengeful and calculating. In the two thousand years before Christ, these gods communicated directly with people and were feared. The Bible, through bad translations and calculated politics, has lumped together both these frightening, powerful gods and the Great Universal Energy as one ruling entity that must be obeyed. Other sacred texts, such as the Tao Te Ching, only speak of the great energy and the humbleness and sacrifice necessary to connect with it. These are books that were not tainted by politics or translation, books meant for enlightenment. The gods of the Old Testament were real, but they were not good, and definitely not holy. May I see the stone again?"

Hadley fished the stone out of her pocket and handed it to him.

"This was one of their stones," he said.

"Whose stones?"

"The gods of the Old Testament."

"You said it was a stone from my ancestors."

"It is."

Hadley looked at the stone cradled in his palm. She couldn't understand why a baby would sleep with a rock and how the rock could be the rock of gods and also the rock of her ancestors.

"I don't get it," she frowned.

His eyes darkened like evening lake water. He looked down at the stone and said with great sadness, "I hope, one day soon, it will make sense to you."

"Why are you sad?"

"I am missing times from long ago."

"I remember times before this life."

"You do?"

"I remember Austria a long time ago. I remember living in the mountains. Is this what you remember, things from old lives?"

"No," he said, shaking his head.

"Sometimes I remember other things, too, but then they slip from me and I can't recall them. They're like a flash of lightning and then they're gone."

"Someday you will remember more clearly," he said.

"When? When will I remember?"

"That is up to you."

"Do you remember all your past lives?"

"I have lived only one life. I am not like you."

She reached for the stone and took it back. "But I thought we were the same, you and me. I thought that was why I came here."

He shook his head and smiled a sad smile. "We are not the same."

She put the stone back in her pocket, disappointed. She wanted to be the same as Issa. She wanted to be the same as somebody.

"Let us meditate," Issa said, slipping down onto the floor next to her. "The answers lie in surrender."

She closed her eyes, gods immediately dancing upon her eyelids. They were huge and luminescent with swords of lightening and wrathful brows. They swirled around her thoughts, in angry tones of red and orange.

Issa took her hand into his and the vision disappeared, a soft pink light clouding around her. His touch was warm with a feathery lightness like the feeling of static on laundry fresh out of the dryer.

I will remember the works of the Lord: surely I will remember thy wonders of old.

49

Brett

Jekyll Island, Georgia

Brett sat across from the dark man.

He was at his desk, elbows resting on a calendar, fingers tapping in a square of light from the desk lamp. His face, once again, was hidden in the shadows.

"You didn't bring her," he said.

She had been waiting to hear his voice again. She watched his tapping fingers, wondered if the tips were coarse or soft.

"She didn't want to come."

His fingers went still.

"I'm not going to haul her here against her wishes if that's what you expect."

He leaned forward so a sliver of his chin came into the light. It was covered in neatly trimmed black hair. A few, she noticed, were silver.

"Do we have a loyalty issue here?" he asked.

"Was my sacrifice not proof enough?"

"One action doesn't serve for eternity. Our daily choices are what prove our purpose."

His voice rasped at her, the shadow hiding his lips.

"If you expect me to bring my sister here against her will, you're going to have to explain to me how that's going to help the Order. If she's a Prophet, then I figure she's more powerful than me. And didn't you say force was a bad option, that it creates resistance?"

"It seems she's already resistant. And don't underestimate the power of cultivation. A trained Talent can be as powerful as an untrained Prophet."

He leaned back into the shadows, taking his hands with him.

"Why do you hide?" Brett asked. "I find it insulting."

He offered a hoarse chuckle from the dark. "And I find you overconfident."

"I would hope you wouldn't settle for less here among the Calderbergers."

"Confidence is a virtue. Overconfidence is a liability we cannot afford."

Brett knew she should be afraid of him, but she felt drawn to test him. "What may seem overconfident, may actually be wisdom."

"Why don't you guess why I hide in the shadows," he said, bringing his hands back into the light and folding them. "If you're correct, I'll tell you."

Brett lit up at the challenge, speaking immediately. "If this were a fairy tale, I would say it was because you are frightfully ugly. But it's more likely you're frightfully powerful, a Prophet yourself, and until I prove trustworthy it's prudent for you to remain in the shadows."

"Perhaps it is both," he said.

"Vagueness," she said, rolling her eyes. "The gift of the Order."

"You are correct to the extent you are able to be. You bring me your sister and I will face you man to woman in the bright light of day."

"You assume gazing at you to be quite a prize, then."

"Oh yes," he said.

The arrogance of his statement made her stomach flutter and tighten.

"Hadley seemed to know I was coming."

"How so?"

"She was sitting in the dark, as if she were waiting for us. She knew what I wanted and was quite clear she wasn't interested."

"You must bring her to us. It's important she's part of the Order."

"If Hadley knows about the Order and doesn't want to be part of it, what does that say about the Order?"

"Go," he said, standing in the darkness and waving a hand in the light. "Your questions are premature. If you aren't clever enough to come up with your own plan to bring Hadley to us, I will devise one and contact you when we're ready."

"No," Brett said. "A plan isn't the problem. It's lack of information. As a group, who *are* we? What exactly am I bringing Hadley to? I need to know our history and our purpose."

He sighed in the darkness. It was a familiar sigh, one her curiosity and determination had provoked many times in her life.

"Come," he said, turning in the shadows and walking toward the couches on the far side of the room.

Brett followed him, his form tall and slender in the dim light.

Once in the shadows again, he lowered himself into the couch, crossed one dark leg over the other and pointed to the couch across from him. "Have a seat."

Brett sat, and he began to speak.

"There are three powerful alliances in the world. We, the Order, are one. the Catholic church is another, and the third is a non-formal group made up of the ultra-wealthy, which we refer to as the money launderers. The three of us are both competitors and allies. Throughout the years, we have all harbored Two Truths. We have hidden them from the Masses and used them to our advantages, all in different ways with different motives. The First Truth is the history of our ancestry. It's this Truth we've begun to reveal to you and will eventually share with you completely, now that you're a Calderberger."

"And the Second?"

"The Second Truth is the more important of the two. It is the secret to our ancestors' powers. We have learned to harness this power by using ancient tools, but we don't understand the power fully. We can't tap into it without these tools, and this makes us vulnerable."

"The other groups, they can use this power naturally?"

He shook his head. "No, they understand it less than we do. And that goes for the First Truth too. Neither the church nor the money launderers know how to test blood, how to confirm ancestry. We are the most advanced of the groups." He paused. "But when it comes to the Second Truth, there are those who are even more advanced than we are."

"Another group?"

He shook his head. "Not a group, individuals."

"How many? Where are they?"

"Those are exactly the questions we ask ourselves. How many? Probably not more than a handful who can use the power at will. But how many are *capable* of channeling the power without tools or tedious training? We predict about a thousand. And *where* are they? Scattered. Hidden. Constantly they elude us."

"Prophets," Brett said.

He nodded in the dark. "Prophets are our key to the Second Truth, the most important Truth. Finding them, bringing them into our alliance, understanding them, is one of the main objectives of the Order."

"Yet your methods are inane," she said. "For such a prestigious group."

He laughed. "I beg your pardon?"

"Well, find a Talent who's a sucker and get her to bring in her sister? That's hardly an impressive methodology."

He laughed again. "It's a little more strategic than that. We use the bloodline to narrow in on likely candidates, and we use a segmentation process for selection, breaking people into types based on their behavior. Someone is either a stagnant or a potential. Stagnants are easily controlled by society. While they may have some degree of rebellion, it tends to be directionless. They usually turn out to be Masses or Carrier Clones, but there are some Talents and Prophets who exhibit the behavior of a stagnant."

"When you say easily controlled by society," Brett said. "You mean us, the Order. That they're easily controlled by us?"

"For the most part, yes. We're the force behind society. This is a huge power in itself. Something it would be wise for you to appreciate."

"And the potentials?"

"Potentials sense they're missing something. They've moved beyond their fear of nonconformity and attempt to educate themselves and to understand their world. Most of them are Talents. Occasionally, one is a Prophet. Sometimes a Carrier Clone will exhibit potential. Although rare, Masses can become a potential as well. Omega cells, while they fast track you to the Truth, aren't a prerequisite."

"So, before I became a Calderberger, I was a potential?"

"Exactly."

"And everyone you sent back before initiation, everyone like my father, will always remain in this first group ... Potentials who never learn the Truth."

"Most of them, yes."

"And my mother?"

"Your mother was a potential, raised by potentials, but she chose to become a stagnant when she dissented."

"And my sisters are stagnants?"

"To date, yes. Although we believe Sara may be a potential. She's recently showing signs."

"*Sara?*"

"There aren't enough signs yet for us to act, but we're watching her."

"What're you watching?"

"It's not important. What's important is to understand we, the Order, aren't the only people who know the First Truth about our ancestry, but we are the only group who has tools to channel the Second Truth. These tools have been protected through the ages, passed down through the secret societies—the Assassins, the Priory of Sion, the Knights Templar, the Rosicrucians, the original Freemasons, the Jacobins. All these groups protected the tools of our ancestry throughout the centuries. We have this advantage over the church and the money launderers. But one day we may lose that advantage. When the power is dependent on a tool, a tool that can be found and owned, it is fragile. But when the power is within, it can never be stolen."

"And you think Prophets have this power within them?"

"We know they do."

"Because they don't need the tools."

He nodded. "Therefore, we must gather as many of them as we can, and we must continue to produce as many of them as we can by mating only with other Talents and Prophets. And in the meantime, we must keep our tools secret, protect them from the church and the money launderers."

"Last time we spoke you said a Talent is one in a hundred thousand. What about a Prophet?"

"One in five million," he said.

Brett sat forward on the chair. "That's only about twelve hundred in existence."

"You see why Hadley is so special then."

"So you're saying the Order is a group of advanced humans who have spent years using a tool to channel a power, and their goal is to become free of this tool and unlock natural, dormant powers?"

"Exactly."

Brett sank back into her chair. "And have we gotten anywhere?" she asked. "In the past three thousand years, have we gotten any closer?"

"What if I told you we haven't? Would you drop out, become a stagnant like your mother?"

Brett found the idea frighteningly appealing.

"We have gotten closer, yes," he said finally. "But the real question is, do you want to be part of the search for the Truth and part of our power, or do you want to just exist and be controlled?"

Brett stared at his dark form. "What if I just exist and *not* be controlled?"

"You can try."

"And these tools? What are they? How many do we have?"

"In time we will introduce them."

"How do I know they exist? All I have is your word. How do I know the power even exists?"

"That is why we don't explain these things so soon. You must experience tastes of the power first in order to believe. Don't forget Noel."

She glanced at the clock above the mantle. Noel would be finishing his afternoon run, getting into the shower. Surely there was more power than this silly desire?

She leaned toward the dark man. "How many Prophets were there among our group of initiates? You brought eleven of us here to the island. Six were initiated. How many of those were Prophets?"

"None," he said. "There rarely ever are."

"How many Prophets are among the Order in total?"

"Thirteen. Fourteen if you bring us Hadley."

Brett didn't bother asking him if he was one of the thirteen. She knew he was. But why didn't the other thousand Prophets migrate to the Order? Where were they? What were they doing? Were they turned off by the dogma? If so, did this further prove that Eli was a Prophet? Had they sent him a letter inviting him to the island and he'd turned them down?

She could ask. The dark man might tell her. But she was afraid what he might do if he saw how much she cared. And anyway, she wanted to get home before Noel got out of the shower.

50

Renee
Cincinnati, Ohio

Issa had agreed to come to dinner and the evening had come. Renee was in the kitchen, panicking about her pasta sauce while Hadley sat quietly in the living room.

Jonas would be arriving soon.

What would this Issa man think? Had Hadley told him about the age difference?

The doorbell rang and she looked up, catching a glimpse of herself in the window.

"You know this is the right thing to do," she said to her reflection.

Hadley went to the door, opening it to the looming figure of Jonas, her tiny blonde head coming just above his waist.

He entered the house and hung his coat on a hook. "Come in," she waved. "I'm in the kitchen."

She could smell him immediately, leather and musk cologne. She went to hug him but pulled back, aware of Hadley watching.

Jonas, noticing her hesitation, took her face in his hands and kissed her. "Hi," he said. "Smells great." He moved to the stovetop, opening the pot lid and sticking his finger in.

"It's still simmering." She slapped his hand. "Keep the lid on it." She turned to Hadley. "What time should we expect Issa?"

Hadley went to the fridge and wrote on her whiteboard. HE'LL SHOW UP WHEN HE'S SUPPOSED TO.

Jonas lifted a bowl off the counter. "What's this?" he asked, sniffing.

"Pesto."

"You make your own pesto?"

"It's easy, just basil, garlic, oil, parmesan. Some pine nuts if ..."

Hadley clapped her hands and rushed out of the kitchen, her socked feet thudding against the wooden floor as she ran to the door.

"Did you hear the doorbell?" Renee asked Jonas.

He shook his head.

They watched her fling open the door to a man framed against the setting sun, black hair dancing about his head in the dim light. He clutched a wine bottle under his arm and a pie dish in his hand. Hadley pulled him inside and wrapped her arms around his waist, closing the door behind him with her foot.

He kissed her affectionately on the crown of her head, and Hadley skipped him into the kitchen and stood him in front of Renee and Jonas. He was slender with brown skin and a long nose.

"This is my friend Issa."

"Issa Asad," he said. "Lovely to meet you."

Renee stared at Hadley. "What did you just say?"

Hadley grinned. "I said this is my friend Issa."

"My God, Hadley. You're speaking!"

"I know," she shrugged. "I can speak when Issa's around."

Renee stood baffled.

Jonas extended his hand to Issa. "I'm Jonas. Nice to meet you."

"Yes. Sorry," Renee said, shaking her head and reaching to take the wine from Issa. "I'm so pleased you could come. I'm Renee, Hadley's mother. Thank you for coming. This is my friend Jonas."

Jonas winked at Issa. "I always get introduced as a friend."

"And what would you prefer?" Issa asked in a friendly tone, a black curl falling into his eyes.

"Boyfriend," Jonas said, taking the pie from Issa.

"Either way," Issa said, smiling, "it is nice to meet you both."

His smile was genuine. Renee liked him immediately. "Come, have a seat," she said. "Sorry if I seem flustered. It's been a long time since I've heard my daughter's voice."

"I thought about warning you, Mom," Hadley said. "But I didn't know if I would be able to talk or not and I didn't know whether I'd be able to speak to you or just to Issa. It's confusing for me."

Renee's nose burned with oncoming tears. She reached for Hadley and pulled her to her chest. "It's wonderful to hear you talk again, darling, whatever the reason." She looked over Hadley's yellow hair at Issa. "Now how did you two meet again? It worries me, the thought of Hadley wandering around the neighborhood."

"I can imagine it would," Issa laughed. "Hearing your daughter has made friends with a strange man." He looked at Hadley fondly. "Hadley came to my door seeking answers."

"Answers?" Renee asked.

"She was interested in the Truth."

"I would like to know more about that," Renee said. "Let me get dinner served and you can explain. What would you like to drink with dinner?"

"May I be so bold as to ask what we are having?" he asked.

"Sure," she said, moving back into the kitchen. "I've made my mother's famous lasagna."

"I will have red wine then, thank you." He pulled the bottle of white from under his arm. "And will leave this with you."

"I have a bottle of pinot noir open. Will that be too light?"

"That would be perfect," he said.

While Jonas helped Renee set out the cutlery, Hadley showed Issa her favorite photos and paintings around the house.

"Hadley s*poke*," Jonas said.

"I know," Renee said. "It's wonderful."

"Isn't it strange, though?"

Renee polished a knife and set it beside a plate. "It would have been naive to think Issa wouldn't bring surprises."

"He's nice," Jonas said. "I like him."

"Yes, me too."

"Thank you for including me," he said, catching her eye from across the table.

Once seated and eating, Renee turned to Issa. "So, Hadley came to you searching for the Truth you say?"

"I don't know how I found him," Hadley said. "I saw his house and felt I should approach it, so I knocked on the door."

"Darling, it's so nice to hear you talking."

"You said that already, Mom. Twice."

"I know. But, really, it's such a surprise! And this Truth you were looking for," Renee asked. "What is it?"

Hadley shrugged. "I'm not sure I knew I was searching for the Truth then."

Renee looked back at Issa. "But you knew she was?"

"Yes," he answered. "Just as I know you are doing the same having me here to dinner."

Renee ignored the comment, placing her napkin on her lap and picked up her cutlery. "Perhaps we could start with you telling us a little about yourself."

"What would like to know?"

"Well, what do you do?" Renee asked. "I mean for work."

"I am retired."

"If you don't mind my saying, you look too young to be retired."

Issa only smiled.

"So, what did you do before retirement?"

"I was a teacher and a minister. I suppose I still am a minister. Although I work from home now, serving only seekers."

"What denomination?"

"I do not follow a denomination. I do not believe faith can be segregated."

Renee sensed his answers were only metaphors for the Truth and that he was only partaking in the small talk to appease her nerves. She appreciated it regardless.

"And you live close by?" she asked.

"Yes, on the corner of Fairfield and Mitcham."

"I know the street,' Renee said. "It's good to know Hadley didn't wander too far. And have you always lived in Cincinnati?"

"I have lived many places before here."

"He has lots of cats, too," Hadley said, using her knife to scrape a bite of lasagna onto the fork. "He has seven."

"Seven cats?" Jonas asked.

"Yes, they just seem to arrive."

"Like me!" Hadley giggled.

"Yes," Issa said. "Like you." He smiled warmly at her.

"You know, Hadley. It's not normal to knock on someone's door and introduce yourself," Renee said.

"Yes, I know Mother."

"I worry you'll knock on the wrong door." Renee looked at Issa. "How does a mother protect her daughter from knocking on the wrong door?"

"You cannot," Issa said. "You can only love her and teach her what you have learned in your own life, and hope she gains wisdom from both."

327

"I'm worried about Hadley, Mr. Asad. She's special."

"I can understand your concern."

"You were right about why I had you to dinner this evening. I'm also concerned about my daughter, Sara. I'm hoping you can help me keep them both from harm."

"You are not worried about the eldest child?"

"I think it's too late to save Brett."

"You cannot save any of your daughters, Mrs. Morgan. They must go on their own journeys."

"Although there's logic in what you say, you'll understand that as a mother I can't accept that. I need you to tell me everything you know, anything that might help."

Issa wiped the corner of his mouth with his napkin. "The answer to how you can help them will mean nothing to you if you don't go on the journey of discovering it yourself, and you cannot go on the journey if you already know the answer. So, you see, I *cannot* tell you everything. I am afraid you are not ready."

Renee's hand went slack and her fork dropped into her salad, sending a crouton rolling across the table.

"What did you just say?" she asked.

"I said, you have to go on the journey ..."

"I heard you." She filled a water glass, spilling some on the table and took a drink. "Who are you *really*?"

"I am not sure how to answer that."

"What you just said about the journey and the Truth, I've heard before. A long time ago someone with the same manner and the same words told me the same thing."

"Why does that worry you?" he asked.

"Never mind," she said. "It's nothing."

"It is hardly nothing," Issa said.

Renee opened her mouth to protest and then hesitated and closed it.

"Go on. This is why you invited me, is it not?"

Renee sighed and glanced at Jonas sitting stiffly in his chair and Hadley beside him, wide eyed, listening.

"A long time ago I asked someone to explain something to me and he responded like you did. Not only did he use the same words, but he said them in the same way, with the exact same certainty and passion." She shook her head. "I've been around enough to know when something isn't a coincidence."

"I know who spoke these words to you. Ernest and I are acquainted."

"Excuse me?"

"Renee," Issa said. "May I call you Renee?" But he continued before she could answer. "You wanted the Truth and I have given you a little sliver of it and see it has upset you. This is exactly why you cannot spring the Truth on someone." He took another bite of salad. "And anyway, I thought you did not want to know the Truth. You decided a long time ago you were not interested, did you not?"

She fiddled with her fork, looking from Issa to Jonas and then to Hadley before finally saying, "Forgive me, Mr. Asad, but I'm just looking for some tips on how I can protect my daughters, nothing more."

"And you think the answers to those questions are not linked to a deeper Truth?"

Renee shrugged.

"All questions lead back to the Truth, to the meaning of life. And yours are particularly closer than most." He took a sip of wine. "Lovely lasagna, by the way."

"Are you part of the Order?" Renee asked.

"No," he said. "I am not a member of the Order."

"Then who are you? Why did Hadley approach your door? How do you know Ernest? Did you know my husband?" The questions fell from her, the words tumbling over each other.

"Your husband came to see me once."

Hadley looked at him. "My dad came to see you?"

"Yes, he and his friend Mr. Weishaup. They were looking for the address of a friend of mine."

"And how did they get your address? Why you?" Renee asked.

"I do not know, and I do not ask. People show up at my door and I accept them."

"Like cats," Hadley said.

He laughed. "Only the people have questions. And when they ask, I answer."

"I'm asking you questions," Renee said.

"And I am trying to answer them."

"I just want to know if you can help me save Hadley."

"From what?"

"From the Order."

"Only Hadley can save herself from the Order. As I alluded to before, we are each in charge of our own journey and only that."

"But you claim to be helping Hadley."

"Because she was open to being involved in the process of her own learning. This allowed me to be part of her journey. Unlike you, who only wants quick answers to what you think are simple questions."

"Time, Mr. Asad, is of the essence."

"No quick answer will enable you to help your daughters. You cannot help anyone with your back turned on the Truth."

Hadley's feet were swinging nervously beneath the tablecloth, brushing rhythmically against Renee's leg. She reached under the table and placed a hand on her knee to stop them.

"It is always more exhausting to fight something than to accept it," Issa said. "If you are ready to accept your fate, then I am here to help."

Renee noticed his wine glass was empty. She scooted her chair back and stood. "I'm sorry. I'm being a terrible hostess. Can I get you more wine?"

"No, thank you. I am fine."

Renee sat back down, closed her eyes and sighed. "It has been so long since I've tried to understand that I don't know where to begin."

"Begin where you left off."

"Where I left off?"

"When did you last stop looking for the Truth?" Issa asked.

Renee thought about a young girl, not much older than Hadley, walking along the ridge of a mountain. "As a child I was curious," she said. "I felt there was a world beyond my parents, beyond me, that was calling to me. That's why I walked into the snow that day. I looked up the face of that mountain, and it was like a door to another world telling me to enter. I wasn't afraid. I didn't even take my ski boots off. I just followed the path."

"Like me," Hadley said. "Like I followed the sidewalk to Issa."

"Yes," Renee said. "I suppose so. And then there he was, standing before me; like no man I'd seen before. I was sure it was he who had called me; that it wasn't another world at all but him and him alone who had called. When he died, my curiosity died too."

She looked at them all. "I suppose Ernest, then, is where I left off."

"To make a young girl think a man can be her entire world is careless," Issa said. "How Ernest would have loved that."

"How did you know him?"

"That is a long story for another time."

"But what does he have to do with all this?"

"He is holding you back. You have to let him go if you want to help your daughters."

"Let go of Ernest? But he's dead."

"Let go of what you believe him to be."

Renee scooted her chair back, scraping it against the floor. "How about the pie you brought? Perhaps some dessert will lighten things up."

She stood and hurried out of the room, collapsing onto a barstool in the kitchen and slumping over the counter.

A hand touched her back.

She turned and saw it was Issa. It was what she'd wanted, for Issa to follow her. To be alone with him.

"Why am I so afraid to let Ernest go?"

"You are confused," he said. "You don't know who Ernest is or what happened between the two of you. It is still too much of a mystery for you to let it go. You need to understand it first."

"And you can help me understand it?"

"It is the first part of your journey."

"Yes," Renee said. "I know you're right."

He looked at her with a soberness that reminded her of her father. How old was he?

A yawn rose in her throat. She covered her mouth.

"Perhaps we should have dessert before it gets too late?" Issa suggested.

"I know where you are now," Renee said. "I will come see you."

"And I look forward to your knock on my door."

51

Hadley
Cincinnati, Ohio

Things were changing, Hadley could feel it. It was more than the fact her mother had met Issa. It was a brooding chaos that hung heavy, like morning mist, about the villa.

I will shew wonders in heaven above, and signs in the earth beneath; blood, and fire, and vapor of smoke.

For the first time, Hadley sought out the spirits for guidance.

Quit being afraid, her father told her. *Fear overrides your gifts.*

She knows that, Mr. Ernest said. *She fears because she loves like I do.*

Hadley didn't think she was anything like Mr. Ernest, but she dared not tell him this.

You, my dearest, are more like me than you think, he said.

She always forgot the spirits could read her mind.

Her father's wings fluttered, and he said, *You think you're so special, Ernest, because you love life and all the earthly tragedy that goes with it. But how about the Truth? How about the peace that comes with that?*

You were nothing but a pawn on Earth, Mr. Ernest said. *What do you know of Truth?*

And you were nothing but a rebel.

Rebellion is juicy and full of the spice of life.

Her father turned away from Mr. Ernest and looked toward Hadley, his wings settling. *What is on your mind, child?*

"I want to remember," Hadley said out loud, surprising herself with her own voice.

Remember what?

"Remember *him*," she said.

Her father cocked his head to the side in curiosity.

She remembered Issa intermittently, like a strobe light. The memories arrived in a strong, bright vision and vanished as quickly as they came. In every vision, Issa had dark curly hair, his nose long and sharp. But in Austria he'd worn the clothes of a pauper, and in Laos he'd been dressed as a missionary. She remembered him best as a professor in Argentina, where each day he'd worn a navy blazer.

He'd always been kind to her, but in Argentina he'd played a larger role. He'd fathered her when her parents were killed. He'd built her a bunk in his office and she'd stayed with him for years. This memory had become quite clear. She remembered how they would sit by a fire in the evening and he would read to her, stories of faraway places and ancient people. He'd given her a book when she married and moved to a faraway land. In the new land, she'd buried the book as an old woman.

"The book!" Hadley exclaimed. "The little red book!"

She looked at the ghost and angel in excitement.

"Where is it?" she asked.

It was lost in the accident, her father said.

He was right. She had had the book with her at the accident and hadn't thought of it since, too caught up with death and her lessons with Issa.

"What did you think when I found the book?" she asked her father's angel, now perched on the dressing table.

That day, when you led me to the ground and pulled out that book, many things changed for me. Not only did I realize I should have been cultivating you all those years instead of Brett, but I realized I didn't want to. Everything I'd believed my whole life suddenly seemed ridiculous. You found something that represented a connection between another life and this one. You found part of the Truth I'd been searching for and you didn't have to pass any test or endure any initiation to find it.

A lot of good that epiphany did, Mr. Ernest said. *Now you're a dead.*

Being dead is only a problem for you. For me, I am finally awake.

And what will you do with this wakefulness? Mr. Ernest asked with a gray smirk.

I will support Hadley.

And after that? After she no longer needs you?

I will move on, increase my vibrations and see what's next. Or I will decrease them and return to the weight of the world. Why don't you do that, Ernest, if you miss it all so much?

Mr. Ernest floated to the window and gazed out at the gray skies.

You can't go back, can you? her father asked the ghost as he flapped down to the floor and stood in front of Mr. Ernest.

The ghost kept his back to them. But his thought was still revealed. That was the problem with being a ghost.

You have lost your power, the angel said. *Your hatred for death has lowered your vibration. You have nothing positive to manifest power from.*

Mr. Ernest nodded.

And the only way to get it back is to give up your obsession with human tragedy.

It seems that way, Mr. Ernest said solemnly.

Why here? Why Hadley?

Even in death you do not see the Truth, Mr. Ernest said.

What Truth?

That Hadley is as much my daughter as she is yours.

Hadley heard the door downstairs open and close. She welcomed the distraction. She didn't enjoy the two spirits fighting and she feared Mr. Mr. Ernest would cry soon. She wasn't interested in his anguish. She was happy. She'd remembered the book and was sure she would soon remember the stone and her ancestors.

I will for their sakes remember the covenant of their ancestors, whom I brought forth out of the land of Egypt in the sight of the heathen, that I might be their God.

She trotted downstairs to see who had arrived, leaving the spirits to their debate.

It was Jonas. He was looking for his coat. He'd left it behind the night before.

"Ah, here it is," he said, winking at Hadley and lifting it from the coat rack.

Hadley smiled back.

"Cat got your tongue again?" he asked.

She nodded.

He draped the coat over his arm and looked at her. "So, you can only talk around Issa, is that it?"

Hadley nodded.

He frowned. "Do you know what I think?"

Hadley shook her head.

He leaned toward her. "I think that's nonsense. I think you could talk if you wanted to."

And with that he gave her a quick kiss on her cheek and backed out the door.

52

Brett
Jekyll Island, Georgia

Brett opened the door to Mr. Emulius smiling at her. Behind her, Noel exhaled loudly. He thought she was wrong to question the Order and this unannounced visit would put him in a panic.

She opened the door wide to show *she* was not worried. "Mr. Emulius, I wasn't expecting you."

"My brother has sent me," he said, glancing over her shoulder at Noel on the couch.

"And your brother is?" Brett asked.

"Kham," he said, pulling his eyes from Noel. "Apparently he finds your questions admirable."

"So, the dark man has a name," Brett said, stepping back to let him in. "And, it seems, a brother."

Mr. Emulius stepped inside. "Your doubt concerns him. He's decided to speed up your induction."

"Oh?"

"He wants you to feel the power we can offer you."

"Why didn't he come himself?"

"He has more important matters to attend to."

"Do you always do his grunt work?"

"I never thought you'd consider yourself grunt work, Brett. What a nice change." He smiled at her and moved further into the apartment. "Humility becomes you."

He continued through the living room and stepped onto the balcony. "Come."

"Noel too?"

"Yes, please," Mr. Emulius said, his eyes scanning Noel's body. "The two of you are a pair now. You'll learn quicker together."

Noel stood, his anxiety gone. The shift in his stance, the return of his arrogant stature, pleased Brett, and she smiled at him as they joined Mr. Emulius on the balcony.

Mr. Emulius spread his arms wide to the sea and, with a dullness that didn't match his gesture, said, "All of this—the land, the water, the buildings—everything is malleable." He turned to them with a quizzical look. "Do you accept this?"

"Malleable?" Noel asked.

"Everything is composed of particles that, once understood, can be manipulated without touch."

"So, you're saying that by seeing objects as a configuration of molecules and atoms, we can move matter with our minds?"

"Yes," Mr. Emulius said. "Brett?"

"I'm listening," she said.

"Now then, I want you to pick something to concentrate on. Anything you want."

Brett chose a wave rolling in off the sea, a small curl of white moving toward the beach.

"Have you chosen?" Mr. Emulius asked.

"Yes," Noel said. "I've chosen the tree, there with the gnarly branches."

"And I've chosen a wave," Brett said.

"Now decide what you'd like them to do. If you could make your object do anything, what would you like it to do?"

Brett immediately wanted to see the wave curl the other way and move *back* into the ocean, where gravity insisted it couldn't go.

"Now focus on your object," he said, "And at the same time find the place inside you where life flows, that place where you feel all the power and joy of laughter and fucking and learning." He gave Noel a sassy look. "Then close your eyes, let the excitement grow and stay with it."

Brett knew this place within herself. Since she and Noel had been having sex, she was more aware of it. What used to spark randomly at her sternum lasted long enough now to awe her. But it was fleeting.

She pictured Noel the way she loved him most, standing naked in the French doors gazing out to sea, his shoulder against the door frame. An image of Eli came too, of him leaning against a wall in their favorite restaurant, waiting for her, watching her intensely as she entered. She remembered the feeling of his unspoken adoration.

With this thought, a light static began to crackle in her sternum.

"Keep your eyes closed and stay with the feeling," Mr. Emulius said, this time his voice closer to her. "I'm going to put something in your hand. Don't be alarmed."

Immediately a cool, smooth, object slid into her hand. It was slick and oily, strangely leathery. The buzz in her sternum disappeared and she opened her eyes.

The object was slightly longer than her palm and tubular, a shiny purple-gray. She wrapped her hand around it, finding despite its metallic look, that it was pliable. She looked at Noel and saw he had one too.

Mr. Emulius sighed. "I guess you weren't as ready as my brother thought."

Brett pulled her eyes from the objects. "Why?"

"Because you opened your eyes."

"I lost the feeling," she said.

"That's what makes me think you're not ready."

"Wouldn't anyone lose their concentration if someone slipped something strange in their hand?" Brett asked.

"Yes," he said. "Nearly everyone opens their eyes."

"Then it's normal," Noel said.

"I would've thought you'd both hope for more than normal." He looked from one to the other. "My brother hoped for more from you."

"Let's try again," Brett said.

"Yes," Mr. Emulius said. "Let's."

He removed the objects from their hands. "Now look at your item of manipulation. Picture what it is you want it to do. Close your eyes and summon back the excitement, the energy of life's greatest pleasures."

Why couldn't they do that with the objects already in their hands?

"It would be easier that way, yes," Mr. Emulius said. "But it's better for you to find the place and hold it than to let the lundicroix do it all for you. The less dependent you are on the lundicroix the better."

"You just read my mind," Brett said.

"No. *It* did."

Brett looked at the objects in his hand. "A lundi-what?"

"A lundi-*craw*. Now pick your item of focus, imagine what you want it to do and *close your eyes*."

She chose another wave and closed her eyes.

The lundicroix slid onto her palm.

"Keep focusing."

It began to grow warm.

"Let yourself be excited and stay with that excitement. Be in awe of the object you've chosen."

Brett contemplated the wave, appreciated it, saw it for the moving hydrogen and oxygen it was. The object vibrated and nestled into her hand and a hum grew in her chest, moved to her shoulders, her arms, her hands. Her eyes watered beneath their lids.

"Allow the object to harness your emotions. As it does, open your eyes, find your item of focus and fixate on it."

Brett opened her eyes and looked at the white caps on the water.

"Now picture it morphing, moving, whatever it is you want it to do, and don't take your eyes off it until it changes with your desire."

She found a wave coming into shore, but as she focused on it the humming diminished and her wave crashed and dissolved on the sand.

"Pick another wave," Mr. Emulius said. "Keep trying."

The object immediately began to cool, and Mr. Emulius removed it from her hand.

Brett closed her eyes and focused. The lundicroix was placed in her palm once more and the buzz of energy began again. But when she opened her eyes, it diminished instantly.

"You must make the feeling of your focus greater than the distraction of the outside world," he said, removing the lundicroix from her hand. "Keep trying. This time with your eyes open from the beginning. For some people, this helps."

Brett gathered her concentration once more, keeping her eyes open. She focused on the wave, became aware of the throat of its curve as it came down from the whitewash, and the angle it held against the wake of the water. She breathed deeply and created the feeling of excitement, willing it to gather and grow.

But the wave kept moving toward her, flattening until it was gone.

Beside her Noel slapped his hand on the railing. "Shit, I moved it! The tree bent. It bent away from the wind. I saw it bend!"

Mr. Emulius smiled. "Gorgeous, Noel. Absolutely gorgeous."

Brett blocked them out and concentrated on another wave. She fixated on the foamy thickness of the white cap, became aware of the crystals of water pressing together, moving against themselves, teaming with molecules. There was a sound to the movement, a sound that matched the breeze blowing past and the fast thump of blood in her veins. Exhilaration welled in her chest. The lundicroix arrived in her hand, instantly warming her palm. The crystals of water changed, the molecules moving to the beat of her pulse, swaying in equal motion. They condensed, rewinding bit by bit until the wave curled backward, moving away from her as the rest of the sea rolled in without it. Her breath expanded and a sensation shot from her abdomen to her heart, up through her throat and between her eyes, releasing a swell of static out the top of her head.

"Holy Mary, Mother of God!" She fell gasping into the railing. "What was *that*?"

"Did you feel that?" Noel asked from beside her. "Did you fucking *feel* that?"

She placed her hand on top of his and squeezed it as she watched the strange sight of her wave petering out and dissipating into the ocean it had come from.

"It will go as far back into the sea as you like," Mr. Emulius said. "All you have to do is keep practicing."

The lundicroix was cooling in her hand. She looked out at the sea, no longer able to see it as anything but the particles which made it. She remembered learning to read as a child and the day when she no longer saw the letters in a word as separate marks but instead saw the word as one entity. She could remember the speed at which she began to read after this and how clever she'd felt, how powerful. She looked past the veranda to the sand on the beach and the bricks of the sidewalk below. She took in the palm tree blowing in the wind. It was the opposite of when she was a child. Now she saw what the objects were made up of, instead of the object itself.

She focused her eyes on a chair on the other side of the veranda. She considered its shape, the simplicity of its structure. The lundicroix warmed and vibrated, nestling into her hand. She willed the chair to her, her body tingling as a bolt of energy shot through her spine. The chair scooted across the tiles and positioned itself behind her. She stared at it in disbelief before falling into it, exhausted.

"You found moving the chair easy, didn't you?" Mr. Emulius asked. "Easier than the wave?"

"Yes," she said.

"It was because you were holding the lundicroix at the moment of your desire. It can tap into the most miniscule plea within you and manifest it for you."

Brett watched as the other chair slid across the veranda and came to rest beside Noel. "Holy shit," he said.

"Yes, it *is* holy. The lundicroix is sacred. It shows us what we're capable of." Mr. Emulius walked across the veranda and looked out to sea. "*Now* do you believe in the Order?"

Brett stared at the churning ocean.

"Isn't this worth protecting?" he asked.

"It's worth the total of everything else," she answered.

"Then go get Hadley," he said. "Her ability goes well beyond this."

53

Sara
Paris, France

It was the evening of their fourteenth day at Germain's. Sara hadn't anticipated they would be there that long. She slumped in the kitchen chair.

"What're you grumpy about now?" Penny asked from across the table.

"I'm sick of being here."

"But we're learning so much!"

"I'm *not* getting it all," Sara said. "I'm a Mass, remember?"

"It's a lot for anyone to take in."

"The only part that's made any sense is that I was born stupid."

Germain came back into the kitchen with a wooden spoon in one hand and a bottle of wine in the other. He was making dinner. Apparently, they were going to have a visitor.

"Shall we continue our talk about the Sumerians?" he asked, holding up the spoon.

They looked at him blankly. They had been talking about the difference between cooking with a Merlot versus a dessert wine when he had left the room.

"Well, where did we leave off?" he asked.

They continued to stare at him. It had been nearly two weeks since they had spoken of the Sumerians.

"Well?"

"I don't remember," Penny said. "I think maybe we were talking about how they disappeared."

He began stirring the vegetables vigorously in the frying pan. "And what do you know about that?"

"There's no more written history about the Sumerians after 2,000 BC," she said. "But there were individuals after this time who tried to keep the Sumerian legends and the stories about the gods alive."

"And who were they?" he asked, flicking the vegetables back and forth, the oil spitting and crackling above the skillet.

"Moses, the Egyptians, the Greeks, Buddha, the Gnostics, Jesus." Penny listed them quickly. "They all knew something they were trying to share and teach, something that led back to the Sumerians."

"Yes," Germain said as a piece of red pepper landed on the wall behind the oven. "After the Sumerians, the Great Sages reigned."

"That was the third era wasn't it? The Era of the Sages. But what about the first two eras? What happened in the those? Who were the Sumerians and where did they disappear to?"

"The second era, the Restoration, is when the Sumerians lived." Germain turned around and waved the spoon at them. "But more important than the Sumerians are the Anunnaki. Nothing will make sense until you understand them. And to understand the Anunnaki, we must go to the first era, rightly called the Beginning."

"Are you finally going to tell us about them?" Penny asked.

"Who do you *think* they are?" he asked, winking.

"Gods of some kind. But obviously not any kind of god we've been taught about."

"The *traditional* idea of God," he said, closing his eyes and sniffing the steam above the skillet, "is not completely fictional."

345

He opened his eyes and sprinkled some pepper. "The belief in a monotheistic being that can communicate and control people through creating respect and fear is real. God has been portrayed over the years in this way for a reason. Can you pass me the turmeric on that shelf?"

Penny went to the spice rack and ran her finger along the spices.

"The more eastern, new-age vision of God as the Great Universal Energy—all knowing, omnipotent, loving, always and forever constant—is *also* true," he said, taking the turmeric from her and sprinkling it on the vegetables. "These are the main two views of God, and if you read Genesis, you will see there is clearly a reference to both a controlling, human-like God and a universal energy-like God. My point is, they are two completely different things. The lack of differentiating between the two, in fact the biblical *amalgamation* of the two, has caused much confusion."

The doorbell buzzed and Germain jumped and dropped the turmeric into the skillet. "Oh my, he is early," he said, picking the jar out of the vegetables. "Sara, can you let him in? Just pull the cord there on the wall behind the door."

Sara saw a faded green rope hanging behind the door and pulled on it.

"And the Anunnaki?" Penny asked.

Footsteps entered below and began up the stairs.

"The Anunnaki are the controlling human-like Gods," Germain said, turning back to the skillet. "They existed in the Beginning, and there were many of them." He put the spoon down and picked up a spatula.

"But what *were* they?"

"Looks like I've arrived before the good part!"

Penny's eyes brightened and a smile spread across her face.

Sara stepped out from behind the door to see Shane Rhodes, tanned and grinning in a bright orange shirt.

"Hello girls," he said. "Looks like you found Germain okay."

"Hello son!" Germain crossed the kitchen and wrapped his thick arms around Rhodes. "I was just starting the girls' next lesson. They have been so patient. You cannot rush these things though, can you?" He clapped Rhodes on the back and pulled him further into the kitchen. "Anyway, fantastic timing! How I have missed you!"

Penny held her hand out to Rhodes and he shook it. "Good to see you again, Penny."

"Sara," he said, putting his hand out to her.

"Why didn't you tell us it was *him* coming?" Sara asked.

"I thought I did?" German said. "Oh, maybe not. But surprises are nice, aren't they?"

"I'm sick of surprises."

"Sara!" Penny looked at Rhodes, embarrassed.

"Go on then," Rhodes said. "Don't stop the lessons. You were talking about gods."

"Yes, Shane, have a seat," Germain said. "I am sure Sara would love to pour you a glass of wine, and then we can continue our discussion while dinner is cooking. Or would you prefer a smoke?"

Rhodes waved his hand. "No, nothing for me. Do continue. I've been waiting years for you to tell me about the Anunnaki. Is today the day?"

"It is precisely why I invited you! But first, how have you been? Where have you been? Do fill me in on your journey."

"I've been staying in Massachusetts, teaching yoga in Provincetown. Yoga on my own doesn't seem to be as effective. It seems only when I teach that the memories are triggered."

"So, you are remembering more, are you? Fantastic! Absolutely marvelous! It is as I predicted then."

"Remembering what?" Penny asked.

"My past," Rhodes said. "I'm beginning to remember how I began."

"Does this have to do with living the Second Truth that you spoke of at the concert?" Penny asked. "I've thought a lot about that."

Sara rolled her eyes.

Germain went back to the stove. "We will discuss Shane's enlightening later. Regarding the human-like Gods we were just talking about, you must ask yourself where they came from."

"Mars," Sara said. "Just like everyone here."

Penny scowled at her.

Germain put up his index finger. "Hold that thought, Sara. And Penny, why don't you sit back down." He motioned to a chair with the spatula.

Penny pulled out a chair and sat.

He gave them all a familiar sideways glance to make sure they were listening before he continued. "Sara is very nearly right. During Earth's ice age, a group of beings, looking much like you, arrived on Earth."

"From Mars," Sara said, laughing. "I fucking told you."

"Not from Mars, Sara, and *do* watch your language."

Sara hadn't sworn in a long time. It felt nice.

"They came from Nibiru," he continued. "The twelfth planet in your solar system."

"So, I was right!" Sara said. "They're aliens."

"Yes, dear. But there is a lot of muck attached to the word *alien*. I prefer we do not use it. It creates terrible prototypical images. You will immediately think the Anunnaki are blue-green and bug-eyed." He chuckled. "The people of Nibiru, the Anunnaki, looked very much like you and I actually." He continued, unaware of the smoking and splattering behind him. "The Anunnaki journeyed to Earth five hundred thousand years ago as Earth and Nibiru came into proximity. You see, the Anunnaki needed an earthly resource and therefore had been planning their trip for many thousands of years, waiting for the planets to align. They also needed a place on Earth that had moderate weather and a good source of water for their basecamp. At the time there were only three options: Mesopotamia, the Indus River valley, and the Nile River valley."

"Mesopotamia," Penny said. "Iraq!"

"Yes, Mesopotamia is now Iraq."

"So, that's why our fathers went to Iraq?" Sara asked.

"You are correct again, Sara. The members of the Order are protective of Iraq because it is the place where the Gods landed. For a long time there was something there, something left behind, that the Order worked hard to keep veiled. That thing is gone now, but they still believe the Holy Land is their best chance of reconnecting with the Gods."

"What was left behind?" Penny asked. "Where did it go?"

Germain's head disappeared into the pantry. "I swear I had some fresh garlic," he muttered.

Rhodes looked from Sara to Penny and smiled.

"Are you just learning all of this now too?" Penny asked.

"About the Anunnaki, yes."

"You know what is so funny?" Germain chuckled, backing out of the pantry holding a garlic bulb. "They are killing people to protect access to something that is around them all the time. The Order thinks the Anunnaki are something much different than themselves, and that immortality is something much different than what it is, so they fail to see either when both are staring them in the face."

"I'm not following," Penny said.

"See how it feels?" Sara said.

"I think you may be getting ahead of yourself," Rhodes said.

"Ahead of myself?" Germain asked. "Well, ahead of you three probably. Okay, then, where were we?"

He turned down the burner, pulled out a chair and sat down. "Yes, there is much to explain before you will understand the irony of it all. Now, back to the story. When the Anunnaki arrived, there was only primitive human life. This was the time of Homo erectus."

"But the Sumerians weren't primitive," Penny said.

"The Sumerians came later. They were descendants of Homo sapiens, created by the Anunnaki."

"So, humans were made by God then," Rhodes said. "Like the Bible says."

"Made them how?" Sara asked.

"The Anunnaki created the first humans as workers and nothing more. Even though the Anunnaki were powerful beings, they were clunky on Earth. The physics here are different than on Nibiru. They could not work as fluidly as they were used to."

"Sorry, Germain." Rhodes interjected. "But what work did they have to do? You haven't told us what the Anunnaki came to Earth for."

"Oh yes, I do get ahead of myself, you are right. Nibiru had a large hole in its ozone layer, one much like what we are creating here on Earth, only much bigger. And the Anunnaki came to Earth to collect a unique material to patch this hole."

"Oil," Penny said. "That's why they picked Mesopotamia over the other two valleys."

"No, not oil. Gold. They came here to collect gold. Nibiru had plenty of oil but little gold. A clever Anunnaki, named Enik, had engineered a way to disperse tiny flakes of gold into the

350

atmosphere so it condensed and created a new protective atmospheric layer, but there was not enough gold for the project. Mesopotamia had the most gold and that is why they chose it over the Indus and Nile valleys. But even Mesopotamia did not have enough gold. After mining it all, it was only about ten percent of what was needed. So Enik moved further across Earth and began to mine in Africa and South America. There was a lot of gold to be found in these places, but the climates were harsh, and the work was hard. They needed help. They tried to capture and train the Homo erectus, but there were not enough of them and they were wild and unintelligent. So Enik decided to create a smarter, more docile creature by implanting Anunnaki sperm into a female Homo erectus."

Germain looked from one to the other before he said, "And he produced a Homo sapiens."

"And let me guess," Sara said. "They named the first one Adam."

"They did actually."

"So, Adam was the first test tube baby," Penny said.

Germain laughed. "In a way he was. Following in the footsteps of their ancestors, humans have learned to do the same. Humans can now create life in a laboratory. But in the beginning, humans could not even procreate. Enik created the first humans to be sterile."

The alarm went off on the stove. "Now, what was that timer for? Oh yes, the bread. Excuse me."

He got up and went back to the pantry. "Enik did not want the Homo sapiens reproducing and becoming pests." He came out with a long baguette. "But that did not turn out to be a good idea."

"Why not?" Rhodes asked.

"Because without the ability to procreate, the will to live was weak and the first humans did not live long. For the first two hundred thousand years, this is how it was. Humans were created in a lab and worked a short life until they died."

"Two hundred thousand years! How much gold did they need?" Penny asked.

"Two hundred thousand years passes quicker than you think." Germain put the bread in the oven, reset the timer and returned to the table. "Let me go back a bit. The Anunnaki were here under the supervision of two brothers. Enik, the engineer I mentioned earlier, and his brother, Enlil. During this time, Enik was constantly creating and recycling humans, but he could not keep up with demand, so eventually he manipulated their genetic code so they could reproduce. This proved clever at first, for they began breeding and living longer and the work continued much faster, but eventually a new problem arose. Can you guess?"

"The Anunnaki began consorting with the humans," Rhodes said.

"Consorting?" Penny asked.

"Fucking," Sara said.

"Really, Sara. There are better words," Germain said. "But, yes, I suppose that's the gist of it. And, obviously, it was not long before children were born half Anunnaki and half human."

"So, the Gods and the humans were mating?" Penny asked.

"That's totally *lit*." Sara said. "They never taught us that in Sunday School."

"Oh, but they did!" Germain clapped his hands together. "Shane, go get the Bible in the lounge. You know where it is."

Rhodes stood and Penny watched him go, her eyes lingering after he'd gone.

Sara slapped her knee. "I was right about the aliens, wasn't I? *And* the fucking."

Penny ignored her and turned to Germain. "So, saying this is all true, wouldn't these offspring be three-fourths Anunnaki? I mean the Homo sapiens, the humans, were already half Anunnaki since they were made from their sperm."

"Yes and no. Physically the humans, although considerably smaller, were similar to the Anunnaki. But they had no Omega blood cells, so mentally and spiritually they were inferior. Enik did this on purpose. Red and white blood cells kept them alive, but Omega cells would have allowed them to deliberate and dream. Deliberation and dreaming are the seeds of power. They would have allowed humans to tap into the great power of the universe. It is these Omega cells that separate a human and an Anunnaki."

"Why didn't he want them to have power?" Sara asked.

"Empowered people won't work as slaves," Penny said.

"Got it," Rhodes said, returning with a Bible. "What verse?"

"Genesis 6:4."

Rhodes sat down and opened the book, flipping the thin pages until he found the verse with his finger. He began to read. "The Nephilim were on Earth in those days, and also afterward, when the sons of God went to the daughters of humans and had children by them. They were the heroes of old, men of renown." He looked up at Germain. "Why don't I remember that verse?"

Germain shrugged and smiled. "Not often one they use in sermons, which is good because it is wrong. It was not the sons of God with the daughters of humans. Anunnaki are androgynous. They are not male or female and they consorted with both male and female humans."

"Why didn't the Bible just say that then?" Sara asked.

"Because humans have forever been fixated on gender, obsessed with having a dominating gender and a submissive gender. The thought of human males being *taken* by a God was unacceptable. All books are a product of their time."

Germain looked at his watch. "Dinner is nearly ready. Shall we eat?"

Sara had forgotten about the food and noticed the room was filled with the wonderful aroma of cooked meat and freshly baked bread. Her stomach growled.

"You girls set the table. I will serve it up," said Germain, moving back to the stovetop. "Shane, can you hold this skillet?"

Sara was happy to move on to something as straightforward as eating dinner. She went to the cutlery drawer and took out four knives and four forks. The silver sparkled in the candlelight and Sara watched it shimmer. Since their day in Paris, she often noticed small, sensual details that had previously eluded her.

Penny was still sitting at the table and Sara placed the cutlery and mats around her.

"Are you okay?"

Penny blinked and looked at Sara dumbly.

"This is the Truth you were waiting for, isn't it?"

Penny nodded, her eyes glazed.

"Come, sit and let us pray!" Germain said, setting steaming plates of meat and vegetables on the table.

He sat down and put his hands out to Penny on one side of him and Sara on the other, turning his palms upward. "Let us hold hands and give thanks."

Sara put her hand in his, her palm immediately warming. A light static moved up her arm, and she was overcome by the smell of the food and the coziness of the room and the soft music floating from the lounge.

"Amen," Germain said, letting go of her hand.

She opened her eyes to the vibrant greens of the vegetables and the bright pink of the meat. She wasn't sure if a prayer had been said or not.

Germain began to cut the roast. "Now eat, my friends."

"So, this is the First Truth then?" Penny asked.

"The beauty of food and good company? No. That is an element of the Second Truth, dear. It is a shame it is such a secret!"

Rhodes laughed.

"I mean the fact humans come from the Anunnaki," Penny said. "Who are a group of beings who came from another planet."

"Oh, yes, that is the First Truth. But like I said to you before, the Second Truth is much more important." He passed the bread to Rhodes. "The funny thing is that the Order thinks the Second Truth is all about immortality. They think the Anunnaki were immortal and are obsessed with becoming immortal themselves. What they do not understand is that immortality is determined by the ability to raise your energy to the highest vibrations, which only a few Anunnaki have ever achieved. And the only way to do this is through appreciation and love and beauty, which are the elements of the Second Truth. It is these essential things that elude the Order." He pushed a piece of meat onto his fork with his knife. "They do not understand that the only way to be immortal is to stop *wanting* to be immortal and learn to appreciate what is in front of you."

He held his empty fork in mid-air, eyes alight with excitement.

"Don't you see how fantastically ironic it all is? You only get what you want when you stop needing it!"

Sara shrugged and bit into her meat, closing her eyes and savoring the taste of garlic and butter and tomato mixed with the salty, blackened beef. She wasn't sure of the irony any more than she was sure of the story.

54

Brett
Jekyll Island, Georgia

Brett and Noel had talked about little but the lundicroix since Mr. Emulius had left them on the veranda the previous day.

They'd sat in silence for over an hour before Noel had brought her a cup of tea and they had begun discussing the feeling of the lundicroix in their hands. What was it made of? How could it be warm and fleshy, cool and metallic all at once? They discussed how its temperature changed with the intensity of the power. Was it *reacting* to the power or was it a catalyst? And then there was the ecstasy, the rush, the release of the telekinesis. What was that? They couldn't explain the feeling.

Many questions followed that evening and the next day. Where did it come from? How many were there? Would they be given one? What would they do if they had one at their disposal?

Now Brett sat with the dark man. He had summoned her to his office, and she was seated, once again, across from his figure in the shadows. One of his hands was exposed on the desk, the palm facing upward, a vein in his wrist pulsing in the light of the lamp. Her eyes followed it to the pale inside of his forearm and to the shadow where his arm disappeared.

"So?" he asked from the darkness. "How did you find your most recent lesson?"

"It was amazing," Brett said. "What *is* the lundicroix?"

His hand closed, the knuckles whitening.

"You haven't even said thank you and you're asking for more. I'll answer *one* question," he said, his hand unfurling. "But after that, we must move to action."

"When do I get a lundicroix?" she asked, quicker than she had meant to.

He reclenched his hand. "My, my. All the information in the world available to you, and all you can think of is getting your hands on that clever little instrument."

"Yes."

"You don't *get* a lundicroix. They aren't something we hand out like grandfather clocks. The lundicroix is an instrument for growing our power, and it must be used in a controlled environment." He massaged his thumb with the nail of his forefinger. "And besides, we only have seven."

She stared at his fingers, the nails like smooth pistachio shells. She wished she'd made her question a request to see his face, to look him in the eye.

"Brett, are you listening?"

She looked into the darkness and nodded.

"Power has the ability to destroy its creator. A lundicroix is a dangerous thing. You're nowhere near cultivated enough to have one at your disposal. Besides, could you imagine what would happen if one of the Masses got their hands on one?"

Brett blinked. "Why would a Mass get their hands on it?"

"If we hand them out like chewing gum, it will eventually happen."

"But a Mass couldn't do anything with it, could they?"

His hand disappeared into the shadows. "Don't underestimate a lundicroix."

"But I thought the lundicroix was tapping into *us*, into our blood. It seemed so, so *organic*."

"Well, you thought wrong."

"You mean people without Omega blood cells can learn to manipulate matter?"

"With the lundicroix they can."

His hand returned, sliding forward on the desk palm down, dark hairs on olive skin.

She wished he would come out of the light and face her.

"Speaking of Masses, we must do something about your sister Sara. She's becoming more of a problem than we'd given her credit for. That's why I've asked you to come here today."

"*Sara?*"

He stretched his arm further across the desk, the other joining from the dark. He twisted one wrist, revealing the inner side of his elbow. "She seems to be following closely in your father's footsteps."

Brett stared at the smoothness of the underside of his arm, noticed how it browned toward the sides. "And what were my father's footsteps exactly? I don't know his story."

"After your father's first week on the island, he was sent away."

"Because he was a Carrier Clone?" Brett asked, interrupting.

"Yes, that is correct. And we made sure he was comfortable and felt important. We got him a well-paid government job and he bred for us, as is customary."

"But he was never told any of the Truth."

"No." His left index finger rose. "No, Carrier Clones don't learn the Truth."

"And I'm guessing he didn't like that?" Brett asked.

"No, he didn't. He was determined to find it out on his own."

"Surely he wouldn't be the first."

"No, many do. We didn't have a problem with his determination to learn the Truth. It happens, and sometimes it can even prove a person's worth and loyalty goes beyond their Omega cells. But your father decided to take what he found to the Masses. He could have come to us. He could have used his determination *here*, demanding to know the Truth, showing he had what it took. But instead, he acted like a typical Carrier Clone. He became overcome with anger and fear and stopped using his intellect. He quit tapping into the authority channels and became careless. He *had* to be stopped. Surely you understand the Masses can't know the Truth?"

"I don't know," Brett said. "I don't know what the Truth is."

"Your father was going to tell them about our ancestors," he said, moving his hands so they lay outside hers. "He was going to give them proof of their existence, and now your sister is trying to do the same."

"Sara doesn't have the ambition for such a thing."

"She's aligned herself with ambition."

"Who?"

"A friend of hers, Penny Weishaup."

Brett shrugged. The name meant nothing to her. "And what would happen if the Masses were told?"

"A theatrical announcement will do nothing but cause disorder. If the Masses want to know, they can. The Truth is discoverable. Not having Omega cells means they'll have to work harder than we do to learn it, to grasp it, but there are many ways to the Truth."

"You're saying they don't deserve to know."

"Brett." He leaned into her as he said her name, teasing her with wisps of his goatee. "Most Masses wouldn't do anything differently if they *did* know. They'd still eat, defecate, and complain."

"Some might embrace it, though. You never know."

"Maybe," he said, falling back into the darkness. "But I promise you, this precious power you've discovered would be diminished if everyone knew about it."

"But the power is dependent on the lundicroix, and there are only seven, so what's there to fear?"

"The power created by the lundicroix is not dependent on the instrument. Telekinesis is possible without the lundicroix. We just haven't figured it out yet. That's why we try to use it as a teacher instead of a portal."

"Okay, fine. But let's not kid ourselves. Regardless of what would happen if Masses knew about it, we're concealing this power because we're greedy. Nothing more. Nothing less."

"And how do you feel about being greedy?"

"I feel fine about it."

"Perfect. Then you won't mind getting rid of Sara for us."

"What do you mean by *getting rid* of her?"

"Killing her."

Brett swallowed then quickly asked, "Why me?" to mask her surprise.

"You've tested us since you arrived. You've questioned and pushed boundaries. We've shown you the lundicroix. Now you must prove your loyalty and your ability."

"Ability to murder?"

"Ability to do what's necessary."

"A man I've never laid eyes on is ordering me to kill my own sister."

He adjusted himself in the darkness.

"Your name is Kham. That's an uncommon name. Is it Hebrew?"

She waited for him to answer but he didn't.

"And your last name is different than your brother's."

She waited for him to answer.

"We have different fathers," he said finally. "Why the interest?"

"I need to know who I'm working for."

"You're working for the Order."

"Yes, but *you* are the one giving the orders." She stood and put both her hands on the desk and leaned into the darkness. "You're asking me to *kill* my own sister. Surely there's integrity in looking a person in the eye during such a request?"

She could hear his breathing, soft and steady.

"I want to see you in the light. I want you to look me in the eye when you ask me to kill my sister."

"I told you that would come only after you bring us Hadley."

"But you've placed a new demand."

"Sit down," he said, standing so his figure loomed over her in the darkness.

She backed into the light but stayed standing.

"I think you should sit down."

"No," she said. "I'll stand."

"It's for you I suggest it," he said, his full goatee coming into the light, his lips appearing, thin and brown with bright pink at the line of his mouth. "It's better if you do."

"I'm fine," she said.

His nose appeared, long and straight, then his jaw, solid and square. His cheekbones came next, chiseled so the light cast a hollow in his cheeks. "I hope you prove stronger than the rest," he said, bringing his eyes into the light.

They met hers with a fierceness she hadn't expected: green like a panther, lashes black and long. His lips curled into a smirk above perfect white teeth and his thick, black eyebrows drew together in an arrow above his nose.

Lightening rushed from her neck to the base of her spine. Her legs wavered beneath her.

He walked around the table, taller in the light and leaner than she'd imagined.

"We need you to terminate your sister Sara," he said looking her in the eye. "And we need you to do it soon."

She looked away. Was it the brightness of his eyes? His handsomeness?

"Okay," she said, bracing herself against the desk. "I'll do what you ask."

"You'll need lessons. You aren't ready yet."

"Will you send your brother again?" She kept her eyes downcast.

"My brother will no longer be needed now that you've seen my face. Now go," he said. "Before you fall over."

55

Hadley
Cincinnati, Ohio

Hadley watched Issa knead cookie dough, his forearms covered in flour as he hovered over the kitchen counter.

"How is it we know each other from a different life but while I'm different in each life, you are always the same?"

Issa wiped his hands on his apron and began to roll the dough with a wooden rolling pin. "How do you know I am always the same?"

"I remember you in different lives and you are always the same, but not me. My hair is sometimes red, sometimes black, my skin is often brown. Sometimes I'm tall and sometimes I'm small."

He looked at her, a hopeful shine in his eyes. "Do you remember such things?"

"Yes," she said. "More since you taught me to meditate."

He smiled and returned to his dough.

"Why do I change, and you don't?"

"I am enlightened, which means I continue to exist. I have only lived but one life."

"You've never died?"

He shook his head, rolling the dough so it spread thinly across the counter.

"And me?"

"Your form dies and returns anew with each life."

"Why can't I remember my lives clearly? Why do they only come to me in pieces?"

"The further you go on your journey, the more your memories will connect." He put the rolling pin down and picked up a cookie cutter shaped like a maple leaf. "You see, each life is a journey. This life, I think, may prove to be an extraordinary one for you." He pressed the cookie cutter into the dough and lifted it.

"Do other people remember their past lives?"

"Not many, no."

"How many do?"

"There are a few I believe will in time. I am not sure how many."

"So, why? Why me?"

He stopped cutting the dough and set the cookie cutter to the side. He wiped his hands on a towel and looked at her.

"You are different because, in your first life, you were born different."

"When was my first life?'

"One hundred and thirty lives before this one."

"That's a lot of lives."

"Yes."

"How was I born different?"

"You were born with high vibrations. Most people are doing well if they slightly increase their vibrations in a lifetime. But you," he smiled, "you were buzzing at birth."

"You mean the spirit I connect with when I meditate, I was born with this?"

"Yes. That is why it is more important you meditate than read the Bible. You see, God is in *you*, not in a book."

"Why was I born with these high vibrations?"

"Because you are a Prophet. One of the earliest Prophets ever born."

"Me? A prophet? But Jesus was the only prophet!"

Issa sighed. "He was not the only Prophet."

"I don't understand."

"Yes," Issa sighed again. "I fear it is too early."

"No! It's *not*. I *can* understand. I *will* understand. Please keep teaching me."

"Of course I will keep teaching you," he said.

"You say I'm a Prophet and that I'm different than others, and Jesus is different than me too, and you are different than me. So, what are you? What is Jesus? What are other people?"

"Yes, yes. Those are important questions." He picked up the cookie cutter and began to press it into the remainder of the rolled dough. "A Prophet is always a Prophet. So today, in this life, even though you may look different than in past lives, you are also a Prophet. This makes you different than other people because other people who are born into this world the first time as Talents or Carrier Clones or Masses do not keep their vibration into the next life. If they manage to reach a high enough level of vibrations though, they can be born as a Prophet in a future life, and once a person manages that, they will be born again and again as a Prophet. There is no going back."

"If they become enlightened, like you, you mean?"

"If they become fully enlightened, they will become much more than a Prophet. Being a Prophet only sets the foundation for enlightenment."

"But what does it mean to *become* a Prophet?"

"It means a person has raised their vibrations enough that they change their physiology. They pass into a new way of living and dying. They are bumped up to a new level of the video game."

"And then they can remember past lives, like me?"

"Yes, but it takes many lives to become a Prophet if you were not originally born one."

He had exhausted the rolled dough and gathered the scraps into a ball.

"How many lives does it take for a Prophet to become enlightened?"

"No Prophet has yet," Issa said. "But I am thinking it is one hundred and thirty."

"And that's why I'm remembering?"

"I think so," he said. "I *hope* so."

"But why was *I* born a with higher vibration than others? Why was I born a Prophet?"

"Because it was in your blood at your first birth. You inherited it."

"I inherited what?"

"There is a pink blood cell, called an Omega cell, which predisposes a person to enlightenment. Prophets, and Prophets only, have three-quarters of their blood made up of Omega cells. This is the threshold for physiological change, for existential transformation. Omega cells create high vibrations, they open us to the portal of the Second Truth."

"And these Masses and Talents you mentioned, they have fewer Omega cells then? And what was the other one, a Clone? What do they have?"

"Half of a Talent's blood cell count is made up of Omega cells, it is a quarter for Carrier Clones. Masses are born with none."

"So, a Mass can't become a Prophet, can't reach enlightenment?"

"None have yet, but they *can* raise their energy. They can change their vibrations. I think we will eventually see a Mass reach enlightenment. It may be thousands of years before it happens, but I believe it will happen."

"How would that be possible without the Omega cells?"

"Will alone can produce Omega cells."

"So, what're my sisters? My mother?"

"Your mother and your eldest sister are Talents. Your father was a Carrier Clone. Sara is a Mass. You are the only Prophet in your family."

"And what're you?"

"I have conquered the challenge of being both of the world and of the spirit. I am fully enlightened."

"Like Jesus?"

"No. Like I said, Jesus and I are different."

"So, what *are* you?"

"It is too early to explain that."

There was a yearning in his eyes that didn't match his words. She sensed he wanted to tell her.

"What is it? Why can't you tell me?"

He shot her a pained warning. She'd never seen his water-green eyes so dark.

"Tell me more about the gods of the Old Testament," she said, changing the subject. "The ones you said were vengeful. I understand the Great Universal Energy. I get that it's the love Jesus speaks of. But the other gods, what about them?"

If our gospel be hid, it is hid to them that are lost.

Issa put his cookies in the oven and set the timer. Then he went out on the deck and picked up his watering can and began watering the flowers. She followed him out and sat next to a cat on the picnic bench and rubbed it under its chin.

"So?" she asked.

"The gods of the Old Testament are not important. The Great Universal Energy is the only thing that matters."

"But you told me to read Genesis!"

"Yes, I suppose I did."

"I want to know who the gods were. Where did they come from? Are they still here? If not, why not?"

367

He sighed. "Curiosity killed the cat."

"But the cat has nine lives."

"Surely eight have been used up?"

"Apparently, one hundred and thirty have been," she said.

He laughed, his eyes lightening.

"Please?" she asked.

He nodded, surrendering to her questions. "The Gods were beings that came to Earth a long time ago, about two hundred fifty thousand years before Jesus."

"Where did they come from?"

"From a distant planet. They came to Earth in search of gold and created humans as laborers, to help them do the work."

"How many did they create?"

"Hundreds at first. Eventually more."

"They were the Nephilim that Genesis talks about?"

"Yes."

"Did they mate with humans like it said in the verse?"

"Sometimes."

Hadley watched one of the cats stalk a bird.

"Are you one of their children?"

"No," he said.

She nodded in disappointment. "So, who were their children?"

"Moses was one. And Noah too."

"Is that why they saved Noah during the flood?"

"Yes."

"What happened to these Gods? Where are they now?"

"They went back home."

"Why?"

"They got what they came for and were done with Earth."

"Did they all go?"

He shook his head.

"How many stayed?"

"Two."

"Only two?"

Issa nodded.

"Why'd they stay?"

"Because they loved the humans. One was old and tired. Earth made him feel youthful."

"And the other?"

"He fell in love with a human and they had a son together."

"Is that in the Old Testament too?"

"No. It is in the New Testament."

"Jesus."

"Yes."

"So, Jesus *is* the son of God!"

"No, he is the son of *a* God."

"Like Moses and Noah."

"Moses and Noah were born of a human and a God. Jesus was born of a Prophet and a God."

"A Prophet like me?" she asked.

"Yes."

The timer went off in the kitchen.

"Your cookies."

He nodded but made no movement toward the kitchen.

"I should go," Hadley said. "My mom said I had to be home by six."

"Okay," Issa said, sullen again.

"I don't want to go. You could call my mom and ask her if I could stay."

"No, no. You must go. Don't be late."

She started to leave.

Hadley

She turned around, surprised at the sound of the thought-voice. She didn't think the ghosts had followed her inside.

Do you still wish to die?

It was Issa, speaking to her with his mind. He looked vulnerable, strangely hopeful and scared.

Yes, she said with her thoughts, not sure if he would hear her or not. *I can't help it. Death was so beautiful.*

"As is life," he said out loud. "Do you want a cookie to take with you?"

He'd heard her! "You can speak to me like the spirits," she said.

"Yes."

"Why haven't you before?"

"Because you were not ready."

"It's because of our Omega cells we can speak like this?"

"Yes."

"So, you have them too!"

He nodded.

"So, our ancestry is the same!"

"Partly, yes. Now you get going. Your mother is waiting."

Hadley went to him and kissed his cheek.

Thank you for teaching me.

56

Renee
Cincinnati, Ohio

Renee didn't ask Hadley what the house number was. Mitcham Road wasn't a long street and she wanted to find the house herself. She knew it was a Tudor with flowers and thought that would be enough.

It was the cats, however, that alerted her to Issa's home. The first one strolled from a bush and pushed itself against her shins, rubbing its head into the cuff of her slacks. It was a large tabby.

"Hello, kitty," she said, bending to pet it, as another one, orange and white, came and nosed her fingers.

Seven cats, she remembered Hadley saying and looked up over the bush to see a brown brick Tudor half-shadowed by the setting sun. At the front door white orchids were bending in the breeze.

Orchids in Ohio? This is definitely the house!

Renee walked up the stone path, taking in the low line roof, the potted plants lining the windowsills and the white shutters shining in the late afternoon light. It was, indeed, a welcoming home.

The stones seemed familiar. A few feet from the front door, she knelt to get a closer look.

They're like Hadley's rock, the one she used to sleep with.

She looked up at the house. It loomed above her, the windows open, ready to reveal secrets she'd long denied existed.

She approached the front door.

She could hear music inside. Scarlatti's *Salve Regina*. It was his last composition, Renee's favorite.

She knocked.

"Coming!" She could feel the thud of socked feet.

The door opened and Hadley stood in front of her.

"Oh," Renee said. "Hello, darling."

"Hi, Mom."

Renee hadn't heard Hadley speak since dinner the previous week and was, once again, taken aback. "Your voice!"

Hadley smiled and nodded.

"I thought I asked you to go to the store?" Renee frowned.

"Oh, yes, sorry. I stopped here on my way. Come in."

"I came to talk to Issa," Renee said.

"He's in the kitchen making pasta. He makes it from scratch. He was showing me how."

"I'm not sure I'm happy about you stopping here when you were supposed to go to the store," Renee said. "You're only thirteen, Hadley. You should tell me if you're going to stop by somewhere."

"Mom, it's safe here."

"That's not the point. Maybe we should *both* go home and talk about this further."

"No, no. You must stay," Issa said, appearing in the entryway with a tea towel in his hands. "Hadley was about to leave."

"Yes, I'll go to the store now," Hadley said.

"And the pasta is done," he said. "I have just cleaned up. Come in."

Renee stepped inside and Hadley brushed by her and out the door.

"You go straight home after," Renee said.

Hadley nodded and skipped down the driveway.

Renee turned to Issa. "I apologize. I should have called first."

"There is nothing to apologize for. You are here and that's what matters."

She slipped her shoes off and pushed them against the wall "The house smells lovely. I didn't know pasta could smell so good."

"Oh no. That is bread you smell. I always bake bread on Sunday. The pasta was a specialty today. Now what can I get you to drink?"

"Just water please."

She followed Issa into the kitchen, where he gestured for her to have a seat at the table. She noticed an old-fashioned cat clock on the wall, its eyes moving back and forth.

"I am glad you came," he said.

"You were right the other night. I am searching for the Truth. But I'm fighting it too. I'm confused."

"It is quite amazing how long you have managed to fight the Truth," he said. "Some of us, due to our makeup, have a harder time avoiding it than others."

"Our makeup?"

"Our biological makeup." He sat her water on the table. "You see, spirituality is closely linked with biology."

"Spirituality?"

"The Truth is, naturally, of a metaphysical nature." He pulled out a chair across from her and sat down. "Getting to the Truth is a spiritual journey, one I have been guiding Hadley on. And you are biologically predisposed to this spiritual journey. As is your friend Jonas."

"Jonas?"

"Oh yes, Jonas too. Do you think your attraction to each other is random? Or that basketball playing of his? Or that fantastic writing of yours that you show no one?"

"How do you know about my writing?"

373

"I can see it all around you. Your talents are like music hovering about your body. Like Ernest. When you were a child you used to see his talents, like fog wrapped about him. Remember?"

"How can you know all this?"

"Before we get into it, would you like some fresh bread?"

"No, thank you. I could hardly eat."

He settled into his chair. "With you, we must start with science. You are a learned woman, a skeptic of spirit, right?"

"Yes, I suppose that's true."

"Would you also agree that revealing truths and explaining spirituality has always been the aim of science? When we do not understand something, we see it as mystical and godly. Once we have studied it and we can label its parts and processes, it becomes scientific and real. But it is still spiritual. Science simply gives us the language."

"I suppose," Renee said.

"You must first understand that you have a special type of blood running through your veins. Some call it the blood of God. Your blood consists of rare blood cells referred to as Omega cells. The few scientists who know of these, call them ingeniacytes."

"These ingeniacytes predispose you to the Truth. Not only do you see signs of the Truth all around you, but you crave the Truth. And somewhere deep inside you, you know the Truth as well. When it is revealed to you, it will feel more like retrieving a lost memory than learning a new concept. You see, the Truth is in your veins."

"Okay," Renee said. "I'm listening."

"Fifty percent of your red blood cells are Omega cells. You are what they call a Talent."

"Who is *they*?"

"Those who understand our ancestry and our blood."

"The Order."

"Not just the Order. There are others who know about this blood."

"I never thought the Order actually possessed any real knowledge. I thought it was a hoax used to create control."

"Is that why you resisted your upbringing?"

Renee traced her index finger along the ridge of a placemat. "I didn't want to spend my entire life working toward something that wasn't real."

"What made you think it was not real?"

"I saw my parents enslaving themselves to an idea. I saw no evidence of any Truth."

"What evidence did you expect to see?"

Renee continued tracing her finger along the placemat. "I would have expected them to be happy, healthy and kind, the things you would think Truth would bring. But they were none of these things."

"That is very insightful."

"Ernest had these things. To me, he had what everyone was looking for. *He* was the Truth."

Issa placed the palm of his hand over the back of hers, stopping her tracing. His hand was soft and warm, his touch fuzzy.

She looked up at him.

"Ernest was a very special man who embodied a slice of the Truth, but he was not the Truth itself."

"And he had these Omega cells?"

He lifted his hand from hers. "Yes. The number of Omega cells a person carries varies. Talents, like I said, have half Omega cells. Your daughter Brett is a Talent, as is Jonas. There are only a small number of Talents in the world."

"And Ernest?"

"Ernest is what they call a Prophet. He has three-quarter Omega cells. Human beings like Ernest are very rare. Hadley is also a Prophet."

Hadley is the same as Ernest?

"It is because of these Omega cells you and Jonas are so attracted to one another."

Renee blushed.

"Every molecule and cell emits a vibration of energy. The Omega cell has a higher vibrating energy field, and this makes it attractive. This heightened energy displays itself in charismatic qualities, and high vibrating cells attract each other, enhancing the intensity."

"And Sara?"

"Sara does not have any Omega blood cells. She will have little desire for understanding the Truth."

"How is it all determined?" Renee asked, curling a corner of the placemat. "I assume it's genetic?"

"This presence of ingeniacytes is an autosomal recessive trait. Depending on the parents, a child can be born with none."

"So, Scott didn't have any then?"

"Scott was a Carrier Clone. He had one-quarter Omega cells. Carrier Clones are often interested in the Truth but usually unable to grasp the metaphysics of it. Carrier Clones have the ability to pass them on, but only when they procreate with a Talent or a Prophet, and even then it is possible a child will be born with none."

"And you are a Prophet too. That's why you speak like Ernest and why I feel so comfortable around you, isn't it?"

Issa shook his head. "I am enlightened, whereas Ernest loves ego and passion and refuses to surrender to the Truth. He thinks if he becomes enlightened, he will lose the rush and drama of being human."

"You speak of him as if he's still here."

"He is here, now, standing behind you."

Renee let go of the placemat and it unfurled back to the table.

"You know it is true," Issa said. "You have always known he was there."

The burn of oncoming tears stung the end of her nose. She sniffed them away.

"And Scott?"

"Scott is not here. He stays with Hadley."

"And Scott knew all this? About the genetics?"

"It was not revealed to him. He discovered it."

Renee crossed her arms on the table and rested her forehead on them, sadness overcoming her. Scott had worked so hard to earn the Truth.

"Why didn't they tell him? I thought he was initiated."

"He was only initiated into Claw and Bones. Claw and Bones members do not learn the Truth. He was never properly inducted into the Order. Only some of the Order learn the Truth."

"And I suppose they killed him for discovering it?"

"They killed him because he was planning to expose it."

Renee lifted her head. "Expose what?"

"He and his friend found something the Order have been hiding for centuries and were going to alert the media."

"What did they find?"

"There are more pertinent questions, Renee."

"I *need* to know."

"And I will tell you. But there are other things you must deal with first."

She put her head back down.

"You know why you have come here today. You know what the first step to the Truth is for you."

Renee sighed and spoke into the darkness of the table. "To understand what I experienced with Ernest."

"Yes."

"I guess I was attracted to him because we share these Omega cells."

"You were especially attracted to him because he had *more* cells than you."

"But he loved me too, didn't he?" she asked, looking up.

"He loved the idea of a young girl being in love with him. He loved you as his last attempt to hold onto life."

"That would mean he didn't really love me."

"And you really loved him? Is it possible you only loved him because he made you feel special?"

"So, does anyone really love another then?" she asked.

"Only when one becomes fully conscious are they able to truly love another."

"So why is he here? Why doesn't he follow someone else?"

"Because you were his last, and because you were a Talent. He had not met a Talent before you. What he shared with you would have been more conscious and more real than what he'd experienced before."

"When he touched me, I filled with light," Renee said.

"Yes, Renee. That was real. Come here." He turned his hands face up and placed them in front of her. "Place your hands in mine."

Renee took off her glasses and wiped her eyes. She laid her hands in his soft, pink palms and he closed his finger over hers.

The lightness began as a warmness between her fingers and slowly spread to her wrist. It traveled up her arms, tingling at the curve of her elbow. It intensified at her shoulders, warm static massaging the curve of her neck. Then it reached her spine and ripped through her body in a wave of brightness.

They sat in silence until Renee finally said, "I feel this with Jonas too. Is it these Omega cells?"

Issa gently pulled his hands away. "It is the energy they create."

Renee nodded. "And Hadley? If she's a Prophet, why do I not feel this with her?"

"Hadley is young; the lightening develops with maturity."

"And the Order? They can create this lightening?"

"Not consistently. They have means to create the consciousness but not the love. Their power is shallow."

Renee looked at her hands. She hadn't moved them since Issa had taken his away. She thought of Ernest there in the room. She could sense him. Why was he still there when she loved Jonas now?

"Because you have not let him go."

"How did you know what I was thinking?"

Issa tilted his head and raised his eyebrows as if to say, *"Surely that does not come as a surprise?"*

"How do I let Ernest go if it's not by loving another?"

"By understanding what happened between you and him, the spell will break."

"So, what happened?"

Issa got up and went to the oven. He pulled the bread out and put it on a cutting board. "You tell me."

"We connected through the Omega cells. We *vibrated* together."

"Yes. That is what happened. Now, what did *not* happen?"

"He didn't tell me all of the Truth. He didn't know all of the Truth."

"And?" Issa sliced off the heel of the bread.

"Ernest was only a beautiful part of something much bigger. There's much more than Ernest."

Issa nodded and sniffed the bread, closing his eyes.

"And I've been entranced by him because I thought nothing would ever compare."

Issa smiled, breadcrumbs in the corner of his mouth. "Exactly."

"And you say Jonas has these Omega cells, that he's a Talent like me?"

Issa nodded, opening his eyes.

"Then I don't want to learn any more of the Truth without him."

"He is ready to learn, Renee. He is waiting for you."

57

Sara
Paris, France

It was a beautiful day, cold with clear skies and a bright sun. Sara, Penny, and Germain sat on a park bench a few blocks from Germain's apartment, warming themselves in the sun and enjoying the smell of burning wood coming from nearby chimneys.

Rhodes was there too. The night before, Sara had dreamed he'd left but awoke to find he was still there.

"You mentioned Anunnaki and humans can become enlightened," Penny said to Germain. "You said it was possible by giving up greed and pride."

"Yes."

"Is that what you've done, Shane?" She looked behind her at Rhodes standing in the sun. "To live the Second Truth?"

"One of the things, yes. I've been visiting Germain for five years now. He's been teaching me the laws of the Second Truth."

"Is he always so painfully slow with sharing?" she asked, laughing.

Rhodes smiled. "He's always insisted on days of normality between his great teachings. I think that is part of the lesson."

"What about you?" Penny asked, turning back to Germain. "When did you become enlightened?"

"Around 20,000 BC," he said. "After the great floods."

"Twenty thousand BC!" Penny exclaimed. "So, you were alive when the Anunnaki were here on Earth?"

"Oh yes, very much so."

"How the hell do you think he knows all of this?" Sara said. "Of course he was alive then, probably as a frog."

Penny glared at her.

"By the great floods, do you mean the forty-day flood in the Bible?" Rhodes asked.

"Yes, that flood. The flood like no other."

"Did the Gods create the flood as the Bible says?" Penny asked.

"They did not create it, but they utilized it. Anu, the king of the Gods back home, was not happy with the creation and existence of humans. He wanted Earth left as it was found. He believed the humans were unnatural, that they would alter the ecosystem. And he knew the imminent realignment of Nibiru and Earth would bring great climatic changes that would wipe out humans. He wanted the Anunnaki to allow nature to take its course. But Enik and Enlil could not do as Anu wished. To wipe out life on Earth, life they had created and seen flourish and grow, life that was spawned from Anunnaki DNA, was unthinkable to them."

He paused, closing his eyes and lifting his face to the sun. "Enik and Enlil had great compassion for the humans."

"So, what did they do?"

"They warned a human and instructed him to build a boat."

"Noah," Penny said.

Germain nodded.

"Why'd they choose him?" Rhodes asked. "What was special about Noah?"

"Noah was Enik's son. Enik had succumbed to the earthly temptation of the Homo sapiens and consorted with a human. Noah was his direct heir and had four children who were all were Prophets, which was rare. Noah and his family were, therefore, a logical choice as much as an emotional one."

"And what happened?"

"The floods came, like nothing I'd seen before. They began with rain, rain that fell for weeks. Rain that brought together rivers and lakes and oceans."

Rhodes rose abruptly. "I remember the rain," he said. "I remember the rivers rising. I remember animals floating, so many animals."

Germain stood and went to him. "Yes. That is right. You were there."

"I was alive during the floods?"

"Yes, you were."

"Did I survive them?"

"Yes, you did."

"What else do you remember?" Penny asked.

"I don't know," Rhodes said, walking away from them.

"Leave him to remember," Germain said, sitting back down.

"But I don't understand," Penny said, looking over her shoulder as Rhodes retreated. "Who is he?"

"Leave him to remember," he said again. "Now, where were we?"

"The floods came and wiped out the humans."

"Most of them, yes." Germain nodded. "And with them, the land was destroyed, thus marking the beginning of the second era, the Restoration. But while the land was reestablished during this time, the humans were pulled apart."

"Pulled apart?"

"You see, to rebuild the land, they had to farm. And farming brought land ownership, which slowly split the land into regions, and in turn, kingships were born. For thousands of years there was much fighting and war between the humans."

"And the Anunnaki, were they still there during this time?"

"Yes, but they were segregated. Anu forbade them from consorting with the humans, insisting they live separately. They were restless. They had the gold they needed, the humans were getting out of control, and the planets were getting closer. They were ready to return home."

"Even Enik and Enlil?" Penny asked.

Germain smiled. "No, Enik and Enlil loved the humans and they couldn't help but help them. One of Noah's descendants showed particular skills and they guided him, helping him to become a leader for peace and order, protecting him and his descendants where they could."

"Abraham," Rhodes said, returning. "The Bible says God promised to make Abraham the father of a great people and said that if Abraham and his descendants obeyed God, in return God would guide them and protect them and give them the land of Israel."

"Yes" Germain said. "And Abraham and his followers did just this. In 2,000 BC, they stopped the wars in Mesopotamia and created the first great civilization."

"Sumer!" Penny exclaimed.

Germain nodded and turned to Rhodes. "Do you remember the days of Sumer, son?"

"No." Rhodes shook his head. "But I know it was around 2,000 BC that Sumer disappeared, which coincides with the Bible's story of Lot's wife turning to salt. Some historians believe Lot's wife witnessed the annihilation of Sumer."

"Yes, they are one and the same. But it certainly was not salt," Germain laughed. "It was an explosion that took out Sumer. Lot's wife turned to see the civilization wiped out by a giant storm of radioactive fallout."

"A nuclear explosion?" Penny asked.

"Yes."

"Caused by what?"

Germain stood and yawned. "It was the exit of the Anunnaki that caused the explosion. Now come, it is getting cold. Let us return to the apartment."

He walked slowly across the street.

"And Enlil and Enik?" Penny asked, following. "Did they go back too?"

"No. They were in love with Earth, with the kin they had created."

"So they stayed?"

"The brothers worked alongside those that survived, as one of them, helping to rebuild again. Centuries passed and eventually no one knew they had once been Gods. For many generations, the Israelites passed along oral accounts of the ancient stories, while the Gods that lived on were overlooked. Finally, the stories were written down as the Old Testament. But the truth of Enlil and Enik, of the Anunnaki, died with Abraham."

"So, Enlil and Enik died on Earth?"

"No, they are still very much alive," he said, opening his front door and holding it aside so they could enter. "They are enlightened now, having mastered the perfect balance of Earth and spirit."

The four of them clambered up the stairs single file.

The fire had burned to red embers. Germain stoked the ashes and added a fresh log.

"So," Penny asked. "They are still here on Earth?"

"Who dear?" Germain asked, lowering himself into his chair.

"Enik and Enlil."

"Oh yes." He lay his head back and closed his eyes, immediately beginning to snore.

Penny looked at Rhodes. "He's one of them, isn't he?"

"I'm beginning to think so," Rhodes said.

Penny stared at Germain. "A living God, sleeping here in front of us."

"*Snoring* in front of us," Sara said. "Hardly looks like a God."

"He would argue that he isn't a God," Rhodes said, pulling a blanket from the back of the couch and draping it over Germain's shoulders.

"Which one do you think he is?" Sara asked. "Enik or Enlil?"

"No idea," Rhodes said, shrugging.

"And what about you, then?" she asked. "What's your story?"

"My story is only just unfolding."

He moved to the fire and lowered himself to the carpet, gathering his legs beneath him and sitting cross-legged, facing the flames.

"Unfolding how?"

He gazed into the fire for a while before saying, "For years I had memories I didn't understand. Glimpses of lives I'd led but couldn't recall. Lately I've been remembering them."

"What do you remember?"

"I remember myself in jungles," he said to the flickering fire. "In rocky valleys, in cities gray with smog. I remember myself tilling land, and as a scholar of law. I remember myself young and dying, and old and vibrant. And today," he said, pausing. "Today I remembered the floods. I remembered how it all began."

58

Hadley
Cincinnati, Ohio

Hadley couldn't stay away from Issa, not now that they could speak without words. She'd always felt they were connected. Now she had proof.

You have been speaking to me without words for months but that hasn't made you happy, Mr. Ernest said glumly from above her as she strolled down the sidewalk toward Issa's.

But you're a ghost.

What's the problem with that?

Hadley shrugged. *You are always depressed.*

I was once full of life, you know. I was once a powerful and capable man.

Issa's house came into view and Hadley quickened her pace with a skip.

Well, you aren't anymore.

I chose death, he said. *You and I have that in common.*

She stopped skipping and looked at him.

I love death, he continued. *You love death. We are the same.*

She shook her head. *No, I live but long for death. You are dead but long for life. We're the opposite.*

We are more alike, you and I, than you know.

A vision came to her of Mr. Ernest standing in the rain, his hair matted to his head and shoulders hunched against the cold.

She was standing in a puddle. She could feel the cool water over her toes and the splatter of drops against her ankles.

The rain began to ease, and the clouds thinned behind him. A sliver of blue spread across the sky, filling Hadley with joy. He leaned down and picked her up, his eyes full of love and hope, and twirled her in the rainless air. Together they erupted with joyous laughter.

59

Brett
Jekyll Island, Georgia

Brett sat with Noel on the balcony. It had been five days since she had left Kham's office. She had told Noel about the discussion and what was asked of her, but she hadn't told him about seeing Kham's face. She was worried what he might see in hers if she did.

For she woke each morning with Kham's face against her eyelids, his smirk imprinted on her brain. Throughout the day he consumed her thoughts. She could taste him when she ate, smell him when she showered, hear him when others spoke. She prayed at night that something might come and slice him out of her head, release her of the fixation. But given the choice, she wouldn't give it up. The craving was a rush, a thrill that had brought new life.

"I can't believe they want you to kill your sister," Noel said.

"Well," Brett said. "I didn't work my whole life to join a group that doesn't *act*."

Noel looked at her. "A month ago, they asked you to bring Hadley to them and you worried about it night and day. Now they want you to kill Sara and you're okay with it?"

"So now *you're* the skeptic."

"Murder adds a new dimension to things."

If only she could tell him murder was not new for her, albeit indirectly.

"One day they might act *against* us," he continued. "Has that crossed your mind?"

"They won't touch us. We're Talents. They spend all their resources trying to find us. They're not going to get rid of us easily. And anyway, I'm not interested in the alternative."

"Which is?"

"Living on the outside."

The congregation siren went off. Its low hum rising through the afternoon air.

Brett looked at Noel and raised her eyebrows. "They're calling."

The assembly hall was full when they arrived, the oldest members seated in front and the youngest members standing along the back wall. She and Noel were ushered in with the other new initiates and led to an empty row of chairs in the second row.

As they sat down, the lights dimmed, and a large screen dropped from the ceiling. A blue and purple planet appeared, slowly rotating toward them until it consumed the screen.

A familiar deep voice began to speak. "Four billion years ago, a wayward planet called Nibiru entered this solar system and collided with a large planet called Tiamat, causing it to crack and fragment." The animated planets appeared as a reenactment, showing the collision.

As the screen lit up the room, Brett searched for Kham. She found him standing in the shadows to the right of the screen. Next to him was Mr. Emulius.

"Some fragments from Tiamat remained in its original orbit. Today they are our asteroid belt. The largest fragment of Tiamat was propelled into a new orbit closer to the sun. Over time this fragment changed and morphed and eventually became Earth. One of Nibiru's moons accompanied this fragment and is now our own moon and satellite. Five hundred thousand years ago, the people of

Nibiru journeyed to Earth as the two planets approached each other. They were called the Anunnaki.

"Their initial landing was in Mesopotamia, known today as Iraq. The combination of archeology and ancient Sumerian texts gives us more than enough proof these facts are true. But as further proof, one of the Anunnaki ships remains in Iraq, in the Holy Land." The screen showed a photo of a large, egg-shaped structure with a purple, rock-like base, sitting in a vast dessert. The coloring of the object was like a lundicroix, its texture equally difficult to define.

"Most of the world's leaders know about the Anunnaki and about this precious artifact. And all who know about it protect this site and this knowledge with their lives. Now you neophytes must do the same. For this power you have begun to experience has been given to us by the Anunnaki. We, all of us here in this room, are their children. Our Sumerian ancestors were the product of the Anunnaki, and their blood still lives in us today through the Omega cells we carry."

Brett pictured Kham's cutting green eyes, his lewd smile and long legs that glided him across a room.

He oozes Omega cells.

"In the Sumerian times, the Anunnaki lived with us and helped us build great cities and architecture. The evidence of this is everywhere, from the Nazca lines to the great pyramids, from Stonehenge to Easter Island, and through stories passed down from our fathers' fathers; stories that we'll share with you." His hands came into the light and gestured to the expanse of the room. "But since the Anunnaki left, four thousand years ago, we have been on a slow decline, fewer and fewer people being born with Omega cells and less and less in touch with our power.

"In the last few centuries, through strategic breeding, we have started to grow again in numbers and are learning more and more how to harness our ancient power via these tools. But we're advancing slowly. We are only just discovering now things that were second nature to our ancestors. There's much we still don't understand. We believe the quickest way to return to this power is to reconnect with our ancestors, the Anunnaki. And we believe our main chance at contacting them lies in this ship."

The previous screen zoomed in on the egg-shaped object, accentuating its odd purple-brown color.

"At the moment, our power is dependent on tools left here by the Anunnaki. Tools that we'll soon show you and teach you how to use."

So, the other initiates haven't been shown a lundicroix yet! Brett smiled. Still first in the class.

"We'll show you the power capable when we align with these tools, but the answer isn't to be dependent on the tools. We must learn how to harness the energy of our Omega cells without the tools, and we must gather enough Prophets and Talents to combine our energies in an attempt to gain the Anunnaki's greatest power."

He paused.

"The power of immortality."

He paused again, the room deathly silent.

When he continued, his voice was deeper and he spoke slower. "All the great scientific discoveries have led us closer, but the Masses pose a threat; they slow us down with their prying. We need order. We can't tolerate distractions. It is everyone's job to make sure there are no more setbacks."

Mr. Emulius stepped forward. "We must keep this power, and the tools that make it possible, a secret." His voice, soft and high-pitched, was a distinct change. "If the Masses obtain access to the tools, or obtain knowledge of our power, it will sabotage our development."

"Throughout the years," Kham continued, "Masses have discovered the existence of the Anunnaki and have, understandably, been angry this knowledge was hidden from them. Many times they have retaliated, and once they managed to destroy something we had spent decades preserving."

The video fast-forwarded. Scenes flashed quickly across the screen, creating a sequence of history. The first was of a silent black and white filmstrip. Brett recognized the scenery as Jekyll Island. There was shooting and bloodshed. The rest of the images, except one in the middle of New York City in the 1930s, were set in the desert. The most modern footage took place around a large steel contraption embedded in the sand. It was smooth and cylindrical and the same metallic purple-gray as the ship. People in the video collected around it, pointing cameras and weapons at it. They yelled at each other frantically. It was hard to tell what they were doing. There was a flash of fire on the screen and the metallic object began to smoke and turn a copper color. Then it exploded, shrapnel shooting in all directions.

"What you just saw destroyed was a giant lundicroix," Mr. Emulius said. "An Anunnaki instrument, an all-seeing telescope, an emotional compass."

A murmur began in the room.

"It was a highly sophisticated and powerful version of smaller tools we'll be teaching you to use," Kham said. "We call them lundicroix as well. But the giant lundicroix, the *only* giant lundicroix, was destroyed. Gone forever due to the meddling of commoners."

Brett sat back in her chair and stared at the blank screen.

A giant lundicroix! She could imagine what it would have been capable of. She thought about Sara. What stupidity had she become involved in?

She looked at Kham's tall figure in the shadows, imagining his cat eyes beneath his angled brow, her sternum swelling with resolve.

I will stop her.

60

Renee
Cincinnati, Ohio

Jonas's sweet-leather smell was still in the room, a ring of moisture on the bedside table from his coffee glistening in the pale light. He had left while the sun was setting, and now it was dark, the only light a sliver of yellow from the half-open door.

But Renee was not alone. Ernest was there. She could feel him quivering in the stillness.

Look at me

His voice was a thin version of what she remembered.

Acknowledge me

She moved her eyes toward his voice. He was at the end of the bed, his image blurry, misty.

With the sight of him came his scent. She breathed in the old, rustic smell, her body growing heavy with remembrance.

She felt no fear, only sadness, and focusing on a strength deep in her sternum, she willed him to her, a dense vapor rising and swelling as she exhaled, her body pulling forward with the power of it.

He was near her now, his hands on her face, huge and calloused, his form coming into focus as she relaxed.

The wrinkles around his eyes were as she remembered them, like crevices in a dry lakebed, his whiskers leftover salt. She placed her mouth on his cheek and tasted him. Even in death he tasted like the earth.

He wrapped the weightless bulk of his arms around her and she embraced him, quivering as she had at fourteen, seeing for a brief moment how it was all the same, then and now, fourteen and fifty-nine, alive and dead.

His breath was in her ear, light and cold.

Love Jonas. Love your daughters.

She could feel him finding his way forward through surrender, his greed yielding to integrity.

Do not turn your back on the Truth. Protect what is beautiful.

He pulled away from her, her body rising with the force of him leaving, her back curving as he grew further away. Then he was gone, and she fell back to the bed with a soft jerk, silence encompassing her.

She lay in the stillness, resisting the urge to convince herself it had been a dream.

How easy to blame delusion.

61

Sara
Paris, France

"It was exciting enough when I realized Germain was a saint, but to think he might be a God!" Penny exclaimed, squinting against the morning sun streaming through a break in the curtains. "And Shane, alive during the floods. Just imagine!"

Sara sat propped against a pillow, watching her. She could hear the clatter of dishes in the kitchen. She guessed it was Rhodes cleaning up.

"I said the Truth would blow us away, didn't I?" Penny asked.

"The man who killed our fathers is still out there," Sara said. "Don't see us getting any closer to finding him."

Penny opened the curtains, light flooding the room, dust dancing in the brightness. "But we're getting close to understanding our fathers' mission."

"So?"

"And the more we learn, the more I feel we're meant to complete it."

"How're we going to carry out a mission our fathers failed at?"

"We find out where they went wrong and learn from their mistakes."

"How?"

"I've always been smarter than my father. It shouldn't be too hard."

"Yeah," Sara said, slumping against her pillow. "You're like Brett. But me, I'm just a Mass."

"Masses are capable too. You heard Germain."

If Sara wasn't careful, Penny would ask Rhodes to help her.

"Okay, then," Sara said, getting out of bed. "When we find out what our fathers were up to, I'll help you accomplish their mission. But then you have to help *me* find the man who killed them."

Penny brushed a loose curl from her eye. "I won't have anything to do with killing him."

"I didn't say we'd *kill* him. Jesus, don't be so *extra*."

"Well, what'll we do?'

"That's where your brains come in."

"Okay," Penny nodded. "Okay, when the time's right."

The door opened and Germain stepped in, rubbing his hands with excitement. "Today I thought I would tell you about the Era of the Sages. What do you think?"

"Yes, please" Penny said.

"Come, then, to the fire. It is warm and ready for us."

They followed him down the narrow hallway, the worn floorboards creaking beneath their socked feet, and sat in front of the fire. Rhodes appeared from the kitchen and sat down with them as Germain jiggled himself into his chair. "The Era of the Sages is my favorite time of life on Earth."

"While there were still wars and human suffering during this era, there was also great freedom. Freedom from the ruling of the Anunnaki and freedom from the church. The Era of the Sages lasted from 2,000 BC right up to Jesus's death. His death marked the end of the era." He paused. "I told you about the things that happened in 2,000 BC, right? The nuclear fallout that wiped out Sumer, the exit of the Anunnaki, the rebuilding by the humans?"

They all nodded.

"Well the Era of the Sages is what followed. It was a special time when enlightened beings prospered and influenced the world. Buddha, Zoroaster, Lao Tzu, Confucius, Aristotle, Socrates. All of these great men practiced the Second Truth during this time, using the power of love."

"Were all these Sages descendants of Noah?"

"Yes, they were, and the prophetic abilities hidden in their genes came to a peak around fifteen hundred years after the exit of the Anunnaki. Between 600 and 400 BC, the largest group of powerful Prophets lived, referred to as the Great Sages. It was the best time on Earth."

He gazed into the fire, smiling.

"But, unfortunately, it did not last," he said, his smile fading. "Because even though the mastery of the Second Truth had improved, fewer Prophets were being born. So not only were the powers less common after 400 BC, but people began to fear the Sages, and this fear affected the following generations. Slowly the Second Truth began to dwindle, and when Jesus died, the Second Truth died with him."

"But why were fewer Prophets being born?"

"Because the Anunnaki had left. The pure source of Omega cells was gone."

"But the Second Truth still lives today. You practice it," Sara said.

"But, as you have already guessed, I am not human."

"You're an Anunnaki," Rhodes said.

He nodded. "Yes."

"Which one?" Penny asked.

"Enik."

"The one who created us?"

"It was not me who created you. I only harnessed the power of the Great Universal Energy. *It* created you. That is why I teach you the Second Truth. It is far more important than I."

"But you are a living God," Rhodes said. "One of only two on Earth!"

"I am not a God. I am an Anunnaki, as common as common in Nibiru."

"So, everyone in Nibiru turns into princes and frogs?" Sara asked.

Germain laughed. "Let us not focus on what I am but on what I am capable of, which is all due to the Second Truth."

"You say the Second Truth died with Jesus, but what about Muhammad?" Rhodes asked.

"Oh yes, you are right. There was a time, a beautiful surprise of a time, when one of Jesus's descendants reached enlightenment six hundred years after he had died. Muhammad, through seclusion and prayer, managed to master the Second Truth and once again inspire the Masses. Muhammad was the last of our Great Sages." He leaned forward in his chair. "But soon, we will have great Sages once again. This is it, my friends. This is the era where the children of Noah will remember. A new era has dawned. The Era of Enlightenment is upon us!"

"Upon us how?" Penny asked.

"The first children of Noah are beginning to remember. And as they remember, they will master the Second Truth; they will become enlightened."

"But what does that mean?" Sara asked.

"It means they will influence the world in a way my brother and I cannot, because we are not human."

"And I'm one of the sons of Noah," Rhodes said quietly. "Aren't I?"

"That is for you to remember, not for me to tell."

"I know that I am," Rhodes said. "But Noah had three sons. Who are the others?"

"And a daughter," Germain answered. "Although she is not mentioned in the Bible."

"So, *four* of us will remember in this lifetime?" He asked.

"Yes, I believe so," Germain said, nodding. "I *hope* so."

"But what will they remember?" Sara asked.

"We will remember our beginning," Rhodes said.

"And that knowledge, that Truth, will open a portal inside you," Germain added.

"But what will this mean?" Sara asked again.

"It will mean Shane and his brothers and sister will have the potential to heal like Jesus and Muhammad; that they will be powerful beyond measure."

They sat staring into the fire for what seemed a long time to Sara.

Finally Rhodes said, "So, the Order is trying to reunite with the Gods, to obtain their power, but the greatest potential lies in the Prophets, not the Gods."

"In you," Germain said. "The greatest potential lies in you and your brothers and sister, in the four children of Noah." His eyes glazed over. "And let us pray they do not realize this, let them continue to chase the Gods."

62

Hadley
Cincinnati, Ohio

Issa was despondent. He sat across from Hadley in his library, one leg crossed over the other while he read an old canvas-covered book.

His lessons were bridging the gap between life and death for Hadley, helping her to understand her place in between. And with that, the things that once made her feel separate from others now made her feel connected.

She didn't have to speak to him anymore. They would talk, sometimes for hours, without speaking at all. But there was still this strange new sadness of his.

Sorrow is better than laughter: for by the sadness of the countenance the heart is made better.

Through the denseness of the room she asked, *Why are you so sad?*

I am wanting something too much and being impatient.

What do you want?

I cannot tell you. That is part of the sadness.

He returned his thoughts to his reading.

Why do you read when you already know what the book says?

I do not read to learn. I read because I enjoy the act of reading. I find joy in the words, pleasure in the language they form, inspiration in the world they create.

And is that why you speak, too?

"That is why I do everything," he said, looking up from his book. "I do it to celebrate it exists."

His talking aloud disappointed Hadley. She preferred the not-talking.

Your desire not to speak comes from your blood, from your innate understanding of greater things. He paused. *But I worry it also comes from your love of death.*

He was right. The more she learned, the less she wanted to stay in a place where she'd conquered the inefficient essentials.

If you want to live in peace here on Earth, you must learn to love life.

Hadley stood and began pacing. *I don't want both the boundless eternity and the limited earthly existence as you do. I want the simplicity of death. I want weightlessness and infinity and peace and lightness!*

"And so, death will find you," Issa said sadly, returning to his book.

She watched him read.

She hadn't looked at him in a long time, not as a man, not as she had seen him when she first met him. He'd become magical to her, beyond human in his wisdom. Now she saw him as the man he also was. She saw the way his back stooped as he read, his thin shoulders rising softly as he breathed, the blades creating a ridge under his shirt. She noticed the slant of his arm coming from his sleeve, the bronze skin turning copper as it caught the light.

Ask me about Jesus.

She raised her eyes to his face. *What?*

He continued to read, offering only his profile, his long thin nose, his lips moving slightly with the words of the book.

Ask me about Jesus.

The thought, though nearly desperate, didn't show on his face, didn't change the finite movements of his lips, yet it filtered through the room and arrived clear in her mind. The longing in his thought made her go to him and place a hand on his arm.

His skin was light and static.

Ask me about Jesus.

But ask you what?

Anything.

"Okay," Hadley said. "Was Jesus the son of God or just a man?"

"Jesus was more than a man," Issa said, putting the book down. "He was a golden bridge stretched from the skies. He brought the Great Universal Energy to the Masses. Because he understood their plight, you see, he could reach them. That was what made him special."

"Special like you."

Issa shook his head. "No, not like me."

A vision of a man came to Hadley. A man not unlike Issa. A man similar in height with the same brown skin and dark hair. He stood on a stormy beach, gray clouds brooding behind him, white caps rushing about his ankles.

"There are many things that made Jesus special," Issa said softly.

"What *was* he?" Hadley asked. "Was he a Nephilim?"

Issa shook his head. "He was the only child ever born of a Prophet and a God."

The vision returned to her. The man approached her and looked in her eyes, his own eyes alight with flecks of emerald and onyx from the moonlit water. The beach was very stormy, the wind blowing his hair about his face in dark wisps. He smiled at her and a powerful churning swelled in her.

She let go of Issa's arm and sat down.

"You see him, don't you?" Issa asked, hopeful.

"Was that *Jesus?*"

"The feeling of gazing on him is indescribable, isn't it?"

Hadley began to cry.

"Why am I crying?"

"It is the combination of awe and pride, joy and grief."

His words rang true, but she didn't understand. "Pride? Why would I feel pride?"

"When you remember fully, you will understand."

"I saw your memory. I shared it with you," she said, excited.

"It was not my memory. It was yours."

"Mine? How can it be mine?"

"Why wouldn't it be yours?"

She sat quietly, pondering, before she said. "I knew *Jesus*?"

"Yes," Issa said. "You did."

Hadley grabbed his hands and held them tightly. "Tell me everything, please."

"I cannot tell you. I can only help you remember."

63

Brett
Jekyll Island, Georgia

Brett pulled herself from Noel's embrace and crept from the bed to the balcony doors, opening them and slipping into the early morning light.

Since seeing Kham's face, the nights had become long and restless.

She went to the balcony and stared out at the calm, blue ocean.

There were no waves, no white caps for her to send back from where they came, only a rhythmic lapping of the water on the sand.

What *was* it about him?

But she knew she was drawn to him because of his Omega cells. The Truth had brought her power, but it had also brought her a fated reality that frightened her.

She used to dream of Eli. Had it been Omega cells then, too? Or had they shared something more? And what was *more* anyway? Weren't shared Omega cells special? Either way, she hadn't thought of Eli since seeing Kham's face. The strength of unfulfilled love was no match for the power of Kham.

She would have to act soon. He'd granted both her wishes. He had shown her power and revealed himself, as she'd asked. But a double major at an Ivy League school had hardly prepared her for the act of murder.

"But it has been twenty years and I've had nothing but a few lucid dreams!"

The voice came from below. Brett stepped away from the railing and into the shadow of the awning.

"I don't know what to tell you," a second voice said.

She flattened herself against the cold stucco.

"But you've been having your visions for twenty years!"

"Something like that, yes."

They were coming closer. She could hear shoes clicking against the sidewalk. She held her breath.

"Surely there's something you do to trigger your visions. Some clue you can give to help me?"

It was Japeth.

"They come after great surges of power."

And Kham.

"Are they clear?"

"More and more every day."

"Maybe you aren't remembering right," Japeth said, his voice growing louder as they passed.

"They aren't the kind of memories you get wrong."

"Your latest vision, you haven't told me about it yet."

"There was a girl," Kham said, his voice fading. "A sister."

"A sister?"

Then their voices tailed off, became indiscernible.

Brett exhaled and slid down the wall, hugging her knees to her chest, Kham's voice lingering in her ears.

After great surges of power ...

64

Hadley
Cincinnati, Ohio

Hadley awaited her death like she once waited for Christmas, with bubbling excitement and lucid dreams. The vision of Jesus had heightened her need to die, making her believe death would embrace her with the powerful feeling that had flooded her when she looked upon him in the vision.

She spent most of her time in her mother's office, bathing in the orange light and dreaming of death.

But she was still alive, her body heavy with the engines of blood and breath. And there was Issa's voice constantly nagging her, whispering in her ear like a fly.

When you remember fully, you will understand.

Where once the Bible had whispered to her, now it was Issa's voice. She swatted at it, but it returned.

It was not my memory. It was yourzzzzzzzz.

And so she found herself once again on the white stones of his doorstep, the rocks of her ancestors.

When he opened the door, she immediately saw the sadness in his eyes. She'd hoped it would be gone.

You have stayed away for over a week. I have worried about you.

It's because I've been wanting to die.

"That is what makes me sad," he said, opening the door so she could step inside.

I want to know more about Jesus.

"Why?" he asked, turning his back to her and entering the library. "If you only want to die." He sat on the bench and picked up a book.

"Because you told me it was *my* memory," she said.

"And it is."

"It's from death isn't it? From when I was dead? He was with me then, wasn't he?"

"On a beach?" Issa asked. "I am not sure there are beaches in the afterlife."

"But the afterlife could be anything, couldn't it?"

"I do not know. I have not seen death. You tell me."

The death Hadley had seen was nothing like life. The weightless light she'd experienced was unlikely to have anything as earthly as a beach. But surely she hadn't seen all that death had to offer.

"I could feel how special Jesus was when I saw him in the vision," she said. "I want that feeling back."

"Do not credit Jesus with everything you felt in the vision."

She looked at Issa in surprise. "Well, who do I credit the feeling to then?"

He tilted his head to the side to infer he wasn't going to tell her.

"Is it his father, the God, I was feeling? You know I've thought about him. You say he stayed because he loved his son."

"Not just his son."

"And Mary?"

Issa nodded.

"Why didn't his father save him?"

"He could not. He did not have that kind of power."

"What happened to his father, to the God, after Jesus died?"

"On one hand he misses his son a great deal. You see he has become quite human-like, living so long on Earth. On the other hand, he grasps that all is one and that he is his son and his son is part of him and there is nothing to miss."

"You speak of this God as if he's still here."

"Because he is."

"Where?"

"I cannot tell you that. But you will understand soon. I can feel it."

"And Mary?" Hadley asked. "Is she here on Earth, in this life?"

"Yes, she is."

"So, Mary was a Prophet?"

He put his book down and uncrossed his legs. "The most beautiful Prophet I have ever known."

He said this with so much admiration that Hadley felt jealous.

"You *knew* Mary?"

"Yes."

She'd only experienced jealousy once before, when Issa had mentioned that other strangers visited him. Like indigestion, it churned once again behind her breastbone.

"She was very special. As she has been in every life she has lived."

Hadley lowered her head. "I don't understand."

You understand. You just don't remember.

The vision of Jesus returned. He was standing in the water looking at her, his eyes full of hope and sadness. His eyes were green, deep and light … like water.

And then she understood, the beauty and enormity of it stopping her breath.

She looked at Issa in astonishment.

You were his father.

Issa's hands were trembling, the lock of hair that always hovered at his brow bouncing softly with his tremors. Hadley could feel his vulnerability. To feel this at the same moment she understood he was a God made her body soften and the jealousy in her breast vanish.

But how is it my memory?

Go back again. Revisit.

The vision came back, Jesus calm and dark in the low light of the water's edge. Benevolence flooded her, behind it a swirling of fear and pride. The waves washed over her feet, the late evening chill biting into the bare skin on her arms. She saw her own feet, thin and aged, the veins dark against her pale, freckled skin. She had only a light gown on. It was wet at the fringes.

"Come out of the water and get warm," she heard herself say.

"I can't, I must go," he said. He reached for her hand and held it, smiling warmly as he backed away. "Let me go, Mother. I have a world to save."

And with those words the Truth of who Jesus was, of who she was, of all the years in between, flashed before her; two thousand years combined into one sharp clear memory that sent her staggering into the bookshelves behind her.

She slid down the bookcase and squatted on the floor.

Issa stared at her.

Did he see an old woman or a young girl?

But she knew he saw neither. He saw her as she'd always been and always would be.

"But I'm only ..."

Yet she didn't know how to describe herself, for at that moment she was much more than she had ever understood herself to be and yet was still herself.

"But I'm only *me*," she said.

Issa squatted and looked her in the eyes. "And Mary was only herself, nothing more."

As he said *Mary*, he took her hands in his, and Hadley saw them together two millenniums ago, the moon full but a sliver, the red rock of the cave bright in the night light.

And she remembered Joseph, and how he had surrendered and left them, and how Issa's curl had caught the moonlight. She remembered how she'd disappeared into him and how he'd disappeared into something else and how they'd become the wind.

"I remember you," she whispered.

"Yes," he said, the sadness in his eyes gone. "You finally do."

65

Sara
Paris, France

"Hah!" Germain exclaimed, pointing to the newspaper on his lap. "They have finally discovered how to use carbon nanotube and boron nitride nanotube-based materials! Fantastic! Soon they will have a cable to the moon. Hah! They will be disappointed with the moon, but how much fun, eh?"

This was more than he had spoken in four days. Even Sara was missing their lessons.

"Tell us," Penny said. "About the moon."

"The moon? Oh, there is not much to tell you about the moon."

"Tell us something else then, anything," Rhodes added.

"Well," he said, folding the paper on his lap. "I suppose you have been patient. What eras have we covered? I have lost track."

"You told us about the Beginning when the Anunnaki ruled, and about the Restoration, when the Sumerians lived, and the Era of the Sages that followed. But what about the final era, the Corruption? What was it about?"

"Awful times," he said, tossing the paper in the fire.

It immediately ignited, brightening the room.

"The Corruption began as a feud between those who knew the Truths. You see, during the Era of the Sages, the Second Truth was openly taught. They wanted to share the beauty of the power of our ancestors in hopes of enlightening the world. But some people, as

413

they learned, became possessive of the Truths. Enthralled by the power, they did not want to share the knowledge, afraid if everyone learned the Truths, their own power would be lessened."

"So, they broke away," Penny said. "And formed their own group."

Germain nodded. "Thus creating the great division between those of love and those of fear, which continues today."

"Our fathers' notes indicated that the Corruption was started by the Catholic church," Penny said.

Germain nodded again. "Yes, that is right. The group that broke away from the Sages became the Catholic church. They formed the church as a means of concealing the Truths."

"How did they do it?" Rhodes asked.

"First, they stopped people looking inside themselves for love and power. One of their first sacraments, the Eucharist, was created to get people to focus on a god outside of themselves, to convince the Masses that love and magic were not human, but godly. Second, they ensured people came together routinely in large groups so they could keep control by insisting that the Eucharist was practiced in *mass*. Third, they conceived beautiful churches and enticing saints to compete with the unadorned, humble Sages. And last, they created the Bible, a book with the right recipe of historical facts and psychological manipulation to create just the right concoction of fear and confusion."

"What do you mean the right recipe?"

"They used the teachings of Jesus in the New Testament to satisfy people's need for love yet juxtaposed it with the fear from the Old Testament to keep them afraid. This fear and confusion not only stifled curiosity for the Truths, but it made the Masses suspicious of the Sages. Their strategy was so successful that in the early days of the Corruption, the Catholics grew in numbers and quickly gained political power."

"I don't understand," Rhodes interjected. "Why would Talents and Prophets feel a need to possess the Truths?"

"Those who broke away from the Sages were mostly Carrier Clones. There were a few Talents among them, but no Prophets. Prophets tend to avoid fear-based endeavors."

"What about the leaders?" Penny asked.

"The bishops were Carrier Clones as well, and a few Talents."

"And the followers of the church?"

"Mostly Masses. The followers of the Sages had a larger percentage of Talents."

Sara crossed her arms. "Great. So, I'm with the assholes then."

Germain laughed. "You are not with any of them, dear. You have not chosen yet."

"Chosen what?"

"What you will do with the Truth."

"Whatever," Sara rolled her eyes.

"It is not *whatever*," Germain said. "It is a *choice* and it is a very important one."

Sara shrugged and rolled her eyes again.

"Now then," Germain said, turning back to Rhodes and Penny. "You might ask what was happening with the Gnostics during the rise of the Catholic church?"

"The who?"

"The Gnostics, the followers of the Sages—the other side of the division."

"Oh, right, yes."

"During the rise of the church, the Gnostics continued practicing the Second Truth and sharing the teachings of the Great Sages in their villages, doing what they could to avoid the church, who was threatened by them. They were a peaceful group who disagreed with the church's domination, and for nearly a hundred years they practiced their powers quietly, mostly undisturbed.

"As their population grew and traveled, different groups of Gnostics formed throughout the continent. One group, the Cathars, practiced their powers too openly for the church's liking, and the church went on a killing spree, exterminating them. After this, many of the Gnostics rose up and formed a new group that was determined to fight back. They called themselves the Priory of Sion. They were the first of a string of secret societies, that would one day become the Order."

"And the Knights Templar?" Penny asked. "They were part of the Corruption, right?"

"The Knights Templar formed later, after a member of the Priory of Sion discovered a set of Anunnaki tools found in a mountainside in Israel, locked in an ark. Whenever a new treasure is found, you will see humans divide."

"In an ark?" Rhodes asked. "You mean the Ark of the Covenant?"

"It has been called many things over the years as it has been lost and found, hidden and dug up. It was never the ark that was coveted, of course, but the tools within it."

"You mean Aaron's rod?"

"Or Moses's staff. A different name for different times."

"They *were* real?"

"*Are* real," Germain said. "But there's more." He pointed his finger at them. "In the thirteenth century, the Knights Templar unearthed a large object, similar to the tools in the ark, in the Persian desert. On examination they realized it was a giant version of the small tools. And, of course, a feud arose.

"And out of the feud the Freemasons were born and became the main secret society for the next four hundred years, possessing the tools and practicing the power made possible by them. During this time the tools became known as lundicroix."

"Tools of the Gods," Rhodes said.

"And, like a baton, they passed from the Freemasons to the Jacobins to the Illuminati, to finally live within the Order."

"And the church? Did they know about these tools too?"

"No, the church continued to control the common man through fear and confusion, caught up in their own quest for power, mostly ignorant of the items harbored by the secret societies."

"Mostly ignorant?" Rhodes asked.

"They heard rumors, some bishops believed the ark existed and that the societies had it, but they never believed enough to find them."

"So, the Order and the church are what is left of the followers of the Great Sages?"

"And sadly," Germain lamented. "Both are a far cry from the original Gnostics."

"It seems they've become what they once rebelled against," Rhodes reflected.

"Yes, humans without Omega blood will always return to a state of fear unless they practice love, which is difficult without an intrinsic understanding of the Second Truth. And with each generation bearing fewer and fewer Prophets, there were fewer examples of love. So, the perversion of the societies was twofold."

"And what of the money launderers?" Penny asked, glancing at Rhodes. "Weren't they part of the Corruption?"

"The money men added a whole new dimension to the Corruption. I never saw it coming—a group that would become so rich they would buy the Truths right off the church and the societies! Scared me, it did."

"And that's when you came out of hiding!" Rhodes said, lighting up. "That's when you appeared as Saint Germain."

"Yes, son, you are correct. I had to do something to try to raise the vibrations of the world. Things were looking grim. I thought if

I could gather attention, I might be able to unite the few Prophets that remained, start to spin things in the right direction."

"So where were all the Prophets during the Corruption?"

"They left the church and the societies as the groups became corrupt. Most lived the Second Truth independently. Today very few Prophets exist in either the church or the Order. They are not able to reach their potential in a low-vibration, fear-based environment."

"Their potential?" Penny asked.

"Prophets are destined to become enlightened. They cannot resist it."

"What about the Claw and Bones of Yale?" Sara asked. "Our fathers were members, and my sister too. Isn't it a secret society?"

"It's part of the Order, their top training ground, the first step of initiation." Germain nodded. "Your fathers were found worthy of the first induction, but they did not pass the second test. They did not have enough Omega cells."

"They were Masses, like me?"

"Carrier Clones," Germain answered.

"So, what was done with them?" Penny asked.

"They were given high status political jobs but kept in the dark about the Truth."

"But why kill them?" Sara asked.

"They got angry at being ousted, didn't they?" Penny asked. "They started looking for answers and got too close to something, didn't they?"

Germain sat back in his chair and picked up his gold tin. "Pretty much."

"They went to Iraq," she said. "Persia."

Germain nodded, flicking open his tin. "They had realized long ago that the Gulf Wars were not about oil. They knew the fighting was over something else."

418

"And they were going to show the world," Penny murmured to herself.

"Yes," Germain said.

"So, they brought their deaths upon themselves then," Penny said, watching him sprinkle green leaves onto a white square of a paper.

"What?" Sara asked incredulously.

"If they were acting out of anger and vengeance, then they were acting against the Second Truth, which would only cause more problems, don't you see?"

Germain looked at Sara. "Something you should keep in mind, my dear."

"How do we act out of anything else?" Sara exclaimed. "Someone killed our fathers and is lying to us all. What're we supposed to do, *pray* about it? Have some kind of *love* party?" Sara stood, angry. "Who did it? Who killed them?"

"It doesn't matter who killed them," Germain sighed. "That is not the point."

"It matters to me," she said, stomping toward bedroom. "If it's what got them killed, then it matters to me. And I'm going to find out who did it, whether you help me or not."

66

Brett
Jekyll Island, Georgia

Brett woke with a sweat, Kham's tiger-eyes fading with a dream. She threw the covers back, the cool air frigid against her damp skin. Noel reached for her in his sleep and she moved away and sat up.

The balcony doors were open, the white curtains billowing in the moonlight. She stood and walked through them and onto the cool tiles of the veranda. The moon was bright, the white caps of the ocean glowing pale blue. She went to the rail and leaned against it, clutching her thin nightgown against her.

A movement caught her eye, a figure at the edge of the water. The leanness of the silhouette and the length of the shadow was unmistakable.

Come, he said.

She looked around her, startled at the nearness of his voice.

Come down and join me.

Was he was using the power to speak to her?

His shadow glided along the shore.

You know you want to.

She looked behind her at Noel sleeping through the curtains.

Come, he said again.

"No."

Ah, so you hate me now.

How had he heard her?

You're the one that asked me to reveal myself. He was walking toward her, his figure growing larger as he approached. *There's no one to blame but yourself.*

She glanced at Noel again. One of his legs was uncovered, his thigh shining in the moonlight. There was a time the sight of it would have moved her.

And you hate me for that too, don't you? For killing that desire.

She turned back to the beach.

He was approaching the footpath.

"You overheard us the other day, my brother and me. I could feel you listening." His words sounded different when he used his voice.

"How did you speak to me from the shore? Your words, they were in my head."

"A lesson for another time," he said. "So much to learn."

"What are you doing here?"

"You were awake with desire," he said, beneath the balcony now. "I could feel it."

She attempted a laugh. "Could you really?"

"Don't deny it." He looked up at her, his eyes bright green in the moonlight.

She looked away. "You were talking about visions," she said. "When I overheard you with your brother. Will I have them too one day?"

"Not in this lifetime, no."

"Why not?" She asked, keeping her eyes averted.

"Because you haven't lived enough lives."

"Enough lives?"

"Never mind," he said.

"Who else has the visions?"

"No one I know of. But I predict there are others."

She brought her eyes back to him. His brown skin was damp from a swim, his hair slick in the moonlight. She imagined him naked, a chiseled line of pelvis, a trail of dark hair, lean thighs.

"You want me," he said. "It's killing you."

"You flatter yourself."

"It'll be easier if you let me have you."

"*Have* me?"

"Until you surrender, your lessons will be jeopardized."

"You should go," she said, forcing herself away from the railing.

He remained beneath her, smirking.

She moved quickly inside and pulled the doors closed.

Noel stirred and sat up. "Brett?"

She leaned against the door in the semi-dark, her breath fast and quick.

"Brett, you okay?"

She went to him, lifting her nightgown over her head and dropping it to the carpet. He drew the covers back and pulled her naked body to his. She closed her eyes, imagining green eyes watching.

67

Renee
Cincinnati, Ohio

Renee and Jonas sat on a park bench. They were in the cemetery again, the tombstones casting long shadows across the grass. Renee's head was on Jonas's shoulder. She could smell the detergent in his shirt as it warmed in the sun.

"I wish my mother had a grave," Jonas said. "It would be nice to have a place to visit."

"Tell me about her," Renee said, touching his arm.

"She was wise and spiritual. She insisted I exercise my spirit. She believed a spirit needed to dance to stay healthy."

Renee pulled her head from his shoulder and turned to him, the sun glaring off his head. "And you chose basketball. And that's why you're so good."

He nodded. "I'm better than the others because I approach the game differently. I don't tap into my spirit to be a good basketball player, I use basketball as a vehicle to nourish my spirit. My mother taught me this."

"I wish I could have met her."

"Me too."

They sat in silence for a few minutes before Renee said, "I went to see Issa the other day."

"I know."

"How do you know?"

"Because you've been different."

423

"I have?"

"You've been quieter."

"He told me some remarkable things about you and me."

"About us?"

Renee nodded.

"Like what?"

"I think you should hear it from him."

"I want to hear it from you."

Renee stood. "Let's walk."

He stood next to her, blocking the sun, and they began to walk.

"I don't understand everything he told me," Renee said, taking his hand. "But I believe him."

"Tell me," Jonas asked.

"He says we carry a unique blood cell. Something not known to the medical world. He says it's linked to a predisposition to the Truth, the Truth being of a metaphysical nature. He calls them Omega cells. Apparently, fifty percent of our blood cells are Omega cells. The Order refers to people like us as Talents."

"What else did he say?"

"He said Hadley has three-quarter Omega cells, which is very rare. She's what they call a Prophet."

"So that's why the Order is after her?"

"Issa didn't say this, but I think so. I think they have tested Brett and they want to test Hadley."

"So, Brett's a Prophet too?"

Renee shook her head. "No. She's a Talent like us."

Jonas picked up the pace and Renee had to stretch her legs to keep up.

"My mother must have been a Talent too, then," Jonas said.

"She could have been a Prophet the way you talk about her."

They came to the corner of Fairfield and Mitcham and Jonas paused, then turned down Mitcham Road.

"Where are you going?" Renee asked.

"You know where I'm going," he said.

Two blocks along, he stopped in front of the neatly trimmed bushes of Issa's Tudor.

"How did you know where his house was?" Renee asked.

He winked at her. "I'm a Talent too, remember?"

Renee smiled. "How do you believe so easily?"

"My mother told me the Truth would find me and when it did, that I shouldn't resist."

"So, she *knew*?"

He shrugged. "She knew something."

"Issa said we're attracted to each other because we're both Talents."

He smiled. "I told you, didn't I?"

Issa opened the door before they reached it, Hadley standing at his side.

She is here all the time! And to think I didn't notice.

"When you decide to avoid the Truth," Issa said, as he gestured them in. "You miss a lot of other things too."

"You read my mind again," Renee said.

"Can he do that?" Jonas asked.

"Apparently."

"Cool." Jonas said, ducking his head and stepping into the foyer. "Renee has told me about the Omega blood cells. I want to know more."

"Come, come," Issa said.

They followed him down the hall and into the library.

"This is Issa's library," Hadley said. "He says all the important books are here."

Renee saw they were alphabetized by the author's last name. She searched the spines for Ernest's name and found one book, pulling it out and holding it up. "Is this the only one of Ernest's books you have?"

"That is his only important book."

"How do you determine a book's importance?" She asked.

"By its consciousness. Before that book, the bell tolled only for Ernest."

Jonas sat on the bench and looked eagerly at Issa. "I want to learn. I want to know what this all means and what we're meant to do with it."

Renee glanced at Hadley and then to Issa. "Does Hadley already know about all this?"

"Hadley has always known," Issa said.

Hadley smiled. "I haven't *always* known, Mom. I'm only just remembering."

"What do you mean remembering?"

"Prophets are different," Issa said, taking the book from Renee and putting it back in its slot on the shelf. "They return to this world again and again, always as Prophets. Their consciousness returns with them, although deeply buried, and if they are open to it, they can remember past lives."

"Do you remember past lives?" Renee asked Hadley.

Hadley nodded.

"And Talents?" Renee asked, taking a seat next to Jonas. "Our consciousness doesn't return with us?"

"It hasn't happened yet, not that I know of."

"When we spoke, you talked about enlightenment. What does it mean?"

"Enlightenment is full consciousness. It is seeing the spirit and energy of the world. It is vibrating at the highest level while maintaining life on Earth. This requires balancing being human and being godly. Many people mistakenly think that godliness is better than humanness."

"And Ernest was the opposite," Renee said. "He rejected godliness."

"Yes," Issa answered. "He was determined to be human at all costs."

"And you," Jonas said. "You are enlightened?"

"Yes," Issa said.

"What is the secret?"

"Time," Issa said. "More time than you can imagine."

"So, what does this all mean?" Renee asked. "Why does the Order want Hadley. Is it because of these Omega cells?"

"They want her because she's a Prophet, yes. And because she's still young."

"What do they want to do with her?" Jonas asked.

"They want to use her powers to help them discover the Second Truth."

"Which is?"

"Love in its purest form, enlightenment itself. It is being one with the Great Universal Energy. It is something that, once a person grasps it, means they no longer need to be part of an elitist group. Exactly why the Second Truth eludes the Order."

"But it doesn't elude them!" Hadley said. "They have this power, this Second Truth. I've seen them use it. They used it to kill my father."

"What?" Renee asked.

"I saw a man on the side of the road. His hands were glowing. He caused the truck to crash into us."

"What you saw Japeth do that day of the accident," Issa said to Hadley, "May have looked powerful to you. But the power of the Second Truth is much greater than controlling objects with your mind."

"I should have been there," Renee said. "I'm so sorry, Hadley."

"It's okay, Mom. You couldn't have saved Dad, and I enjoyed dying."

Renee shook her head. "You say the strangest things, Hadley."

"So, Hadley is no use to them?" Jonas asked. "Not like they think?"

Issa smiled. "No, she is not."

"So, they kill people to protect something that will always elude them?"

"They kill to keep the First Truth from the Masses, the Truth about our ancestry and the Omega cells. And this, in a sense, is a service to mankind."

"A service to mankind?"

"Each person has a choice whether to know the Truth or not, and most people choose not to know. To know is to be responsible for your own existence. Few people want that responsibility. Careless living is its own joy. Who are we to tell them what they do not want to know? Who was Scott to tell them? The Truth is there. If they want to find it, they will make their way to it."

"Is that what Scott tried to do?" Renee asked. "Tell the Masses about the Truths?"

"That was his plan, but he never had the chance."

"Because they killed him."

"You husband was killed because he found something ancient and important."

"What did he find?"

"The last remaining ship of our ancestors."

"A ship? What kind of ship?"

"Our ancestors are called the Anunnaki. They came here a very long time ago from another planet. What Scott found was a spaceship."

Renee laughed. "A *space*ship?"

"How long ago?" Jonas asked.

"What did they look like?"

"They arrived during the end of the Ice Age. They are similar to humans. Humans are their offspring."

"How did Scott find this ship?" Renee asked.

"He uncovered information and followed the clues."

"What did he do when he found it?"

"He was going to use it as proof of the Anunnaki. He was going to tell people the Truth."

"So, my dad," Hadley said. "Brought his death upon himself."

"I am afraid so. He was focusing on the anger of being left out and brought those vibrations right back to himself."

"You get what you focus on. That's the Second Truth!" Hadley shouted.

"It is part of it."

"And if we choose to know the Second Truth, to focus on it, then what? What will happen?" Renee asked.

"Eventually you will be at one with the universe. You will become powerful and all knowing. You will be at peace and connected to all things. You will be of God."

"And we'll leave this world," Renee said softly. "Exactly what Ernest feared."

"If you allow your vibrations to become too high for this world, then yes. But I am still here. I have learned how to be both of God and of the world. It is this balance that is the secret to enlightenment."

"So, if you aren't a Prophet then what are you?" Jonas asked.

"I am an Anunnaki," he said, folding his hands neatly on his book. "I am what is left of your ancestors."

68

Sara
Paris, France

Sara was in Germain's bathroom brushing her teeth when she saw it. It was lying inside the medicine cabinet next to his shaving cream.

She took it out and lifted it to the light. It was metallic purple with a gray sheen, cylindrical, not much longer than her toothbrush and about as wide as a quarter. She placed it in her palm and it pivoted, coming to rest between her thumb and forefinger.

She jumped back, startled, but it remained firmly in her hand.

A tingling sensation moved up her arm, filling the hollow of her armpit, spreading to her shoulder, rising the length of her neck. She closed her eyes and a kaleidoscope of pictures danced on the back of her eyelids. She saw a desert and ships and tall people dressed in dark clothes. She watched as the doors closed and the ships lifted into the air. As they rose, they left giant holes behind them in the sand, holes slick with oil, their surfaces swimming with purple and pink.

"It is a lundicroix," Germain said from behind her. "The Anunnaki's idea of a telescope."

Sara turned around, the object fixed to her palm.

"It is able to collect your energy and turn off your mind," he said. "An easy way to connect to the Great Universal Energy. I used to use it all the time before I became enlightened."

He lifted it from Sara's hand. "The Anunnaki created it to help them manage the physics of Earth." He held it up to the light and smiled. "Funny. I no longer need it, but I miss the ritual of using it."

"The oil," she said. "The ships made the oil in Iraq."

"Except the oil you saw was not fuel for their ships; it was the *byproduct* of Anunnaki fuel. When the ships left, they blew great holes into the ground."

"And my father, he knew this? He saw these holes?"

"There is more than oil there. There is still a ship. A ship with holograms and computers and everything you need to prove to the Masses they are the children, the creations of beings from far away."

"And our fathers found the ship?"

Germain nodded. "It was left behind for Enlil and me. In case we changed our minds."

"Where's the man who killed my father?" Sara asked, taking the object back from him.

"It does not matter who the man is."

"I want revenge," Sara said, wrapping her fingers around the instrument.

"Revenge will not serve you the way you hope."

"Where is he?" she asked the object. "Where's the man who killed my father?"

Sara opened her palm and the light spread through her arm. She closed her eyes and saw two tall men standing in a dark room shadowed by a bookcase. They were in deep discussion. One had a light, feminine voice and the other was gruff and raspy. The vision widened and she saw a woman, young and blonde, sitting on a couch in front of them.

The woman turned toward the light and Sara opened her eyes in surprise, a quick rush of blood flooding her head.

"It is better if you come back gradually," Germain said.

"Brett." Sara clutched the lundicroix to her chest. "I saw Brett."

"Sara, please give me the lundicroix." He held his hand out to her. "You are not ready for its power. Work with me, let me show you how to use it properly."

She shook her head. "This can lead me to my father's killer, can't it?"

"That is not how it is meant to be used."

Sara backed away from him.

"It will not go well, Sara. Please give it to me."

"No," Sara said.

"You have a chance," Germain said. "A chance to protect yourself from evil, to protect happiness, to protect the joys you experienced in Paris. Give me the lundicroix."

"You could just take it," Sara said laughing. "If you really wanted it, you could just float it from my hands into yours like you did with that painting."

Germain nodded. "Yes, I could."

"So why don't you?"

"Because I want you to choose to give it to me. The power of choice is more powerful than the lundicroix."

Sara thought of what it would mean to give it back to him, how it would involve learning and how Penny would learn quicker than she would. She thought of Rhodes's bright smile and how he and Penny would laugh with their new discoveries.

She loosened her grip on the object and opened her palm, knowing Germain wouldn't take it from her.

"How can I find this man?" she asked the lundicroix, closing her eyes as the lightening began to spread through her.

She saw Brett on the beach with one of the tall men. They were facing the water, both of their hands glowing like the man from the side of the road at the accident. Then the vision moved away until Brett and the man were only dots on a small curved coastline. The beach grew longer and longer as Sara flew high above them, seeing that the coast was an island and that the island lay to the east, in the Atlantic Ocean.

She opened her eyes, alive with new knowledge.

When she turned around, Germain was gone.

69

Brett
Jekyll Island, Georgia

It was a gray day, the kind that neither rains nor clears. The island was quiet, most of the initiates away on projects and Noel in Florida, training. Brett was sitting on the veranda looking at the wall of monochrome in front of her, a throw wrapped around her shoulders and a cup of tea in her hand. The ocean was gray. The sand was gray. The water was gray. She longed for something to break the monotony.

She sat up, clutching the mug to her chest.

She could do it. She could break the clouds.

She inhaled and stared at the flat gray cloud stretched in front of her, the lightness immediately brewing with the intent of manipulation. She grew warm as it moved through her body. She saw the cloud for the cluster of molecules it was. She stared at the minute connections, focusing on them steadily. She exhaled, her breath like two hands reaching into the cloud and spreading the grayness apart.

The edge of the clouds whitened, and a line of blue appeared, beaming a stripe of pale, yellow sun onto the sand.

She had done it without the lundicroix!

"Beautifully done," a voice said behind her.

A chill moved down her spine. She shivered.

"That is, of course, how you'll kill your sister."

"I would have eventually come to that conclusion on my own," she said, taking a sip of her tea without turning around.

"No doubt you would have."

"Then why the invasion?"

"Invasion is awfully dramatic. I did knock."

Was he inside or was he on the veranda?

"Do you want me to leave?" he asked.

Brett wanted nothing more than to look at him, but she remained staring at the clouds. They were beginning to thin at the edges and flatten back over the sky.

"Brett," he said, closer. "You've seen me. It's done."

The sound of her name on his voice quickened her breath.

"You must deal with the consequences."

He was so close now she could feel the heat of his body behind her. He placed his hands on her shoulders, his thumbs warm and coarse against the flesh of her neck.

The grayness reclaimed the last slice of sky.

"And what're the consequences?" she asked, turning around to find him in faded jeans and leather sandals.

There was a casualness in his eyes that surprised her. She looked away.

"There is but one consequence, Brett."

There it was again, her name on his lips.

"You must look at me when I speak of it."

She rose her eyes to meet his. They sliced through her, bright green in the stark grayness.

"The consequence is that you want me like you've never wanted anything in your life." His pink lips spread into a smile. "And that's also why you hate me."

She pulled her eyes from his, aware it was more than his eyes that drew her in. It was the sneer, the line of the jaw, the brown neck, the vein that rose from his shirt and disappeared in his shoulder. It was the raspy voice. It was the status. It was the power. It was all of it combined.

"I'm the only one who can teach you what you need to know, and you won't be able to learn from me if all your energy is used resisting your desire."

She braced the chair behind her, keeping her eyes locked on his.

"The only answer is to submit," he said.

"How?" she asked with a whisper.

"Let me have you."

"Surely it could be more of a union?"

"A union happens between equals." He placed his hands on her hips. "And I'm more powerful than you."

She closed her eyes.

"If it's any consolation, it has nothing to do with gender," he said, turning her away from him so she was facing the sea. "Whoever has more Omega cells has the control."

He walked her to the banister, one hand at the back of her neck, the other on her hip. He took her earlobe in his teeth, the stubble of his jaw rough against her cheek.

He wasn't gentle, but he was graceful, the clouds thinning and parting, the sun coming through full force with his release and, to her surprise, hers.

70

Hadley
Cincinnati, Ohio

Hadley had spent the last few days in quiet reverie, contemplating her many lives. She didn't remember them in a linear way. She remembered them instead in pieces, seeing herself at a distance in a busy city or from afar on a rolling hill. Sometimes the vision was from her own vantage point and she saw her hands, young and smooth, picking grapes off a vine or her legs beneath her, running on a dusty road.

These memories brought many emotions, and grief was not the least of them. She found each memory, each life, held its own lessons and tragedies that she wanted to clutch to her breast and keep close in this life.

Issa was on the deck, busy sanding the picnic table. He was surrounded by sawdust that rose like gold glitter in a stream of sunlight. She watched his graceful movements, marveling in the love he had for his work.

She saw him differently now, as a friend and a God, and sometimes, in flashes, as a lover. These later memories frightened her for they were dense with an earthly love she hadn't experienced in this life. She longed to touch him but knew it was not yet time.

He looked up and met her eyes. "There is no rush, Hadley. I have waited thirty lives for you to remember me. That alone will suffice me for another thirty if need be."

She pulled a cat onto her lap. "I lived lives before I was Mary, didn't I? I remember things that feel older."

"You lived many a life before Mary. Nearly a hundred."

Hadley thought of this for a while. "And I've lived thirty since?"

"Yes."

"So, I've lived one hundred and thirty lives and you've lived only one?"

"Yes," he said again, smoothing his hand over the surface of the table and blowing the dust so it rolled in a pale, yellow cloud away from him.

The cloud brought the memory of a sandstorm. She watched from above, seeing herself on a camel as a wall of sand rose in front of her like a giant wave. There were others with her, and they dismounted their camels and began to dig furiously into the sand. The camels kicked up dust and a child began to howl. Then the vision left her.

Hadley hugged the cat, waiting for the grief to subside. The children crying had been her grandchildren and they had not survived, nor had she. She trembled in mourning.

Issa came off the deck and across the lawn and placed his hand on the crown of her head. A warmth massaged her scalp and spread through her ears and jaw, chin and neck, settling in her shoulders.

He knelt beside her. "Do you often suffer with your memories?"

"Not always. Sometimes they're beautiful."

"I cannot imagine what it must be like."

"The most painful vision, and the most beautiful, was the one I had of Jesus on the beach, walking backward away from me. I didn't want him to go." She paused. "Where was he going?"

"Away to see the world, to learn and mature so he could fulfill his destiny."

"How long was he gone?"

"Thirteen years."

"Where did he go?"

"To Asia, to study the ways of Buddha. He taught as much as he learned, leaving love and healing in every village he visited."

"You went with him?"

"Yes."

"Why didn't I go?"

"It was not a trip for a woman, not in those days. You were inconsolable for many years."

She shivered. "I don't I want to remember that."

"No," he said, removing his hand from her head and sitting down next to her.

"Will it always be like this now for me? These visions?"

"I don't know. Only one other Prophet has remembered, and I was not with him when he did."

"How many lives did that Prophet live?"

"The same as you."

"One hundred and thirty?"

"It seems that is how many it takes."

"Do I know him?"

"He has been with you in every life. He is your first father, the man who gave you your genes."

She knew who he was referring to. She'd always known but never understood. "But *my* father gave me my genes in this life."

"You already existed by then, you only filled the shell he gave you. It is Ernest who gave you your Omega cells, ten thousand years ago."

Another vision came, of a man framed in the doorway of an earthen house beside a weathered woman in a gray dress. He was tall and broad and not at all dissimilar to the ghost of Mr. Ernest. Hadley looked down to see her own young hands, brown and dirty under the nails. She'd been working that day. She could feel dried sweat and grit on her skin. Behind her was laughter and she turned to see three boys playing on a dusty road.

Noah, the woman said. *Gather the children.*

"Ernest was Noah," Hadley said quietly. "In my first life."

"Yes," Issa said.

"But Noah didn't have a daughter."

"Not in the Bible, no. Most women were left out of the Bible."

"What was her name?"

"Zeruah."

"Zeruah," she repeated. It didn't feel familiar. "And the brothers. Do they remember? Are they here, like me, in this life?"

"They are."

A vision of rising waters came to her in a rush. She was on a boat inside a small shelter. The rain was spraying through the cracks in the door.

"The flood!" she said, reaching out and holding onto Issa's knee as if it would ground her from the violent rocking of the boat.

Hadley heard the knocking of jars and saw her father disappear behind a small door.

"The jars!" she said. "We took all the animals' DNA in the jars, so we could re-create them. Those were our instructions. We didn't take real animals!"

Issa nodded. "That is right."

She blinked as the vision disappeared. "Who gave us those instructions? Was it the Anunnaki? Are they the ones who saved us?"

"Yes, they saved you and your family."

"But why us?"

"Because Noah was the only Prophet to have four children who were also Prophets. This was so rare we saw it as a sign."

"*You* were the God that spoke to Noah?"

"One of them, yes."

"And Moses? Did you speak to Moses on Mt. Sinai?"

"Yes, with my brother."

"You told the Israelites Earth was yours and they should follow your rule?"

"I was not yet enlightened," he said. "We felt we had to create order."

Hadley looked at Issa, trying to imagine him as a God. "Were you and your brother in the clouds when you spoke to Moses and Noah?"

Issa laughed. "No. We faced them eye to eye, but we created a bright light and wind for effect."

"How?"

"We had tools that helped with such things."

"Then why didn't you stop the flood?"

"The tools were not strong enough for that kind of power."

"Things are much different once you understand them," Hadley said quietly.

"It was a long time ago. We are all different now, the Gods *and* the humans."

Hadley pushed the cat from her lap and scooted to Issa, laying her head on his shoulder. She watched the sun drop behind the maple tree, beaming golden rays through the branches and onto the lawn.

71

Brett
Jekyll Island, Georgia

Brett had spent every morning with Kham for the past two weeks. He was the teacher she'd been searching for her. He instructed with a mixture of precision and dry passion that made sense to her. There was no drama in his lessons, no unnecessary protocol or etiquette.

She learned fast, and the lundicroix, when placed in her hand, was no longer a distraction but a comfort. It had become an extension of herself. She was now able to summon her power instantaneously with her desires. She could control anything.

Except him.

He took her when he wanted her, the only warning a narrowing of his eyes and a rise in his shoulders, like a sleuthing cat coming upon prey in the jungle. Sometimes he would seize her immediately and passionately, other days he would watch her like this for hours, both savoring the anticipation.

While she hated the submission he triggered, her respect for him grew. She learned not to arrive at his office with expectations because he was unpredictable. Instead, she arrived with faith, because until now she had never met anyone she could count on to impress her.

He sat propped at the end of his desk, one leg hanging from it and the other braced against the floor. He was holding his elbow with one hand while the fingers of the other lay delicately across his lips. This was what he did when he was deep in thought.

He hadn't touched her for three days and she longed for him.

"You're almost ready," he said. "There's but one lesson left."

"Whatever it is, I'm ready."

His green eyes brightened. "Oh, I don't doubt that."

She watched for a narrowing of his eyes or a rise of his shoulders, but he offered neither.

"You're aware of the Winter Ball?" he asked.

"Yes," she said. "But I wasn't planning on going."

He released himself from his pensive pose and came to her.

She braced herself for his touch, but he stopped and placed his hands behind his back. "You'll go to the ball," he said.

"But why?"

"I'll see you there," he said, motioning to the door.

"The ball is on Christmas Eve. That's two weeks away. Will there be no lessons until then?"

"There's nothing left to learn but what the ball has to offer. Now go."

Back at her apartment, Brett found Noel in the office he had made out of the second bedroom. He sat swiveling between his three computer screens.

Since he had returned from Florida, she rarely found him elsewhere.

"Hi," he said without looking up, his face blue from the reflection of the screen.

She entered the room and opened the window. "It's stuffy in here. Have you been in front of those computers all morning?"

"Yes," he said, running his finger horizontally along a screen, his lips moving as he read.

"It looks like I'll be going to the ball," she said.

He looked up. "Oh?"

"Apparently there's a lesson for me to learn there."

"At the ball?"

She nodded.

"That should be interesting. Do you want me to go with you?"

"It would be odd if I went on my own."

"I'll go with you," he said, turning back to his computers and beginning to type.

"It's a masquerade ball. I'll order our costumes. Any requests?"

"No," he said. "You choose."

She considered ordering a sheer and translucent costume, something that showed her back, or perhaps something low in the front that would accent the slope of her breasts. She knew Kham would be there, dancing among the crowd behind a mask, and she entertained herself with the idea he would be overcome by her beauty. But she knew he only took her when he wanted to tame her, or when he felt a connection with her intellect. Physical beauty as a sole motive was beneath him.

She chose a long green gown with white gloves that stretched to her elbows and a peacock-feathered head dress. For Noel she chose a white suit with black lapels and cuffs and a white mask on a stick.

"The less dress you choose the better!" Noel hollered from the other room.

She glanced through the door at him, remembering how she'd once loved his affection.

72

Hadley
Cincinnati, Ohio

Hadley was sitting on the floor in Issa's library when the books caught her eye. There were several of them, all hard bound and leather, some gilded. A collection of Holy Bible translations. There was an American Standard and an English Standard, a Revised Standard and a New Revised Standard, a New American Standard and a New International, a Common English and a Lexham English, a Good News Translation and a New Living Translation. And there was something called a Douay-Rheims and a Holman Christian Standard. And last, rising taller than the others and more worn, was her favorite, the King James.

She removed it from the shelf. It was heavy and the spine was cracked. She thought of her grandmother and the sound of the King James on her lips. She had enjoyed the stories of the Old Testament, but she had cherished the stories of Jesus. She had cried sometimes at their beauty. Had she somehow known then, sitting on her grandmother's lap, that these were stories of her own son? Had she wept from a longing for the past, or from the beauty she'd been part of creating?

She ran her hand across the cover with sorrow. She had found the Truth and, in so doing, had lost her religion.

A red ribbon ran a third of the way through the gold lined pages. She opened to the page marked. It was the book of Psalms. The fray of the ribbon ran across chapter 119, verse 45.

And I will walk at liberty: for I seek thy precepts.

She closed her eyes and shut the Bible, meditating on the idea put forth by the psalm, losing herself and the verse as she became alert and soft with the nothingness of where she came from. And as she fell further into the void, she found she was not Zeruah or Mary, not daughter or sister, not girl or woman, not Hadley at all.

The further she went from herself, the more awake she became, and a knowing encompassed her; a knowing that she would live, that she would not choose death in this life or the next; a knowing that she would reunite with her brothers and they would understand her and relate to her power. She became so awake that the light within her warmed her eyelids. She could feel it move to the crown of her head. She sat with it in silence, disappearing into the hot brightness.

When she returned from her meditation, she said to herself, "I must find my brothers for they, too, are living their one hundred and thirtieth lives."

The nebulous form of Mr. Ernest hovered above her.

Be still, he said. *Your brothers will find you.*

73

Renee
Cincinnati, Ohio

It was late evening as they walked home, hand in hand, the sky turning from blue to purple as the streetlights came on.

"Do you think it's odd we're so content?" Jonas asked.

Renee didn't answer; she'd come to know when he was starting a long thought.

"Lately we have been exposed to extraordinary information," he said. "We frequent the house of a God who, I might add, is also from another planet. Your daughters are in imminent danger. Our veins pump with alien blood. And we are now aware we have lived many lives and will live many more. Yet we stroll on an autumn evening as if nothing is different."

The wind was cold. She let go of his hand and put her arm through his, pulling herself against his warmth.

"Regardless of this new knowledge," Jonas continued. "I've never been so content."

"Nor have I," Renee said.

"We haven't discussed what Issa told us."

"How does one discuss such things?"

"Yes, maybe we don't need to. Maybe we're content because we now have the answers to life."

"Do we?" Renee asked.

"Well, don't we?"

"We know where we come from," she said. "We understand the origin of some of our behaviors. But we don't know *why* we're here."

They walked in silence until Jonas said, "Maybe we're simply here to stroll the streets and philosophize."

Renee pulled him closer, pressing her body to his. She marveled more at the pleasure of Jonas's company than any of the Truths. Nothing satisfied her more than listening to him contemplate aloud or watching the colors of his face change with the setting sun.

What did I do before him? Where did all my time go?

"I once read something," he said. "That claimed the test of first-rate intelligence was the ability to hold two opposed ideas in mind at the same time. Maybe we're here for a purpose and we're also here just to exist. Maybe both are true."

"Or perhaps our purpose is to find the balance between them," she said.

"But if you balance them, then both cease to exist."

"Yet something altogether better is created."

Jonas sighed. "Maybe we're just here to love each other."

"As worthy a mission as any."

74

Sara
Cincinnati, Ohio

Germain had not mentioned the lundicroix since their moment in the bathroom, and Sara had endured another month of conversations by firelight, each night retiring early to consult with the lundicroix.

It had given her a new confidence, brought back to her a rush of rebellion and with it a happiness she had forgotten. It was like having her phone back, but better.

She did not speak to Penny or Germain about it. How could she explain to them that returning to her anger, to the hatred they claimed was wrong, was its own kind of happiness? She couldn't, not without a clever rebuttal that would ruin her high.

Thus, she had been quietly letting her confidence grow as they discussed history and Truths and dined on good food. She was convinced the lundicroix would tell her when and how she should make her move. And the time had come. The lundicroix had not only shown her that Brett would soon leave the island and go somewhere with the tall man, but it had helped her find her phone in a box in the bottom of the pantry.

So with the lundicroix tucked safely beneath the underwire of her bra, she called a taxi in the darkness of the early morning, whispering awkward French into the phone, and quietly carried her suitcase down the long stairway and out the tall doors they had entered two months before.

She watched the gas lamps quiver as she waited for the taxi to arrive, thinking of the morning they had headed into Paris and how she'd been nervous following at Germain's heels. Today, although Paris was cold and gray, *she* was in charge.

At the airport she purchased a flight to New York and then on to Charleston. She felt no guilt when she used Penny's credit card to book the flight and signed with Penny's squiggly, loopy "y". She walked easily through the security check point at Charles de Gaulle and slept soundly on the flight to New York, waking relaxed and at ease about changing flights. She was confident nothing could go wrong with the lundicroix cradled against her breast. And on the flight to Charleston, she had thought of nothing but holding it in her hand and feeling its warmth spread up and throughout her body.

As she exited the plane, the lundicroix became slick against her skin. The air was hot in the airbridge, beads of perspiration forming at her hairline and her clothes clinging to her as she walked. But the lobby soon embraced her with a blanket of ice-cold air, and she shivered in relief.

It was crowded, people flowing in from gates at every corner. She pushed through the stream of travelers, moving swiftly to the bathroom, and hurried into the furthest stall, leaning down to check if there was anyone in the stall next to her. Not convinced, she stood on the toilet and peered over the wall at the empty stall. Satisfied, she sat down on the seat, reached into her shirt, and pulled out the lundicroix.

Immediately it warmed in her hand, spun gently, and nestled itself into her palm. She let her head tilt back as the weight of her body relaxed against the seat. The lightening slowly spread from her hand to her elbow, from her elbow to her armpit, and on to the nape of her neck, where it rose to encompass her face and warm her ears.

A vision formed before her, a vision of a brown house with a large wooden door. It was dusk and the house was glowing yellow with the light from inside. Sara could hear laughter, *familiar* laughter. She peered in a window but could only see the blanket of warm yellow light. There was a chuckle above the laughter, a deep chuckle she knew well, and there was a tiny, fairy-like giggles she knew even better. They were laughs she was surprised to hear in the same room.

The lundicroix reacted to her confusion, widening the view so Sara could see a white stone path circling the house. It took her to a small square window that was too high for her to peer through and floated her into the air, the lightness collecting in the hollow arch of her feet as she rose. Parallel with the window, Sara could see Brett and the tall man arguing. Behind them, a gathering of people.

Sara heard the deep roar of Germain's chuckle and the whisper of Hadley's giggle once more before she opened her eyes and found herself staring at the semi-rusted metal lock of the stall door.

She looked at the lundicroix in her palm, her heart sinking at the thought that, despite her best efforts Germain and Penny, had found Brett first.

She curled her hands back over the lundicroix and shut her eyes.

"Show me where the house is," she whispered.

The vision came immediately, taking her high above the house where she could only see the white stone path and brown tiled roof. She saw a street sign with a name and a freeway in the distance.

She opened her eyes.

"Cincinnati."

She slipped the lundicroix back beneath the underwire of her bra and stood, sure that what she had seen was the future, sure that Germain had not yet arrived in Cincinnati. It was the lundicroix that knew this and what it knew, she knew.

She rushed from the toilet stall, past women lined up by the sinks, and hurried out of the restroom.

She would not be the last to arrive.

75

Brett
Jekyll Island, Georgia

It was Christmas Eve. Brett and Noel stood before the great hall in the late afternoon sun. The ball had started at noon and the celebrations could be heard from inside. Brett looked at Noel beside her, his dark strength and Greek charm highlighted by the tuxedo. She slipped her arm through his as they entered the hall beneath the high stone archway decorated with red and green ribbons that whispered against their faces.

The hall was alive with color and laughing voices and the sound of shoes clicking against wood floors. There was a brass band on stage, the musicians moving about the wooden frame, flailing their instruments rhythmically from side to side. A group of women, arms linked, were kicking up their dresses to the beat. Behind them were hundreds of people in costumes and masks.

"Where have they all come from?"

"From everywhere," Noel said. "Members and their families come to the island every four years for Christmas. It's the largest social event of the Order." He shook his head and smiled at her. "People have been arriving for the past few days. Haven't you noticed?"

"No," Brett said.

"Maybe that's why you were told to come along. To improve your social skills."

A man dressed in a black tuxedo and a white cravat appeared from the crowd with a tray of salmon and caviar. He spun it playfully on his index finger and glided the tray to Brett's chest. "Hors d'oeuvre, my lady?"

Brett considered the white gloves stretching to her elbows and declined.

"White gloves are no reason to go hungry," said a husky voice from behind her.

She turned to find Kham looming above them in a top hat, a black satin mask hanging from the brim. Behind him were four women dressed in a collage of sapphire, turquoise, and silver.

"Good evening," Kham said, tipping his hat to Noel. He turned to Brett. "Surely the lady has the power to eat a piece of salmon without soiling her gloves?"

"The lady prefers not to waste powers on trivial matters," Brett retorted.

"Ah!" He lifted a black-gloved finger, the satin swooshing and offering a glimpse of his jaw. "Then she's yet to learn her powers are limitless and thus unable to be wasted."

Behind him the women snickered, and Kham moved backward into the crowd, pushing them with him.

"I suppose the masquerade is all for him," Noel said.

"What do you mean?"

"The masks allow him to join in."

"Oh, right."

"Why does he hide his face anyway?"

Brett shrugged. "Shall we get a drink?"

"Don't avoid the question."

She cocked her head at him.

"I know you've seen his face."

She raised her eyebrows.

"You forget, I too am a Talent."

She smiled and nodded.

"So, what does he hide?" he asked, taking her arm and walking her toward the bar.

"His power. He holds his power in his eyes."

"He isn't horribly ugly and scarred then?"

"He is, perhaps, the most beautiful man I've ever seen."

Noel stopped in front of the bar. "You're attracted to him then."

"Yes, and I hate the fact of it."

"And yet you learn from him."

"He's a good teacher."

"I bet he is. Two gins, please. Neat."

Brett investigated the crowd. It was impossible to miss the top hat sticking above the other hats, its phallic height both alluring and offensive.

The bartender placed their drinks on the bar and Noel handed her a gin.

"Do you want to play twenty-one?" he asked, moving back into the crowd.

"Twenty-one?" Brett asked, following him.

"Apparently there are blackjack tables through the back doors. No money required."

"What fun is there in gambling without money?" she asked.

"You don't gamble with money."

"No?" she sipped her gin, letting it pool on the back of her tongue, savoring the weight of it before swallowing it.

"You gamble with power and knowledge. You can even gamble with your future ... and your life, if you're so daring."

"Have you gambled like this?"

"Yes, in Florida."

The top hat caught her eye again and she turned to watch it move through the mob toward the back of the hall, a hive of turquoise garlands and silver bands fluttering behind it. She lifted her gin to her mouth, keeping her eyes fixed on the bobbing black hat approaching the back doors, and tipped her glass so the last of the gin slid along the back of her throat. Its vapor rose to her nose with a bite.

"Let's go then," she said.

The back hall was smaller than the front but no less grand: high ceilings lined with arched beams; narrow windows loomed two stories high, dressed in thick red curtains pulled back by golden ropes. Two rows of mahogany tables covered in red velvet ran the length of the room, each manned with a sexless figure in a tuxedo.

As the wooden doors closed behind them, the music and laughter from the front hall was abruptly silenced. Although several people were congregated around the tables, their voices were low, a mere murmur in the great room. Kham's lady friends were gathered at a front table, their laughter soft and giddy.

"The tables are all the same," Brett whispered. "Is there no choice in games?"

Noel shook his head. "Only blackjack is played on the island. But the tables aren't all the same."

Brett noticed some were more crowded than others. "What's the difference?"

"The difference is what's at stake."

"You mean how much you want to bet?"

"Not how much. *What* you want to bet. The tables at the front are your less risky options. Only knowledge is wagered at these."

"What kind of knowledge?"

"Secrets about the Order, or yourself, or about someone else. Political secrets, historical secrets. These tables are mostly harmless."

"And the others?"

"The next row of tables, wager missions and jobs. The two behind those gamble with power, although you must have power to risk, so usually only patriarchs sit at those. And there in the back, In the shadows, is a table where you can gamble with life."

"With whose life?"

"Your life if you want. Apparently, it's quite a rush. But usually it's with the lives of the Masses."

"Have you done this?"

Noel shook his head. "You have to be invited to the table of life."

Brett glanced at the dark table in the back, two figures leaned over it.

"It would be the perfect table for *him*, wouldn't it?" Noel said with a smirk, motioning toward Kham.

"Shall we gamble then?" Brett asked, having no doubt whatever lesson she was meant to learn would happen in this room.

Noel led her to a table in the front with four men gathered around it. As they approached, she noticed the tuxedoed figure was Mr. Emulius.

"What's he doing manning a table?" she whispered.

"Secrets and lives are at stake. Did you think they'd have servants working them?"

He pulled a chair out and she sat down. The chair, like the table, was covered in red velvet. It was soft against her arms, reminding her of the coffin at initiation.

Mr. Emulius offered them a nod. "Welcome to the table of knowledge. What is your wager?"

The four men turned toward the newcomers. Brett recognized one of them as a fellow initiate named Roger. Two others were twin brothers who had graduated from Yale directly before her. The other was a man in his fifties named Fredrick. She didn't know much about him except he'd lost his wife a few years before and apparently hadn't left the island since.

One of the twins tapped his fingers twice on the table and said, "A piece of evidence in the case against the Governor of Missouri."

"And the rest of you?" Mr. Emulius asked, hovering the cards above the table.

"Dirt on Claw and Bones," the other twin said. "There are a few new methods that aren't happening to protocol."

"I know of a new Prophet they've found in Ohio," Roger said.

"The facts about what happened in room number 605 in 1982," Fredrick said, taking a sip of his bourbon.

"And what would you like from the newcomers?" Mr. Emulius asked.

Noel leaned into Brett and whispered, "When you join a table, the existing players choose your wager."

"Your mission in Florida," one of the twins said, looking at Noel. "If you lose, you tell us what it is."

"You can't wager missions at this table," Mr. Emulius said.

"Okay, then," Fredrick said. "You'll both tell us what your sacrifice was at initiation."

"Is that allowed?" Noel asked.

Mr. Emulius nodded and began to deal.

Brett removed her gloves and placed them on her lap, trying to look calm. Their *sacrifice*?

She would have to ensure she won.

She focused on the cards as they fell in front of her, the power from her sternum swelling as she willed them transparent. For a flicker of a moment she saw a spade, then a club. But without the lundicroix, the vision was weak.

A figure approached Mr. Emulius in the dim light. Brett looked up in time to see the flash of a green eye behind a silk veil and then he was gone, back to his table. She could hear his entourage welcoming him back, could feel the pauses when he kissed their cheeks.

She stared at the cards on the table, trying to focus. A king, an ace, and a five.

Had those women seen his face?

Noel had twenty-one. The twins were holding at eighteen and nineteen. Roger and Fredrick took another card. Fredrick folded.

The ladies' voices were on the move. A lacy dress brushed against Brett's leg. Out of the corner of her eye she watched Kham lead them to an adjacent table and pull out chairs for them, placing his hand on each shoulder as he did. Brett tried to get a glimpse of their faces, but she could only see sequins and feathers. There was one still standing, a large girl dressed in a turquoise gown. It was Donna Lawson from her class at Yale, another initiate.

Kham led the girl to the far side of the table and pulled out a chair for her, his hand lingering on her wide turquoise-clad shoulder. He leaned in and whispered something through his veil, then seated himself next to her so Brett could see them between the back of the other women's heads.

Mr. Emulius had dealt nineteen and the twins were revealing their knowledge.

Brett looked back at Kham. Donna was laughing, her throat open and turned to him.

"... and so now the Governor is trying to blame it on the Order!" one of the twins was saying.

He placed his hand on her bare shoulder.

"... and now the Governor has disappeared!"

His finger twirled a curl of hair.

Brett pushed her chair back and stood.

"Sit down," Mr. Emulius said. "We're mid-play."

"The game is finished," Brett said.

"Wagers are being shared, my lady. Sit."

"I'm not interested in the Governor of Missouri."

"Perhaps you should be."

Noel gestured to her chair. "Sit down, Brett."

She sat back down.

Fredrick began to speak about room 605, having drawn too high of a card on his last deal. He spoke of a scandal within the Order, of murder in the room.

Brett looked back at Kham. His arm was around the girl, their noses touching through the fabric of his veil. Like the lightness at the moment of creation, the jealousy spread through her. Heavy and green instead of light and yellow, it crept into her limbs, expanded to her fingers, hardened her nails. She imagined herself approaching the table and grabbing the girl, slapping her. The violence surprised her

She willed Kham to look at her, to acknowledge her, even if just a wink. This pathetic need made Brett even more furious.

He was nibbling on her ear now. Donna's eyes closed, her lips parted.

Brett imagined her fist through his veil, cracking his perfectly straight nose.

A waiter arrived with a tray of drinks, signaling the end of the round.

Brett stood. "Drink anyone," she asked, pulling a glove over her trembling fingers as she headed to the bar.

Was he watching? Would he follow her?

She approached the bar and ordered a gin, drinking it like a shot and ordered another.

A hand slipped around the back of her neck and she turned to find Noel.

"I've seen you watching him," he said.

She leaned over the bar, her hair falling around her drink. "I can't help it."

"You've slept with him."

"Yes," she said into her empty glass. "Once I'd seen his face, it was all over."

"I bet you asked him to reveal himself, didn't you? I know you. You would have pushed it, insisted."

She remained staring into the glass.

"You gave up *our* power when you did that."

She offered him a sliver of a glance through her hair.

"The power we created existed because we were equal," Noel said. "You'll never get that with him."

How could she explain the thrill of the submission, the excitement of the obsession?

"If it's any consolation, I hate it," she said. "I hate *him*."

"You only hate him because he's more powerful than you. That's why I thought you'd resist, why I thought you'd be different."

"Different than what?"

"Than all the others."

"What others?"

"Jesus, Brett. Do you think you're the only one?"

She pulled her hair out of her face. "Who else? How many others?"

Noel looked away. "Everyone, Brett."

"What do you mean, *everyone*?"

"Eventually he reveals his face to everyone. It's his job to tame us."

Brett digested this for a moment. "What do you mean *everyone*?" she asked again.

"Everyone. Women *and* men."

She signaled to the bartender for another drink.

"And you thought it was your big secret," he said, shaking his head.

"Does he ..." But she couldn't make herself use the word.

"Fuck everyone?" Noel asked. "Only some."

The bartender set another gin in front of her.

"I'm sure he's quite good," Noel said. "Which explains your recent loss of interest in me."

"You said everyone," Brett said. "Does that include you?"

"He revealed himself to a group of us one night."

"But you asked me what I thought he looked like?"

"I was testing you."

"So, you've seen his face?"

Noel nodded. "For days I wanted to be next to him, sit across from his green stare."

"But you didn't surrender."

"I went to Florida soon after. He's coming."

"What?"

"He's coming over here."

Brett looked over her shoulder. Kham's tall swagger was moving toward them.

He walked past her and approached the bar.

"A bottle of champagne, please."

Noel walked away, shaking his head, and she stood frozen, facing the open hall, wishing she had a gun, imagining how it would feel in her hand.

A cork popped and Kham moved down the bar toward her. She remained still, hoping he would walk past her, hoping he would press himself against her, hoping neither.

He stopped in front of her, holding two glasses in one hand and the bottle in the other. His black satin veil was tucked in the rim of his hat, his green eyes smirking. He raised the glasses, offering her one. "You've passed your last test," he said. "Isn't it fantastic, this rage?"

"*What?*"

"The power that lies in your wrath! Isn't it fabulous?"

"Fabulous?"

"Yes! My dearest Brett, *this* is what will allow you to kill!"

His eyes were bright with excitement. He reached around her and set the glasses on the bar and filled each, holding a glass out to her. "We must celebrate. Skill alone never creates a successful murder."

"In case you missed it, my rage isn't directed at Sara."

"Rage is rage, my dear. Once you've borne it, once you've experienced its darkness rise in your sternum, once you've had visions of violence, you'll be able to call on it again. Finally, you have all the ingredients necessary to see out your mission. Now raise your glass."

She turned away from him, his brilliance riling her further.

He leaned into her. "All your life you wanted to be around power," he whispered. "You wanted to be impressed by a power greater than your own. And now that it's before you, you can't stand it." He lowered his eyes so she could see nothing but green, his glass still in the air.

She couldn't bring herself to toast him.

"Suit yourself, sweetheart. I'm not at a loss for women to celebrate with." He tucked the bottle under his arm and began to walk away with the full glasses. "And there's a more important party looming later that I must attend. If your wrath serves you well, I may see you there."

He winked at her and gave his head a shake, so the veil came back down over his face.

Brett headed for the veranda. Although she walked with poise, inside she was stumbling, groping the tables to hold herself up. When she arrived at the double doors, she opened them and fell into the cool evening air, letting the door close behind her.

Kham was wrong. She didn't want to just be in the midst of power, she wanted to be power*ful*, to be the *most* powerful. And yet she was only a Talent, her threshold for power determined by her genes, while he was a Prophet, destined for greatness. She hated him because she envied him.

The door opened and Noel came onto the patio.

"And the jilted lover appears," she said.

He pulled a cigarette from his breast pocket and placed it in his mouth, leaning into the flame of a burning torch on the rail. His face turned orange-red as the cigarette lit. He took a long drag and pulled it from his lips. "You okay?"

"I'll get over it."

He exhaled a cloud of blue smoke. "It's as awful as they say, isn't it?"

"What is?"

"Unrequited love. Common in theory, devastating in reality."

"I don't love Kham."

He took another drag off his cigarette. "No?"

She thought of Eli, the way he used to watch her across the room with soft eyes. She thought of the algorithm they had solved together in the library late one night, the way his hand had hovered on hers for a moment, how their eyes had met.

Had she killed organic love for power?

She imagined Eli flying, the force of the Second Truth filling the hollow beneath hidden wings.

"Brett?"

She blinked. "He mentioned a party tonight, something I'm meant to attend. I need to find out where it is."

"I saw him leave out the back door. Headed toward the hangar."

"Did he say where?"

Noel shook his head.

"Japeth will know."

"His brother went with him, something about a family reunion."

"I need to find out where they've gone."

"We'll find out, don't worry."

"We?"

"We're partners," he said. "Have been for longer than you'd like to admit." He withdrew his cigarette and dropped it to the ground, stubbing it out with the toe of his shoe, then reached into his pocket and pulled out a lundicroix.

PART IV

Reunion

76

Ernest
Cincinnati, Ohio

Ernest's first vision came to him on his fourth birthday. It had been a windy day and a hot breeze was coming from the lakes to the east, blowing his long curls into his face. With the breeze had come a memory of himself as an older boy, standing breathless atop a dry hill with long hair looping about his head. The boy in the memory had been running in the hot air but, despite his effort, had been getting nowhere fast and was exhausted. Ernest remembered he'd been going to fetch water. He remembered the feel of damp hair against his bare back, and an unquenchable thirst.

After that day, the memories became more frequent but remained insignificant until one day, nearly twenty years later, when he was sitting in a café in Montparnasse watching heavy rain flood the Seine. As the waters rose to meet the cobblestones, he remembered, suddenly and with great clarity, the eminent floods of his first life. He remembered his children and his wife climbing the plank of the ark. And he remembered the Gods who had chosen him to live.

He'd been barely twenty-four that day in Paris, and this unexpected Truth about his ancestry added to his new literary fame, instantly imbued him with a new kind of arrogance and magic. The world and its possibilities came alive, and Ernest lived from thereon in a chaos between sacredness and sin, fascinated

469

with life but lured always by death and darkness. Now his first daughter, in her one hundred and thirtieth life had remembered the floods too.

He sat perched atop a bookcase in Issa's library, looking down on the golden crown of her head as she read by the window. Voices came from the kitchen, light and deep and young. Issa, Renee, and Jonas were making crème brûlée.

Scott was in the library with Hadley and Ernest, balanced on a low shelf, a wing resting lightly on a weathered copy of a Ken Kesey novel. Ernest and Scott hadn't spoken for weeks. Ernest found Scott dull and tiresome, and the fact death didn't alleviate a person of these traits irritated him.

There was a knock on the door.

Below him, Hadley's head turned toward the sound, the light shifting from her hair to her profile. He watched her nose wrinkle and her head cock to the side. Despite the many different faces, she'd existed in throughout the years, this dog-like expression of curiosity had managed to live through them all.

She looked up at him purposefully, something she rarely did, and he smiled at her. *You know today is the day, don't you?*

She nodded.

Renee came from the kitchen. "Do you want me to get that?"

Hadley shook her head and stood. "I'll get it."

She moved toward the door, and Ernest floated down from the bookcase and glided behind her.

Ernest knew there would be several visitors arriving, but he didn't know who would show first. He enjoyed the human feeling of anticipation and leaned forward as Hadley opened the door.

A man with skin like a boy stood at the steps, his hair dark blonde and eyes light brown. He looked both old and young and beamed good health.

Shem! Ernest said, passing through Hadley.

470

He tried to embrace the young man but obviously couldn't. Instead he passed through him and landed on the white steps on the other side of the door.

Oh, to touch again! He lamented.

Hadley giggled.

"Hello!" the man said. "You must be Hadley."

"Hello, Brother."

He opened his arms wide and embraced her.

Come children. Enjoy each other before Kham turns up. Ernest said, floating back into the house. *For drama will surely arrive when he does.*

"As well as Japeth," Shane said.

Ah! So, you can hear me?

And I can see you, Father.

Tremendous! Now tell me, what do you know of them, these brothers from your first life? Have you spoken to them? Are they remembering yet?

"I haven't seen them."

Why do you use voice when you don't need to?

"Voice is of life and I am alive."

"Come," Hadley said. "I will speak as you do. Let's talk of our remembrances. What do they call you in this life?"

"Rhodes," he said. "Shane Rhodes."

"I am Hadley. But in my most important life I was called Mary."

"You were Zeruah first," Rhodes said, sitting on the solitary bench. "I remember your birth. Mother didn't cry out like she did with our brothers. There were only murmurs on the other side of the door, and then the cries of a baby came. I remember wondering if it was because you were a girl she didn't cry out." He smiled at this, then added, "When Kham was born the whole village heard her scream."

Ernest had been away for Zeruah's birth, but he recalled his wife telling him the same. He remembered the candelabra flickering on the hearth as they ate dinner and his wife told the family of the painless birth. The girl child had been swaddled in sheepskin by the hearth, and the boys and their mother had been across the table with pewter bowls of mutton broth.

"Zeruah," Hadley said. "The name doesn't bring any memories."

"It will. I didn't remember my first life for many years."

Shem, Hadley said in thought. *It's similar to Shane.*

"Yes." He smiled.

When did your memories first start?

"Nineteen ninety-five."

Ernest watched them talking, the spirits of his first children alive in different bodies. *What is parentage? They had my genes in their first life. But do they, sitting one hundred and thirty lives later as Shane and Hadley, share my blood?*

"Certainly, they do," a voice said behind him.

Ernest turned to see a wide man with an equally wide grin standing in the door frame. Behind the man was a young girl with wild, red hair and plentiful freckles.

Ernest didn't recognize the girl, but he knew the man well. It had been the last face he'd seen before he pulled the trigger and made himself a lifeless vapor of longing.

The man stepped into the house and stood in front of Ernest, looking him in the eye. He was equal in height to Ernest, but wider in the middle instead of the shoulders. He placed his hands affectionately on either side of Ernest's head. "You may have lost your stature, my son. But you never lost your presence. What I would do to kiss you on the forehead, to feel the aged skin of your face against my palms. But, alas, you have robbed us both of that, my dear boy. One hundred and thirty lives and you insisted on eliminating your options in the exact life in which your glory was being revealed to you. The tragedy!"

You don't know what it's like to be born a half God in a world of ungodliness.

"Oh, Penny, do you hear this nonsense?" The man turned to the red-haired girl. Should we take him for a day in Paris and show him how godly the world is?"

"I don't know who you're talking to," she said.

"Oh, certainly you do not! I am sorry. It is my son, Noah. Well, what is left of him at least. You cannot see him because he chose to put an end to his life and will never know the joy of living half God and half human. But I assure you he is here. He is here as Ernest, though, not Noah. Ernest was his last life. Noah was his first and I will always think of him as Noah. He was once Victor Hugo too, you know. I preferred your writing in that life," he said, turning back to Ernest. "It was your best work. Anyway, names do not matter, nor do bodies."

"And you must be Hadley," he said turning to her. "Or shall I call you Zeruah, or Mary is it? Certainly, you must pick Mary! No?" He patted her golden head and before she had time to respond said, "This is my friend Penny."

"Hello," Hadley said. "Do I know you from one of my lives? You are familiar."

"I'm Penny Weishaup. I met you earlier this year at my father's funeral."

"Oh yes, so it was this life. And who are you?" Hadley asked the man. "I feel I should know, that I *do* know you."

"That, Hadley, is the Anunnaki of Anunnakies," Issa said, coming into the room. "The God who created man, who saved the humans! Enik, it has been too long!"

"Enlil, you old fool!"

They embraced. One round and white, the other lean and dark.

Issa looked up and saw Rhodes and Penny. "You are just in time for dinner. We have made crème brûlée for dessert. I think we have finally mastered it! Come to the kitchen; meet Renee and Jonas. They will be so pleased to meet you all."

77

Ernest
Cincinnati, Ohio

Ernest knew before the knock came that Kham was near. In every life Kham had been near. In every life he'd kept his first name. And in every life he had been immoral, living a fun, sultry kind of debauchery. Ernest knew his second son was the shameless side of himself and he wondered what the memories of this one hundred and thirtieth life would bring for Kham. Had he begun to remember?

When he knocked, the humans didn't hear, for they were deep in post-dinner reverie, bellies full of pasta and minds content with wine. Ernest wanted to spread his wings over them and protect them from his son's conceit. But he didn't have wings and Scott's would never span the distance. He hovered instead above their gilded laughter.

Issa and Germain heard though, and both glanced at him with solemn, knowing looks.

Invite the lad in; he is one of us, Issa said silently.

Cushion his entry though, won't you? Germain added.

The others, unaware of the Gods' distraction, laughed at a joke Rhodes was telling. Ernest watched Renee as she threw her head back in amusement. There was a change in her since she'd met Issa. She was settling into a harmony of human and spirit that Ernest had not allowed himself to master.

He left them and floated into the entryway.

Behind the solid front door, he could see Kham and Japeth, the second and third sons of his first life. He willed the door slowly open, remaining above.

It was nearly seven and the sun was only a glow of light behind them on the horizon.

"Is anyone there?" Japeth asked in the light feminine voice that had followed him through all his lives.

"Yes," Kham said, his emerald eyes shining in the darkness. "Only you can't see him."

Ernest admired the strength and beauty of his second son, his brown skin and the angled leanness were consistent with the chiseled form he'd had in his first life.

"Hello, Father."

So, you have remembered then, Ernest said.

"Yes."

And you can see me?

"Vaguely."

"Who are you talking to?" Japeth asked, following his older brother through the door. "There's no one there."

"Oh, but there is."

"Where?"

"It's another ability of the awakening," Kham said, taking his coat off and handing it to his brother.

Kham turned toward Ernest. "It's interesting that Japeth and I have remained brothers throughout each life and Shem has always existed separately. I don't remember Shem in any memories but the first. Why is that?"

Japeth was always unable to resist your charm. Shem was smarter.

Is Shem here? Kham asked, stepping into the house.

Wait, Ernest said. *Why have you come? I must know your intentions.*

I want to see them, Kham said, answering with his thoughts and reminding Ernest he was only one life behind him.

And still alive, Kham added sharply.

Ernest flinched at the insult and smiled as the old human feeling of competition stirred in his misty soul.

I want to see them all, Kham continued. *I want to see the living Gods, my grandfather and great uncle. I want to see my brother who has rejected the Order and the Talents that elude the Order. I want to see the child Prophet that birthed Jesus thirty lives ago, my own sister.*

But for what end? Ernest asked. *You are hardly sentimental. Why today? Why now?*

Kham turned to Japeth. "It's a shame you can't hear this. Our father, Noah of the great ark, fears what I might do to his precious family of Gods and Gods' blood."

"I'm afraid I don't understand," Japeth said.

"Of course you don't. But one day you will."

Why are you here? Ernest asked again.

Well, for the show, of course. I've been among the ancestors of Gods and I've been amid murder, but I've never been in the presence of both Gods and murder all at once ... and over crème brûlée! How could I miss it?

If Ernest were human, he would have punched him.

I won't cause any havoc beyond what was going to happen anyway, Kham said. *I've done my planting. I'm just here to watch the harvest.*

Ernest knew death was imminent. He could always smell a kill before it happened, sense it like a beast in the wild. Kham couldn't hurt the Gods. But Renee, she was still human, only a Talent.

I won't touch her, Father.

How can I trust someone who thinks of it all as a game?

If it's any consolation, I, too, have a last conquest.

Renee was not a conquest.

Wasn't she? We are not really all that different, you and I.

477

Ernest lunged at the young man, craving to feel his neck in the grip of his hands. Instead, he went through him and out the other side. He stopped and faced the open door, seeing lights in the distance as a car turned onto the street.

You infer she is your last, Ernest said, turning around. *Does that mean you plan on embracing your enlightenment?*

Enik and Enlil have found a way to be part God and part human, Kham said. *You have found a way to avoid the choice. I will find a way to be all God. I will relinquish my humanness.*

How ambitious of you.

To achieve this, I must give up the rush of falling in love. For when they are bright and independent, they enchant me. I become weak. Therefore, the daughter of your precious Renee will be my last love. And as a finale, tonight I will watch her murder with precision. Thanks to my teachings, he added.

A car slowed at the end of the driveway, its lights illuminating the front lawn.

And her timing is exquisite.

Ernest wasn't sure whether that had been his thought or Kham's.

The vehicle came down the driveway. It was a truck, the rising moon shining on the square angles of the hood. It stopped and turned off, the lights dimming as the door opened. A black heel appeared on the running board, a slender leg with a hint of green fabric above the calf. Brett's blonde head slowly rose from behind the door.

"What's *she* doing here?" Japeth asked.

"Seeing out her mission. Shall we go in?"

"We haven't been invited," Japeth said. "We've merely been standing in the hallway while you snicker and gesture at some phantom Noah. Really, it has been an odd evening all around, I must say."

"We don't need an invitation. They're expecting us."

"And who is they?"

"Our long lost grandfather and uncle."

"Our grandfather has been dead for thirty years, and as far as I know we don't have an uncle. Dear brother, I fear you are losing your mind."

"The notable part of that comment is 'as far as you know,' which isn't far at all. Now let's go inside."

"Without me?" Brett asked, standing on the white stone path, her green dress flaring in the night breeze.

"Hello, Brett," Kham said.

Ernest watched him take her in, surprised to see affection in his eyes.

Noel stepped from the shadows behind her.

"Noel," Kham said. "How unexpected."

"I don't like to miss a party."

"And we wouldn't want you to miss it," Japeth said. "A pleasure to see you."

Kham moved to kiss Brett on the cheek. She turned away from him and moved into the house, taking her coat off, and handing it to him.

He gave her coat to Noel and followed her down the hallway toward the sounds of soft conversation and clinks of cutlery.

Ernest knew Brett's arrival would cause angst for Renee, but he didn't realize how much until he saw Renee's face tighten when Brett stepped into the kitchen and her eyes grow heavy with the misery that comes with loving someone you fear.

"Hello, Brett," she said, standing.

"Don't get up, Mother," Brett said and smiled at Hadley. "Hello, little sister. I suppose you knew I was coming?"

Hadley nodded.

Issa scooted his chair back and rose. "Hello. My name is Issa. This is my home. Welcome." He put his hand out and she shook it.

"Thank you. I apologize for the intrusion. I was hoping to find my sister Sara here."

"What do you want with Sara?" Renee interjected.

Brett ignored her and turned to Jonas. "I'm sorry, have we met?"

"This is Jonas," Renee said. "Jonas, this is Brett."

Jonas nodded in her direction.

"And you are who, sorry?"

"Your mother's boyfriend," he said.

"Right," Brett said, confused.

"And this is Issa's brother Germain." Renee gestured to Germain. "And his grandson, Shane Rhodes. And Penny Weishaup, daughter of Clara and Peter Weishaup, I'm sure you remember them?"

"Yes, hello," Brett said.

"Would you like to introduce us to *your* friends?" Renee asked.

Brett turned to the men behind her. "This is Kham and Japeth, brothers of the Order. And you've met Noel."

They came forward and Renee looked at Kham, her eyes locked on his.

Jonas rose and extended his hands to the men. Ernest knew it wasn't politeness that sent him to his feet, but primal instinct.

Kham and Japeth didn't notice Jonas; their eyes were on Rhodes.

"My, my," Kham said. "If it isn't the long, lost brother."

Shane Rhodes, who was once Shem, smiled his perfectly healthy smile, his eyes bright with humor. "Welcome, brothers."

Kham winked at him. "We shall catch up later. I'm keen to hear of your enlightening. We'll compare memories." He glanced down at Hadley. "And the little one here, I don't think we have been introduced?"

"You know very well who Hadley is," Renee retorted, still staring at him. "Let's not play games. Now would you like dinner? There's plenty left."

78

Ernest
Cincinnati, Ohio

Night had fallen and the blackness outside was pressing in on the yellow warmth of the house. The group had moved on from dinner and were congregated in the library with dessert wine. Issa had lit the gas fire beneath the south side bookcase and brought in the kitchen chairs and a velvet chaise from the bedroom. The once solitary leather bench now sat against a bookcase.

Noel and Penny sat on the bench speaking of the Order. Jonas was talking to Japeth, who was more interested in the length of Jonas's fingers than the story of his recent enlightening. Rhodes stood alone against the bookcase, his elbow resting on *The Agony and the Ecstasy* and his glass of Caluso Passito propped against the spine of *Atlas Shrugged*. Scott hovered above, his wings half spread and fluttering softly to keep himself levitated. Ernest found this nervous treading of air irritating but understood Scott's anxiety. Murder was, after all, looming.

Brett and Kham stood beneath the small square window staring each other down like two pit bulls in a ring. Brett was doing her best to appear as though she was done with him, but everything about her was still his. She stood distorted, her head pulled away but her neck open and vulnerable, her feet firmly planted in defense, but her pelvis twisted in invitation. Ernest had never seen two humans so passionately embraced without touching a hair. He envied them. Few things in life were as exhilarating as sexual tension and surely nothing in death.

Hadley sat on the chaise, Issa and Germain standing on either side, casting the shadows of Enik and Enlil over her. Both were so much more than Anunnaki now. Ernest could remember them as the Gods of old. He could remember the way they came to him as the skies were looming black in the distance and told him to build his boat and save his family. There had been egotism in their voices then, an infatuation with their power that was gone now. Ernest missed this old kind of godliness. He preferred it to the unassuming righteousness of enlightenment that had softened them both.

Hovering on the outskirts of the scene, Ernest couldn't help but relish the beauty of the evening reunion of Gods and humans, ghosts and angels, brothers and sisters. The diversity of emotions fused into a tapestry of colored light before him; the bright yellow of hope, the deep green of jealousy, the hot pink of lust, and the dark brown of revenge all swimming in the white translucent love that filled Issa's house.

His reverie was disrupted by a knock on the door, his hazy form rising to the sound of humanity arriving.

Hadley stood. "It's Sara!" she said, as if it was a surprise birthday party for her sister and not an impending disaster.

Easy, child, Ernest said.

Renee rushed to the door, and through the walls, Ernest watched her open the door and pull Sara to her.

"Sara!" Hadley ran and joined their hug.

Sara pulled away from her mother and looked at Hadley. "You're talking!"

"Yes," Hadley said. "I'm in the process of enlightening. I've remembered who I am!"

"Christ, not you too."

"Sara, honey. We've missed you," Renee said. "Your friend Penny arrived, and I was worried when you weren't with her. Where have you been?"

"Penny?"

Sara moved past her mother and toward the voices, pausing at the entrance to the library.

"Hello Sara," Penny said, standing up.

"What're *you* doing here?" Sara asked.

"Looking for you."

"Why?"

"We had an agreement, remember?"

Sara looked at the crowd of familiar faces, confused. "Did we?"

"I was going to help you find the man that killed your father. We were going to do it together."

"Your curiosity about the Truth was slowing me down," Sara said, finding herself again. "I can do this by myself. And I will."

"Using the lundicroix is not doing it by yourself," Germain said.

"Are you hungry, Sara?" Renee interjected. "Would you like something to eat?"

"No, Mother." Sara's eyes fell on Brett and Kham in the shadows at the back of the room.

Issa came forward and offered Sara his hand. "Welcome, Sara. I am Issa and this is my home."

"Sorry for just showing up." Sara brushed shaggy black hair from her eyes. "I've come to see my sister."

Issa nodded.

Germain stood and put his arm around Issa. "This is my brother, Sara. This is Enlil."

Sara shook Issa's hand without registering the name and moved into the room, walking past Jonas, Japeth and Rhodes and stopping in front of Brett.

"Hello, Brett," she said, her eyes resting on Kham, who's eyes were shadowed by the bookcase.

"What're you doing here?" Brett asked.

"I've come to see you."

"Me?"

"I've come to tell you the truth about *him*." Sara pointed at Kham, her eyes scanning the length of his body with contempt.

"About Kham?"

"There's something about him you should know."

Brett laughed. "There's nothing you can tell me about him that will surprise me."

"What if I told you he murdered our father?"

Brett shrugged. She'd hoped for something softer. Something that inferred a weakness in Kham would have been the only thing to surprise her. "I suppose I would believe you."

"You would?"

"I'm sure he's killed a number of people. It's possible our father was one of them."

"And you don't care?"

"No."

"*No?*" Sara asked incredulously.

"No," Brett repeated.

"What the fuck's wrong with you?"

"You're drunk, Sara. Maybe you should sit down."

"I had a few shots of whiskey and it's a big deal, but someone kills our father and you don't care?"

"Our father brought it upon himself," Brett said, twisting away from Sara, her yellow hair fanning out across her back as she reached into her coat. "Just like you're bringing *this* upon yourself."

She turned back around, a gun in her hand, pointed at Sara.

"Jesus, Brett!" Renee gasped from the other side of the room.

Jonas stepped in front of her, his hands instinctively out from his sides as if to block a basketball instead of a bullet. The Gods pressed close to Hadley, squeezing her between them and Noel and Penny crouched on the bench, frozen by instinct.

"Stop her, Kham," Rhodes said. "These are our kin."

Kham came out of the shadows. "Is this your plan, Brett? Shooting Sara in front of your family?"

Brett didn't answer, the gun firmly on Sara.

"After all our lessons, you're going to do it like this?"

"No, not like this," Brett said, turning from Sara and pointing the pistol at Kham. "Like *this*."

Kham cocked his head, forcing a smirk.

"Mother," Brett said. "Please take Hadley out of the room."

Renee stepped around Jonas and rushed to Hadley. "Sara, you come with us too."

"Forget Sara," Brett said. "Get Hadley out of here."

Renee pushed Hadley toward Jonas. "Go with Jonas." She looked back at Sara. "I'm not leaving this room without you, Sara."

Brett stepped closer to Kham, aiming the gun between his eyes.

Kham laughed. "You're not seriously going to shoot *me*?"

Issa moved toward Brett. "You don't need to do this, Brett. It is his one hundred and thirtieth life. He will remember who he is soon. He will rectify his ways."

"He's already remembering," Brett said, the pistol still pointed at Kham. "He's having visions."

"Yes," Germain said, stepping beside Issa. "But he has not had time to process what he is remembering. There is still so much for him to learn."

"Listen to them," Kham said. "You don't know who I am."

"I know enough."

"These men, Brett, are the last Anunnaki," Kham said. "They're Gods living among us. They're the power you are looking for."

Brett glanced at Issa and Germain.

"These are the men who have mastered the Second Truth. They're the ones who elude the Order."

She stared at the Gods, looking from one to the other while keeping the gun firmly on Kham. "Prove it."

"Put the gun down, Brett, and we will show you."

Brett shook her head. "Show me now."

The Gods glanced at each other knowingly and stepped up behind her, each placing a hand on one of her shoulders. Ernest felt their hands as if they were on his own shoulders, lightening gathering at the nape of his neck. It traveled to the base of his skull and came forward, warm and solid, a dense cloud of static covering his ears and flowing over his cheeks. It rose to his eyes and gathered at the hollow above his nose and with it came five hundred thousand years of Truth in one thick-layered vision of land, people, Gods and war.

Brett closed her eyes against the pressure. Ernest could feel her synapses connecting as she began to know, a low hum vibrating in her body, in his body.

The room was silent. Not a person or God moved.

Brett opened her eyes slowly, Kham still at the end of her gun. "Well I certainly don't need you anymore then, do I?"

"We can learn together. It's the next chapter, don't you see?"

She shook her head. "I won't be controlled by desire. That's not what I signed up for."

He laughed nervously. "It's exactly what you signed up for."

"No," she said. "I signed up for power, and I got rage."

"You won't do it," Kham said. "You won't kill the only person who's ever impressed you."

"Watch me," Brett said, the gunshot cracking through the room.

Renee shrieked and Japeth ran to his brother.

But it wasn't Kham who went limp and dropped to the ground. It was Brett.

The gun fell first, slipping from her hand and hitting the wooden floor. She clutched at her throat, blood bubbling at the corners of her mouth and Ernest watched as the colors in the room turned to murky blues and blacks. Hadley was wailing in the other room; a high pitch howl of grief that matched a distant siren. There was music too: Edward Elgar's Cello Concerto was playing in the background and a radio alarm went off somewhere down the hall.

Brett collapsed to the floor and Kham stumbled backward, staring at Sara in disbelief, her father's .22 still smoking in her hand.

"Oh, Sara!" Germain exclaimed. "Don't you remember Paris? Don't you remember the taste of the cinnamon pastry and the music coming from the window and the children's paper boats? My dear child, you have said goodbye to it all now! And you," he turned to Kham. "Death does not escape us, my boy, nor does love."

Renee rushed to Brett, pressing her hands against the wound on her neck. Scott appeared, landing on Brett's hip, his wings spreading over Brett and Renee like a blanket. Through his wings, Ernest watched Renee close her eyes and slowly draw in a breath, her shoulders rising as her lungs filled. Then he watched her open her eyes and remove her hands from Brett's wound, a pale light forming at her forehead pulsing to the rhythm of the veins in her blood-stained wrists. Lightness condensed and spread from her, the room growing warm and bright. A faint, high-pitched purr began as a ray of light streamed from Renee's brow and gathered on the wound. The purr grew into a loud hum and the light swelled brilliant and white until both disappeared in a deafening flash, and Renee stumbled backward, shaking.

Beside her, Brett breathed peacefully, her bleeding stopped.

"Sara," Renee said softly. "Please put the gun down."

Dumbfounded, Sara dropped the gun to the floor.

Renee went to her and took her into her arms.

"*I* wanted to kill him, Mom." Her words were muffled by sobs and the fabric of Renee's shirt. "I couldn't let *her* do it."

"It's okay," Renee said. "I've fixed it."

"You have fixed nothing," Germain said. "Each person creates their own fate. You have only changed the course momentarily. Sara's decisions will bring her back to the same place, again and again, until she makes a change within."

"You're wrong," Renee said. "She'll remember the light. She'll remember the love." She pulled away from Sara and held her at arm's length, looking at her before pulling her back into an embrace and kissing her. "Helping someone, loving someone, sets an example. It plants a seed. And that's never wrong."

Ernest stared at the good and the bad gathered before him in the form of his creators and kin. Renee with Sara in her arms. Brett on the floor breathing calmly, Kham at her side, Shem and Japeth standing over him. Noel knelt at her other side, his hand on her arm. Jonas stooped in the doorway with Hadley and Penny behind him. The great Anunnakies in the middle of the room, arms folded, facing him. Scott fluttering above.

A tear slipped down his cheek and he reached up and touched it, pulling his finger away to see it glisten in the light of the room. It was a real tear.

"If you can tell a God he is wrong," Ernest said to Renee. "Then maybe I can try living again."

Everyone in the room turned toward him.

"Who is it?" Noel asked. "Who is the voice?"

"It is the ghost of my first son, Noah," Germain answered.

"As in Noah's ark?"

"More importantly, the eldest human ancestor to all of you."

"I can see him," Japeth said, approaching Ernest. "I can see his form."

"Me too," Penny said.

"I've always seen him," Hadley added.

Rhodes stepped forward and addressed the Gods. "What is the meaning of this reunion? Why are we here, all of us together?"

"Each of you are enlightening. It is that journey that has brought you here," Germain answered.

"And your energy," Issa added. "Like molecules and atoms, your Omega cells are bound together."

"It could be said that you vibrated here," Germain chuckled.

Issa smiled. "Collectively, there is enough power in this room to alter the course of humanity. And enough to destroy it."

"If you work together through love," Germain said, "you will bring enlightenment to all human beings. If you work together through fear, you will see the demise of human beings."

"And if you separate and fight each other, you will do nothing." Issa paused. "It is a choice for each of you and for all of you."

"Even for *me*?" Sara asked quietly from her mother's arms.

"You are the most important person here, Sara," Germain said. "You have the least gift for enlightenment and yet are still capable. If you can learn to choose love over fear, you will have the key to enlightening the world."

"You're saying we should enlighten the Masses?" Kham asked.

"Enlightening the Masses is exactly what you must do. It is essential for the survival of humans. For those of you who choose to be part of this transformation, the reward will be great."

"But the motive for each of you will be different," Issa explained. "Some of you will do it for the challenge, others because you believe it is the right thing to do. A few of you will do it out of compassion and some will simply be driven by curiosity."

"But the reasons do not matter," Germain said. "It is the choice to act that matters."

"And do you know what each of us will choose?" Renee asked, looking from one God to the other.

"No," Germain said, his eyes sparkling. "But we are looking forward to finding out."

Acknowledgements

This is an ambitious novel that no doubt has fallen short in some places. Attempting to weave sixteen themes into four characters spanning 500,000 years was always a ridiculous endeavor. But thanks to many people, I managed to stay dedicated to the idea and created the book I always dreamed of, the Bohemian Rhapsody of novels (as my good friend Liz calls it).

Several brave souls volunteered to read the manuscript. Thanks to those of you who took the time to critique it: Damien Barr, Sam Cormack, Mel Escott, Andrew Fraser, Hamish Hodgson, Belinda Jeursen, Caroline King, Deirdre Kirk, Jill Kuyper, Shelley Lovegrove, Katherine McCusker, Jill and Brian McNaughton, Sarah Paterson-Hamlin, Juan Pellegrino, Holly Quigley, Lola Reynolds, and Ciarán Tully.

Special thanks to Adam Barker, who took an interest in the book at a critical time of waning motivation, and not only offered sound insights but persuaded several of the above to read it as well, all of which offered valuable perspectives. Liz Blakemore took more interest in this book than I had any right to expect and has kept me going on many a dark day. Her enthusiasm and can-do attitude never cease to amaze me. Thank you, Liz! Thanks also to my sister-in-law, Nicole Bonomini, who encouraged me through the horror-house of querying agents; to Lee Cowan for saying it was *"proper brilliant"* on a day when I was sure it would be better used as toilet paper; and to Susan Coffman for starting me on my writing journey.

Thanks to both my editors, Donna Blaber and Caroline Simpson, who combed through the manuscript with care and dedication. This was not an easy book to edit, with multiple dialogue styles, several historical references, and reincarnated characters. Thank you for your persistence.

And thanks to Tony, my wonderful husband, who would rather suffer a cold, rainy day with a broken tractor and flooded paddocks than read a book. Thank you for staying awake while I read aloud to you in the evenings, for accepting the frequent solitude needed for my creativity, and for steadfastly believing in me.

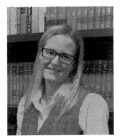 *Two Truths* is Dana C Carver's first published work. She has written two other novels, *Meeting Eve* and *Quatro*. She has a degree in psychology, with post-graduate studies in physiology, and a certificate in creative writing. She is also a certified personal trainer and performance coach. While originally from Columbus, Ohio, USA, she has lived in New Zealand since 2003. Her website is www.danaccarver.com.

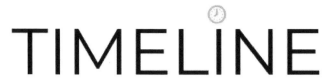

TIMELINE

Eras of the Two Truths

The Beginning

Anunnaki appear- **500,000 BC**

Homo Sapiens created- **300,000 BC**

Procreation enabled- **100,000 BC**

The Great Flood- **10,000 BC**

The Restoration

9200 BC- Farming bears kingship

6500 BC- Abraham called by God

4100 BC- Sumerian civilization appears

2000 BC- Sumer destroyed

The Era of the Sages

Zoraster- **1500 BC**

Moses- **1200 BC**

Greek Philosophers- **500 BC**

Buddha- **400 BC**

Jesus- **00**

The Corruption

AD 30- Catholic church formed

AD 1200- Priory of Sion formed

AD 1450- Freemasons formed

AD 1700- Rothschilds rise

AD 1740- Saint Germain appears

AD 1830- The Order is established

AD 1990- Gulf wars begin

AD 2000- The Era of Enlightenment

While some events are true, this is a fictional timeline
Most dates of true events are historically debatable, and all have been rounded for the sake of simplicity

Made in the USA
Monee, IL
07 December 2021

84164404R00271